Treatment of
Psychological Distress in
Parents of Premature Infants

PTSD in the NICU

Treatment of
Psychological Distress in
Parents of Premature Infants

PTSD in the NICU

Edited by

Richard J. Shaw, M.D.

Sarah M. Horwitz, Ph.D.

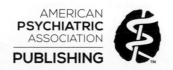

AMERICAN
PSYCHIATRIC
ASSOCIATION
PUBLISHING

Manufactured in the United States of America on acid-free paper
25 24 23 22 21   5 4 3 2 1

American Psychiatric Association Publishing
800 Maine Avenue SW, Suite 900
Washington, DC 20024-2812
www.appi.org

Library of Congress Cataloging-in-Publication Data
Names: Shaw, Richard J., 1958 July 1- editor. | Horwitz, Sarah McCue, editor. | American Psychiatric Association Publishing, publisher.
Title: Treatment of psychological distress in parents of premature infants : PTSD in the NICU / edited by Richard J. Shaw, Sarah M. Horwitz.
Description: First edition. | Washington, DC : American Psychiatric Association Publishing, [2021] | Includes bibliographical references and index.
Identifiers: LCCN 2020032232 (print) | LCCN 2020032233 (ebook) | ISBN 9781615373208 (paperback ; alk. paper) | ISBN 9781615373659 (ebook)
Classification: LCC RC552.P67 (print) | LCC RC552.P67 (ebook) | NLM WM 172.5 | DDC 616.85/21—dc23
LC record available at https://lccn.loc.gov/2020032232
LC ebook record available at https://lccn.loc.gov/2020032233

British Library Cataloguing in Publication Data
A CIP record is available from the British Library.

Contents

Contributors

Tonyanna C. Borkovi, M.B.B.S,
Division of Child and Adolescent Psychiatry, Stanford University School of Medicine, Stanford, California

LaTrice L. Dowtin, Ph.D., LCPC, NCSP, RPT
2018–2019 NICU Psychology Fellow, Department of Child and Adolescent Psychiatry and Neonatology, Stanford University School of Medicine, Palo Alto, California; Owner, PlayfulLeigh Psyched, LLC, Hyattsville, Maryland; Co-Director, Infants, Toddlers, and Families Department, Gallaudet University, Washington, DC

Soudabeh Givrad, M.D.
Assistant Professor in Clinical Psychiatry, Division of Child and Adolescent Psychiatry, Weill Cornell Medicine; Director of Maternal-Infant Psychiatry Program, Associate Director of Sackler Infant Psychiatry Fellowship, New York Presbyterian Hospital-Weill Cornell, New York

Susan R. Hintz, M.D., M.S.(Epi)
Robert L. Hess Family Professor, Division of Neonatal and Developmental Medicine, Department of Pediatrics, Stanford University School of Medicine; Attending Neonatologist, Medical Director, Fetal and Pregnancy Health Program, and Co-Director, The Johnson Center for Pregnancy and Newborn Services, Lucile Packard Children's Hospital Stanford, Palo Alto, California

Margaret K. Hoge, M.D.
Fellow, Department of Pediatrics, Division of Neonatal-Perinatal Medicine and Division of Developmental and Behavioral Pediatrics, The University of Texas Southwestern Medical Center, Dallas, Texas

Sarah M. Horwitz, Ph.D.
Professor, Department of Child and Adolescent Psychiatry, NYU Grossman School of Medicine, New York, New York

Emily A. Lilo, Ph.D., M.P.H.
Assistant Professor of Community Health, Division of Health and Exercise Science, Western Oregon University, Monmouth, Oregon

Angelica Moreyra, Psy.D.
NICCU Psychologist, University of Southern California University Center for Excellence in Developmental Disabilities, Children's Hospital Los Angeles, Los Angeles, California

Melissa Scala, M.D.
Clinical Associate Professor of Pediatrics, Division of Neonatal and Developmental Medicine, Stanford University School of Medicine; Medical Director, Inpatient Infant Developmental Care, Lucile Packard Children's Hospital, Stanford, California

Daniel S. Schechter, M.D.
Director of Perinatal and Early Childhood Research and Senior Attending, University Service of Child and Adolescent Psychiatry, Lausanne University Hospital, Lausanne, Switzerland; Senior Lecturer in Psychiatry, Geneva University Faculty of Medicine, Geneva, Switzerland; and Adjunct Associate Professor, Department of Child and Adolescent Psychiatry, New York University Grossman School of Medicine, New York

Stephanie Seeman, Psy.D.
Clinical Psychology Postdoctoral Fellow, The Motherhood Center, New York, New York

Richard J. Shaw, M.D.
Professor of Psychiatry and Pediatrics, Stanford University School of Medicine; Medical Director, Pediatric Psychiatry Consult Service, Lucile Packard Children's Hospital, Stanford, California

Daniel Singley, Ph.D., ABPP
Board Certified Psychologist, The Center for Men's Excellence, San Diego, California

Krisa P. Van Meurs, M.D.
Rosemarie Hess Professor, Division of Neonatal and Developmental Medicine, Department of Pediatrics, Stanford University School of Medicine; Medical Director, NeuroNICU and ECMO Programs, Lucile Packard Children's Hospital Stanford, Palo Alto, California

Emily Wharton, M.S.
Clinical Psychology Doctoral Candidate, PGSP-Stanford Psy.D. Consortium, Palo Alto University, Palo Alto, California

Tiffany Willis, Psy.D.
Licensed Clinical Psychologist, Division of Developmental and Behavioral Health, Section of Psychology, Division of Neonatology and Fetal Health, Children's Mercy; Assistant Professor, Department of Pediatrics, University of Missouri—Kansas City School of Medicine; Owner of Hope Love Heal, Therapy and Consulting, Kansas City, Missouri

Preface

Richard J. Shaw, M.D.
Sarah M. Horwitz, Ph.D.

Our interest in the psychological issues affecting parents of premature infants started in 1996, when we first conducted an unfunded investigation into the topic of acute stress disorder in parents of premature infants (Shaw et al. 2006). With a skeleton research crew, and the personal experiences of a student who had himself experienced the death of a premature infant, we identified the magnitude of the psychological reactions of parents of premature infants—both mothers and fathers—in the neonatal intensive care unit (NICU). Although the importance of postpartum depression was at the time widely known, PTSD was less recognized. The model of a premature birth as a psychological trauma resonated deeply with our clinical experience and with the experiences of our patients. Drawing on the work of Margaret Stuber and Anne Kazak in the field of pediatric oncology, we were able to expand our views of medical PTSD as incorporating the frequent and repetitive traumatic medical experiences encountered by parents in the NICU, often on a daily basis (Kazak et al. 1998). Our use of the term *continuous traumatic stress disorder* perhaps best encapsulates our conception of the parental NICU experience (Eagle and Kaminer 2013).

Although trauma has been one of the foundations of our work in the NICU, we have also relied heavily upon the concept of bereavement (Kübler-Ross 1969). In our clinical work, we have repeatedly noted the importance and magnitude of the grief and guilt felt by parents of premature infants, starting with the loss of the expected pregnancy and birth experience and evolving into the loss of the idealized infant. An early pioneer who recognized the importance of these profound issues for parents is Margaret Miles, who described the concept of the *alteration in the parental role*, which has helped provide a larger context for the psychological reactions of our patients (Miles et al. 1989). Her analysis of specific stressors in the NICU, including the parental role, have been codified in her widely used research scale, the Parental Stressor Scale: NICU (Miles et al. 1993).

We are also grateful for the early work of Rebecca Bernard, Ph.D., who, during her National Institute of Mental Health (NIMH)-funded T-32 fellowship at Stanford University, first developed an intervention model based on the principles of trauma-focused cognitive behavioral therapy (TF-CBT). In a small pilot study, Dr. Bernard was able to show that a brief four-session intervention was effective in reducing symptoms of psychological stress in mothers of premature infants (Bernard et al. 2011). These data helped springboard our first NIMH application for an R-34 grant to conduct a full-scale randomized controlled effectiveness trial. We were fortunate to secure that funding and are grateful to the reviewers of that application and the program officers at NIMH for recognizing the potential importance of the proposed intervention. Our intervention incorporated material from the cognitive processing therapy manual (Resick et al. 2017), modified to address the specific language and experiences of parents in the NICU. The manual also relied heavily on the concept of *infant redefinition*, incorporated throughout the intervention with the goal of helping parents positively reinterpret their perceptions of both their infant and their own parenting abilities. The results of our brief six-session intervention exceeded even our own expectations. Treatment resulted in significant reductions in symptoms of maternal anxiety, depression, and PTSD at both 1 and 6 months following the intervention (Shaw et al. 2013, 2014).

With the end of our research funding, our intervention, despite its success, was left dormant, even though other investigators and clinical programs have expressed interest. It was not until 2 years ago that we were able to reactivate our program through the generosity of our neonatology colleagues, Krisa Van Meurs and Susan Hintz, in the NICU at Lucile Packard Children's Hospital at Stanford. Although the benefits of psychological consultation in the pediatric setting are well established, a gap often exists between the demand for these services and funding. With financial support, we have embarked on our longstanding goal to develop a group-based intervention model for parents of premature infants, adapting our manual of individual TF-CBT. Our collaboration with Hongyun Gao at Fudan University in Shanghai first raised the potential benefits of scaling and implementing our intervention in a group format to target more parents. Our experiences in piloting the group intervention have so far been overwhelmingly positive and have started a culture shift in our NICU by helping to reduce feelings of parental isolation as groups of mothers continue to socialize and provide each other support after the six-session intervention.

The focus of this book evolved as we started to appreciate the importance of describing a more global approach to psychological consultation in the NICU. This approach involves integrating interventions that begin prior to the infant's conception and extend well beyond the NICU hospitalization, as well as integrating the expertise of the entire NICU team. In Chapter 1, Drs. Van Meurs and Hintz provide a context and review of the medical aspects of the NICU environment and the neurodevelopmental consequences of prematurity. Long-term mental health issues in adults with a history of prematurity raise questions about the genesis of these issues from the dual perspective of biology and environment, including parent–child relational issues. The data also emphasize the importance of early intervention, both before conception and in the NICU. In Chapter 2, we review the common psychological reactions of mothers of premature infants, including specific risk factors associated with maternal psychological distress. We also discuss the relationship between parental posttraumatic stress and infant outcomes as it relates to such issues as breastfeeding, maternal–infant interaction, attachment, and infant development. The concept of the vulnerable child syndrome (VCS), first described by Green and Solnit (1964), as an outcome of parental trauma helps make a case for the potential larger impact of early intervention on infant health and development.

Our decision to dedicate a separate chapter to the unique experiences of fathers acknowledges the greater recognition of issues that have historically been neglected. In Chapter 3, Dr. Dowtin and colleagues describe the form and prevalence of symptoms of paternal psychological distress. They also outline the curriculum for a group-based intervention specifically designed to address fathers' concerns.

Integrating the expertise of the entire NICU team is a core concept for our program. Chapter 4 addresses developmental care interventions that overlap with interventions more narrowly focused on parental psychological distress. This chapter also reviews parent–infant psychotherapy and efforts to address problematic aspects of the parent–infant relationship, including the impact of prematurity on attachment.

Chapters 5 and 6 describe our intervention model in both the individual and group therapy formats. Chapter 5, in particular, offers a detailed description of how to implement the treatment in the NICU setting, using excerpts from our treatment manual. Although lengthy, we believe this chapter is essential reading for clinicians who would like to implement our interventions in their own clinical programs. Lucile Packard Children's Hospital at Stanford will be offering training to assist with the dissemination of the interventions in the near future.

To assist clinicians interested in learning how to deliver this intervention, the treatment manual and related handouts are available at www.appi.org/Shaw. Readers may also contact the editors of this book for further information about training resources.

We are fortunate at our medical center to have the support of our enlightened pediatric colleagues. However, we are also cognizant of the fact that funding for psychological interventions in the pediatric setting rarely captures the interest of the health care system without clear financial implications or improved infant health outcomes. In Chapter 7, Dr. Hoge addresses VCS in more detail. Limited research has shown that VCS is associated with adverse developmental outcomes in children as well as overutilization of health care resources. Application of the trauma model to the concept of VCS provides a framework to understand how parental behavior is altered in the context of trauma. Dr. Hoge uses this model to reconceptualize ways of measuring and quantifing VCS and offers an innovative new scale that she is currently piloting at University of Texas Southwestern. Our contention is that demonstrating the ability of low-cost psychological interventions to reduce health care costs and improve infant outcomes is necessary to make the case for our work. Chapter 7 outlines just such an intervention currently being piloted and tested by Dr. Hoge. Finally, in Chapter 8, we discuss how to implement a psychological intervention program in the NICU that includes screening the parents of premature infants for symptoms of psychological distress.

This book is, to our knowledge, the first of its kind to outline a comprehensive programmatic approach to psychological consultation to the NICU. However, we also acknowledge that our ideas are still in development. We hope this book will encourage a more systematic consideration of the issues of parental psychological distress and its implications for infant development. We look forward to exciting new developments in the field that we anticipate will be forthcoming in the coming years.

References

Bernard RS, Williams SE, Storfer-Isser A, et al: Brief cognitive-behavioral intervention for maternal depression and trauma in the neonatal intensive care unit: a pilot study. J Trauma Stress 24(2):230–234, 2011

Eagle G, Kaminer D: Continuous traumatic stress: expanding the lexicon of traumatic stress. Peace and Conflict Journal of Peace Psychology 19(2):85–99, 2013

Green M, Solnit AJ: Reactions to the threatened loss of a child: a vulnerable child syndrome. Pediatric management of the dying child, part III. Pediatrics 34:58–66, 1964

Kazak AE, Stuber ML, Barakat LP, et al: Predicting posttraumatic stress symptoms in mothers and fathers of survivors of childhood cancers. J Am Acad Child Adolesc Psychiatry 37(8):823–831, 1998

Kübler-Ross E: On Death and Dying. New York, Macmillan, 1969

Miles MS, Carter MC, Riddle I, et al: The pediatric intensive care unit environment as a source of stress for parents. Matern Child Nurs J 18(3):199–206, 1989

Miles MS, Funk SG, Carlson J. Parental Stressor Scale: neonatal intensive care unit. Nurs Res 42(3):148–52, 1993

Resick PA, Monson CM, Chard KM: Cognitive Processing Therapy for PTSD: A Comprehensive Manual. New York, Guilford, 2017

Shaw RJ, DeBlois T, Ikuta L, et al: Acute stress disorder among parents in the neonatal intensive care nursery. Psychosomatics 47:206–212, 2006

Shaw RJ, St John N, Lilo EA, et al: Prevention of traumatic stress in mothers with preterm infants: a randomized controlled trial. Pediatrics 132(4):e886–e894, 2013

Shaw RJ, St John N, Lilo E, et al: Prevention of traumatic stress in mothers of preterms: 6-month outcomes. Pediatrics 134(2):e481–e488, 2014

Acknowledgments

This book is the culmination of many years of collaboration that began with our initial consultation work in the NICU at Lucile Packard Children's Hospital (LPCH) at Stanford. In the course of our work, we have been privileged to have the support and expertise of mentors and colleagues from multiple institutions across the United States. There are innumerable people who we wish to thank for their encouragement and support. We cannot mention them all, but we hope that they know how much we appreciate them.

In particular, we would like to acknowledge Dr. Thomas DeBlois, a fellow in child and adolescent psychiatry in the Division of Child Psychiatry at Stanford University School of Medicine. Dr. DeBlois, as a result of his personal experiences in the NICU, made the first suggestion to research PTSD in the parents of premature infants. With a small cadre of volunteer research assistants, he conducted the initial studies that have been the impetus for all of our future work.

We have been especially fortunate to have the unwavering support of our pediatric colleagues in the NICU, among them the Chief of Neonatology, William Benitz, and David Stevenson, Associate Dean, as well as William Rhine, Krisa Van Meurs, and Susan Hintz. Their recognition of the importance of addressing the psychological issues of NICU parents has been key to the development and implementation of our various interventions. We also acknowledge Robert L. Hess and his family and their generous support of perinatal-neonatal research through their endowment of the Rosemarie Hess Professorship and the Robert L. Hess Family Professorship in the Division of Neonatal and Developmental Medicine at the Stanford University School of Medicine. The advances toward better understanding of the profound psychosocial stressors for parents of premature infants and the ongoing efforts to develop interventions to improve outcomes of high-risk infants and their families could not have moved forward without this support.

We have also been fortunate to benefit from funding from the National Institute of Mental Health through the R-34 mechanism to implement our first randomized controlled trial establishing the effectiveness of our trauma-focused approach to treatment interventions. We thank our project manager, Emily Lilo, and our statistical consultants, Cheryl Koopman, Booil Jo, and Amy Storfer-Isser. We also acknowledge the invaluable contributions of the LPCH NICU nurses, including Ann DeBattista, who provided input into the design of our study materials, and the NICU social workers, Emily Perez, Rachel Arrelano, Candy Taylor Ceballos, and Marlyna Stewart, whose support was instrumental in the implementation of our study. At LPCH, we also thank Nicholas St. John, Karen Weyman, and the staff from the Department of Family Centered Care and the Division of Developmental and Behavioral Pediatrics. We also acknowledge our colleagues, Bernadette Melnyk, Nancy Feinstein, and Eileen Fairbanks, from whose work, COPE for HOPE Inc., we drew when developing our treatment manual. Patricia Chamberlain at the Oregon Social Learning Center provided valuable guidance for our intervention.

In the Department of Psychiatry and Behavioral Sciences at Stanford University School of Medicine, we are deeply grateful to the chair, Laura Roberts, who is also Editor-in-Chief at American Psychiatric Association (APA) Publishing and has supported our work in both logistical and inspirational ways. We thank the Ambassadors for LPCH (www.ambassadorslpch.com) who have so generously provided funding to help establish a NICU psychologist position that has in very concrete ways enabled us to continue our work.

We also acknowledge our postdoctoral students, Rebecca Bernard, Angelica Moreyra, LaTrice Dowtin, and Erin Armer, who have helped implement innovative new clinical services in the NICU. Practicum students from the Palo Alto University/Stanford Consortium, many of whom have completed their dissertation work in the LPCH NICU, have also enlivened our discussions and made it possible for us to implement our research agenda. We thank Carrie Sweetser, Julia Corcoran, Annie Leibowitz, Emma Williams, Stephanie Seeman, and Emily Wharton, among others. Maria Ocampo and Jason Tinero, contributed to the development of the intervention model described in our chapter "Postpartum Psychological Experiences of Fathers of Premature Infants." Tonyanna Borkovi featured not only as a coauthor but also assisted in the formatting and production of the numerous tables, including the New Revised Vulnerable Baby Scale, and assisted with editing the chapter on VCS.

We are deeply indebted to our editor at APA Publishing, Jennifer Gilbreath. Her meticulous attention to detail, careful editing, and thoughtful guidance throughout this process have been quite extraordinary. Rick Prather, our Production Manager at APA Publishing, was responsible for the cover design, layout, and formatting of the many figures and illustrations. We are especially grateful to John McDuffie, publisher of APA Publishing, for his support, and to Erika Parker, acquisitions co-ordinator.

Finally, we express our deep gratitude to the families with whom we have worked in the NICU. Their generosity in sharing their often painful and harrowing stories has formed the foundation upon which we have built our ideas. Our experiences of jointly witnessing their trauma and growth have inspired and motivated us in our aim to integrate psychological care for parents during their child's NICU stay. Our hope is that this book will continue to inspire other researchers and clinicians to further these goals

CHAPTER 1

Medical and Neurodevelopmental Consequences of Prematurity

Krisa P. Van Meurs, M.D.

Susan R. Hintz, M.D., M.S.(Epi)

Infant mortality is an important measure of the overall health of a population. It is measured as deaths in the first year of life per 1,000 live births. With approximately 4 million births annually in the United States, more than 22,000 newborns died in 2017, giving the United States an infant mortality rate of 5.8 deaths per 1,000 live births. Despite steadily declining infant mortality rates, the United States ranks well below other developed countries; Japan and Sweden have some of the lowest infant mortality rates, with 2.0 and 2.5 deaths per 1,000 births, respectively.

The five leading causes of infant mortality in the United States are birth defects, preterm birth and low birth weight, pregnancy complications, sudden infant death syndrome (SIDS), and injuries (Figure 1–1). In 2016, preterm birth and low birth weight accounted for approximately 17% of infant deaths. For this reason, reducing preterm birth is a national public health priority. *Preterm birth* is defined as birth prior to 37 weeks of gestation, and low birth weight is defined as birth weight <2,500 g. Low birth weight can be due to prematurity or to fetal growth restriction, also called small for gestational age (SGA). Preterm births can be subdivided into several categories depending on the infant's weight or gestational age at birth (Table 1–1). Preterm birth rates decreased from 2007 to 2014 but have risen since. Currently, 1 in 10 babies is born prematurely in the United States. The gestational age breakdown of premature infants is mostly made up of babies born between 32 and 36 weeks' gestation, while the minority are babies born at <28 weeks' gestation, or extremely

1

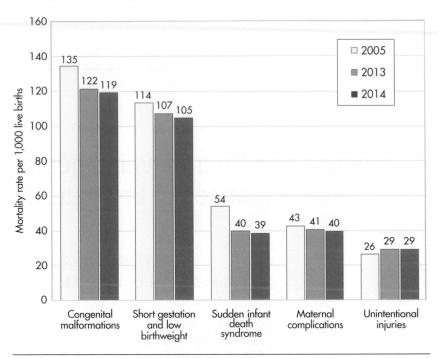

FIGURE 1–1.   Infant mortality rates for the five leading causes of infant death in the United States, 2005, 2013, and 2014.

Source. Centers for Disease Control and Prevention, National Center for Health Statistics, National Vital Statistics System. Available at https://www.cdc.gov/nchs/nvss. Accessed September 1, 2019.

preterm (EPT) (Figure 1–2). The rates of preterm birth vary by maternal age, with higher rates in the youngest and oldest mothers. The overall decrease in prematurity between 2007 and 2014 was attributed to a decline in all age groups; however, a reduction in the proportion of births to younger mothers was noted over this time period. Overall, birth rates declined in all age groups except in women ages 40–44 years (Figure 1–3). These changes were attributed to teen pregnancy prevention efforts and the changing maternal age distribution. The rates of prematurity and low birth weight also vary with race and ethnicity, with higher rates among non-Hispanic black women (Figure 1–4).

Medical Complications of Prematurity

The earlier in pregnancy a baby is born, the higher the risk for death, complications of prematurity, later health problems, and a longer stay in a neonatal intensive care unit (NICU). Due to advances in neonatal in-

Table 1-1. Terminology

Term	Definition
Extremely preterm	<28 weeks of gestation
Preterm	<37 weeks of gestation
Late preterm	34 to <37 weeks of gestation
Term	37–41 weeks of gestation
Post term	42 weeks of gestation
Low birth weight	<2,500 g
Very low birth weight	<1,500 g
Extremely low birth weight	<1,000 g

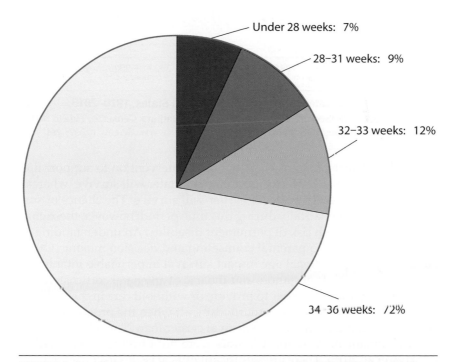

FIGURE 1–2.   Preterm births by gestational age in the United States, 2017.
Source.   Centers for Disease Control and Prevention, National Center for Health Statistics, National Vital Statistics System. Available at https://www.cdc.gov/nchs/nvss. Accessed September 1, 2019.

tensive care, even babies born very prematurely can survive. The borderline of *viability* is defined as the gestational age at which the infant has a

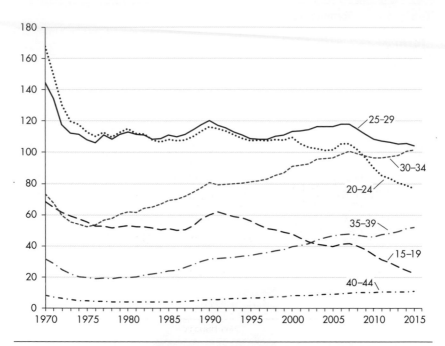

FIGURE 1–3.   Birth rates by maternal age, United States, 1970–2015.

Source.   Centers for Disease Control and Prevention, National Center for Health Statistics, National Vital Statistics System. Available at https://www.cdc.gov/nchs/nvss.

reasonable chance of survival. With active intervention to support life, most infants born at 26 weeks' gestation and later will survive, whereas almost none born at 22 weeks or earlier will survive. The chance of survival increases dramatically during this time period; however, these children also have a high risk of permanent disability. An understanding of this risk is essential to parental counseling and decision making. Other factors beyond gestational age impact survival in periviable infants, including sex, multiple gestation, and the use of antenatal corticosteroids. Decisions regarding whether to provide or withhold care in the delivery room and the NICU are particularly difficult when the prognosis is unclear. Data from U.S. studies on survival earlier than 23 weeks' gestation are problematic because most infants were not provided resuscitation (Rysavy et al. 2015). There are significant ethical issues to consider. Current recommendations from U.S. professional societies (American College of Obstetricians and Gynecologists and Society for Maternal-Fetal Medicine 2017; Cummings and Committee on Fetus and Newborn 2015) suggest the following: 1) if there is no chance of survival (birth earlier than 22 weeks), then attempted resuscitation offers no benefit and should not be initiated; 2) resuscitation should be considered in consul-

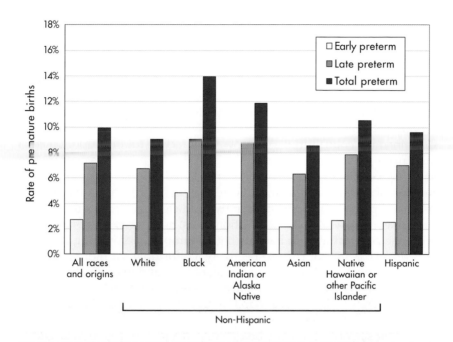

FIGURE 1–4. Rates of premature births by maternal race and ethnicity, United States, 2017.

Source. Centers for Disease Control and Prevention, National Center for Health Statistics, National Vital Statistics System. Available at https://www.cdc.gov/nchs/nvss.

tation with parents for births occurring between 22 and 24 weeks' gestation; and 3) joint discussion between parents and members of the obstetric and neonatal teams prior to high-risk birth will promote optimal decision making. Another important concept is that intensive care can be withdrawn if significant complications occur.

Causes of Prematurity

The causes of prematurity are poorly understood despite decades of research and clinical trials. Understanding of risk factors is limited, and interventions to prevent prematurity have had little impact. The birth of a preterm infant has significant emotional and economic cost for families and implications for health insurance, education, and other social support systems. The annual economic burden associated with preterm birth in the United States was estimated in 2005 at $26 billion (Behrman 2007).

Spontaneous preterm birth is responsible for two-thirds of all preterm births, while the rest are considered medically indicated to avoid or minimize maternal and or fetal complications such as maternal pre-eclampsia and intrauterine growth retardation. Spontaneous preterm birth is usually associated with preterm labor and spontaneous rupture of membranes. Risk factors associated with preterm birth include medical, genetic, environmental, and socioeconomic factors. Those previously identified include prior preterm birth, multiple gestation, use of assisted reproductive technology, tobacco and substance abuse, infections, extremes of BMI, low socioeconomic status, cervical anomalies, short intervals between pregnancies, and early elective delivery. One study examined the contributions of known risk factors for both spontaneous and medically indicated preterm birth in five high-income countries to see how well preterm birth might be predicted based on various combinations of known risk factors (Ferrero et al. 2016). Previous preterm birth and preeclampsia most strongly predicted preterm birth for individual women, while on a population basis, nulliparity and male infant were the risk factors that had the highest impact, accounting for 25%–50% and 11%–16% of risk, respectively. Unfortunately, more than 65% of preterm births lack a biological explanation, underscoring the importance of research that is focused on identifying the underlying biological causes of preterm birth. The March of Dimes began a campaign in 2003 to increase awareness of prematurity and decrease the preterm birth rate. Their scientific advisory board created a research agenda targeting six overlapping categories: epidemiology, genetics, disparities, inflammation, biological stress, and clinical trials (Green et al. 2005). Preterm birth is widely recognized as a common but complex disorder in need of a multipronged research effort that will ideally lead to specific interventions that reduce the rate of preterm birth.

Survival of Premature Infants

Advances in neonatal intensive care over the past several decades have improved perinatal care practices and care of extremely low birth weight (ELBW) infants. Survival rates are known to increase steadily with increasing gestational age; however, ELBW infants continue to contribute disproportionately to the burden of neonatal mortality. Changes in perinatal practices were tracked in an observational study performed by the National Institute of Child Health and Human Development (NICHD) Neonatal Research Network (NRN) (Stoll et al. 2015). In this study, survival in the period 2008–2012 was 8% at 22 weeks and increased to 94% at 28 weeks (Figure 1–5). After 28 weeks' gestation, survival rates were in excess of 90%. This study also investigated the changes in survival for the entire cohort born at 28 weeks or earlier and by gestational age over time. Survival was unchanged for the entire cohort between 1993 and 2008, and after 2008 it varied by gestational age. Significant increases in survival were seen in babies born at 23 and 24 weeks, with smaller im-

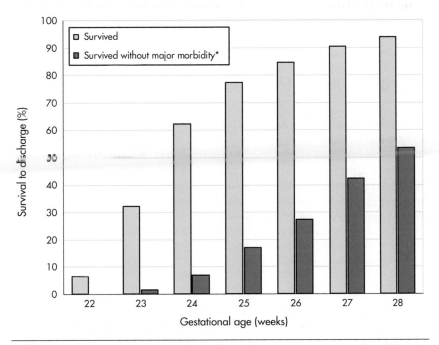

FIGURE 1–5. **Infant survival to discharge by birth year and gestational age.**

Major morbidity was defined as one or more of necrotizing enterocolitis, infections (early onset sepsis, late-onset sepsis, or meningitis), bronchopulmonary dysplasia, severe intracranial hemorrhage, periventricular leukomalacia, and retinopathy of prematurity of stage 3 or greater.

Source. Stoll et al. 2015.

provements at 25 and 27 weeks. No changes were seen for babies born at 22, 26, and 28 weeks' gestation.

Variation in survival rates of ELBW infants between hospitals is present and unexplained. Differences in hospital practices regarding the initiation of active care versus comfort care after birth may be responsible. A retrospective study of ELBW infants born between 2006 and 2011 at 24 hospitals in the NICHD NRN found that among infants who were born at 22, 23, and 24 weeks' gestation, hospital rates of active treatment varied widely, whereas most hospitals provided active treatment to babies born at 25 weeks and later (Rysavy et al. 2015). For babies at 22 and 23 weeks' gestation, the hospital rate of active treatment accounted for 78% of the variation in survival.

The cause of death in ELBW infants was studied between 2000 and 2011 by the NICHD NRN (Patel et al. 2015). Overall mortality declined during this period, and the timing of deaths was evenly distributed between early death within first 12 hours of life and death occurring between 12 hours and 28 days of age. Deaths were most commonly due to immaturity, respiratory distress syndrome, and infection. Deaths due to pulmonary causes, immaturity, infection, and CNS injury decreased over the study period, whereas deaths due to necrotizing enterocolitis (NEC) increased.

Morbidities of Prematurity

Birth prior to 37 weeks' gestation, particularly for ELBW infants with a birth weight <1,000 g, is associated with immaturity of multiple organ systems and myriad short- and long-term consequences in the NICU and after discharge. Common morbidities of ELBW infants include broncho-pulmonary dysplasia (BPD), late-onset sepsis, NEC, severe intracranial hemorrhage (ICH), periventricular leukomalacia (PVL), and retinopathy of prematurity (ROP) (Figure 1–6).

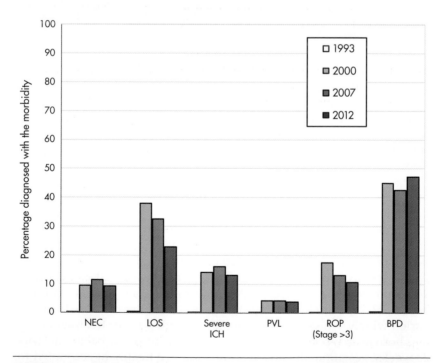

FIGURE 1–6. Neonatal morbidities for infants born at gestational ages 22–28 weeks.

BPD=bronchopulmonary dysplasia; ICH=intracranial hemorrhage; LOS=late-onset sepsis; NEC=necrotizing enterocolitis; PVL=periventricular leukomalacia; ROP=retinopathy of prematurity.

Source.   Adapted from Stoll et al. 2015.

RESPIRATORY SYSTEM

Respiratory Distress Syndrome

Respiratory distress syndrome (RDS), formerly known as hyaline membrane disease, is the major cause of respiratory distress in premature infants. The primary abnormality is surfactant deficiency that causes high surface tension leading to decreased lung compliance, instability of the alveoli at end expiration, and low lung volume. These abnormalities result in atelectasis, causing ventilation and perfusion mismatch, intrapulmonary right-to-left shunting, and hypoxemia. Surfactant deficiency also causes inflammation and respiratory epithelial injury, resulting in pulmonary edema and increased airway resistance. The incidence of RDS increases as gestational age decreases. A study from the NICHD NRN found that 93% of infants born ≤28 weeks' gestation had RDS (Stoll et al. 2010). It can also be seen with a lower frequency in late preterm infants, defined as infants born between 34 weeks' and 36 weeks, 6 days' gestation. Male sex and white race each increase the risk of RDS. The clinical symptoms of RDS present within the first minutes or hours after birth and, if untreated, progressively worsen over the first 48 hours until endogenous surfactant production increases. Tachypnea, nasal flaring, grunting, and retractions are present, and chest radiographs show a diffuse, reticulogranular, ground-glass appearance with air bronchograms and low lung volumes. The natural history of RDS is significantly modified by antenatal steroid use, treatment with exogenous surfactant, or the use of continuous positive airway pressure (CPAP). Antenatal corticosteroid therapy should be administered at 23–34 weeks' gestation to women who are at risk of preterm delivery within 7 days. Randomized controlled trials (RCTs) of antenatal corticosteroids have consistently reported a significant reduction in the incidence of RDS, moderate to severe RDS, and the need for mechanical ventilation as well as a decrease in the risk of intraventricular hemorrhage (IVH), NEC, and mortality (NIH Consensus Development Panel on the Effect of Corticosteroids for Fetal Maturation on Perinatal Outcomes 1995). The benefits are not affected by fetal sex or race. A large randomized trial studying the use of antenatal steroids after 34 weeks and up to 36 weeks, 6 days found that antenatal betamethasone administration significantly reduced the rate of neonatal respiratory complications (Gyamfi-Bannerman et al. 2016). Exogenous surfactant previously was recommended at or shortly after birth for preterm infants with RDS regardless of the use of antenatal steroids or of gestational age (Engle and American Academy of Pediatrics Committee on Fetus and Newborn 2008). Systematic reviews of RCTs concluded that surfactant replacement therapy significantly reduced the incidence of RDS, pneumothorax, pulmonary interstitial emphysema, and death (Suresh and Soll 2005). More recent trials and meta-analysis of prophylactic surfactant versus prophylactic stabilization with CPAP and selective use of surfactant have shown that the CPAP and selective surfactant group had a significantly lower risk of death or BPD (Rojas-Reyes et al. 2012). Of note, babies born at 24 and 25 weeks' gestation benefited the most. In addition, preterm infants treated with early CPAP had a decrease in the length of mechanical ventilation and lower use of postnatal corticosteroid therapy.

Apnea of Prematurity

Apnea is defined as cessation of breathing for ≥20 seconds or a shorter period when accompanied by bradycardia <100 beats per minute, cyanosis, or pallor. It is due to immature respiratory control. Apnea may be further classified as *central*, with cessation of breathing effort; *obstructive*, with lack of airflow usually at the pharyngeal level; or *mixed*. Apnea is common in preterm infants, and the incidence increases as gestational age decreases. It occurs in all premature infants born <29 weeks' gestation and decreases to 20% of infants born at 34 weeks' gestation (Henderson-Smart 1981). Apneic events were shown to resolve by 37 weeks' postmenstrual age in 92% and by 40 weeks' gestation in 98%. Infants born at lower gestational ages were more likely to have longer persistence of apneic events (Eichenwald et al. 1997). The Collaborative Home Infant Monitoring Evaluation study documented that extreme events resolved by 43 weeks' postmenstrual age in premature infants (Ramanathan et al. 2001). No data have suggested that apnea of prematurity is associated with an increased risk of SIDS, although the risk of SIDS is higher in premature infants. Apnea of prematurity is treated most commonly with methylxanthines, and caffeine is used due to its longer half-life and high therapeutic index. A large trial of caffeine use for apnea or to facilitate extubation found that caffeine-treated infants had a shorter duration of mechanical ventilation, lower risk of BPD, and improved neurodevelopmental outcomes at 18 months of age (Schmidt et al. 2006). Other treatments used for apnea of prematurity include CPAP or high-flow nasal cannula in combination with caffeine therapy. Management of apnea in newborns approaching discharge varies, but the usual requirement is for infants to be free of spontaneously occurring apnea and bradycardia for 5–7 days prior to discharge.

Air Leaks

Pulmonary air leaks occur when air escapes from the lung, with rupture of overdistended alveoli dissecting along the perivascular connective tissue sheath, resulting in pneumothorax, pneumomediastinum, pulmonary interstitial emphysema, and pneumopericardium. The incidence is highest in preterm infants with lung disease requiring positive-pressure ventilation. Mechanical ventilation is most apt to increase the risk of air leak when it involves high peak inspiratory pressure, large tidal volume, or long inspiratory time. Air leak can be asymptomatic, noted on routine chest radiograph, or can present dramatically with sudden clinical deterioration. Treatment for pneumothorax, the most common form of air leak, involves needle aspiration of the air, often followed by chest tube placement. Small pneumothoraces in asymptomatic or minimally symptomatic newborns who are not on positive-pressure support may be observed without specific treatment.

Bronchopulmonary Dysplasia

BPD, also known as chronic lung disease, is an important cause of morbidity, affecting more than 25% of very low birth weight (VLBW) infants and approximately 40% of ELBW infants. Lung development is interrupted by preterm birth, and alveolarization and normal lung growth are significantly impaired even without supplemental oxygen and mechanical ventilation. Genetic factors, intrauterine and postnatal infection and inflammation, and oxidant stress are some of the other potential causes of impaired lung development leading to BPD (Higgins et al. 2018) (Figure 1–7). The definition of BPD has changed since the 1990s. The definition used most commonly is oxygen use at 36 weeks' postmenstrual age. Rates of BPD have been increasing in recent years, likely due to the survival of smaller and less mature infants; a large observational study found an increase in BPD from 32% in 1993 to 45% in 2008–2012 (Stoll et al. 2015). Certain factors such as intrauterine growth restriction increase the risk of BPD.

Optimal management strategies to prevent as well as treat BPD have not yet been determined. Many interventions have targeted BPD prevention; however, most have had limited success. Caffeine is one intervention shown to significantly decrease BPD, whereas inhaled nitric oxide did not demonstrate a benefit in BPD prevention, despite biological plausibility. Less invasive approaches to respiratory management following birth are logical because babies have lower rates of BPD when they are never intubated. A large trial of CPAP versus intubation and surfactant found no significant difference in BPD or death; however, the CPAP group did have significantly less need for intubation and fewer days of mechanical ventilation (Finer et al. 2010). In addition, follow-up studies found less clinical lung disease at 2 years of age in the CPAP group (Stevens et al. 2014). Most infants receiving respiratory support improve over time. As pulmonary function improves with growth, they can be transitioned from mechanical ventilation to CPAP to supplemental oxygen delivered via cannula. However, different patterns of respiratory disease are seen in the first 2 weeks of life in ELBW infants. If clinical deterioration with need for mechanical ventilation occurs during this time period, the risk of BPD increases significantly (Laughon et al. 2009). Some infants require long periods of mechanical ventilation

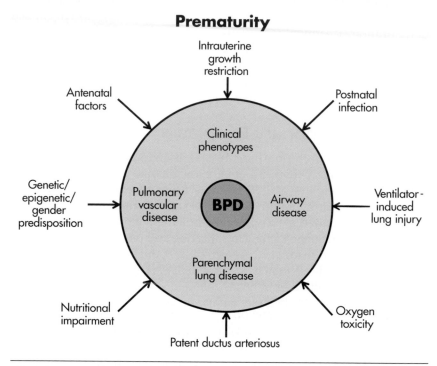

Prematurity

FIGURE 1–7.   Multifactorial etiology of bronchopulmonary dysplasia (BPD).
Source.   Reprinted from *The Journal of Pediatrics*, Vol. 197, Rosemary D. Higgins, Alan H. Jobe, Marion Koso-Thomas, et al. "Bronchopulmonary Dysplasia: Executive Summary of a Workshop," 300–308, Copyright © 2018, with permission from Elsevier.

and are at high risk for adverse long-term outcomes, including poor growth, chronic respiratory morbidities, pulmonary hypertension, and poor neurodevelopmental outcome.

CARDIOVASCULAR SYSTEM

Patent Ductus Arteriosus

The ductus arteriosus, which connects the pulmonary artery and the aorta, is an essential structure in fetal life; however, its persistence after birth becomes problematic in premature infants. After birth, when pulmonary vascular resistance drops, a patent ductus arteriosus (PDA) allows a left-to-right shunt, causing excessive pulmonary blood flow and ductal steal that results in decreased perfusion to other organs. A persistent PDA has been linked to adverse outcomes, including BPD, impaired renal function, NEC, IVH, and death. Elimination of ductal flow can be attempted using cyclooxygenase inhibitors or surgical ligation. Indomethacin prophylaxis after birth for ELBW infants was found to decrease the incidence of severe

IVH, but it did not result in improved neurodevelopmental outcomes (Schmidt et al. 2001). Surgical ligation can also result in both short- and long-term adverse outcomes, including vocal cord paralysis, cardiorespiratory decompensation, BPD, ROP, and neurodevelopmental impairment (NDI). RCTs have not confirmed that either treatment strategy improves outcomes, and for this reason, treatment of a PDA remains a controversial topic in neonatology with wide practice variation (Benitz 2010, 2011; Malviya et al. 2013). Current practices favor selective later treatment over routine early treatment; however, the timing, criteria, and specific method of treating the duct have not been determined.

Hypotension

Extremely preterm infants who are critically ill often experience hypotension after birth. There are no widely accepted definitions for normal blood pressure, and this has led to significant practice variation. Treatments for hypotension include volume boluses, blood transfusion, and vasoactive drugs and are used with the belief that blood pressure is a proxy for tissue perfusion and that by increasing blood pressure, tissue perfusion will improve and adverse outcomes will lessen. Laughon et al. (2007) studied blood pressures in 1,507 newborns between 23 weeks' and 27 weeks, 6 days' gestation and the use of treatments for hypotension. He found that 80% of newborns received treatment for hypotension, and the lowest blood pressures were seen in the lowest gestational age babies and increased with chronological age. Lower birth weight, male sex, and higher severity of illness were associated with treatment, although institutions varied significantly in their use of therapies for hypotension. Batton et al. (2013) prospectively studied blood pressure and treatment of hypotension and found that 55% received treatment for hypotension. Surprisingly, treatment was also administered to 28%–41% of infants without hypotension. Treated infants were significantly more likely than untreated infants to experience adverse outcomes, including severe retinopathy, severe IVH, or death. In a follow-up study, infants given an antihypotensive therapy had a significantly higher rate of death or NDI when compared with the untreated group, and this difference could not be explained by other markers such as severity of illness (Batton et al. 2016).

INFECTIONS

Prematurity places infants, particularly ELBW infants, at risk for infection due to immaturity of the immune system as well as for prolonged hospitalization and invasive procedures, such as endotracheal intubation and use of intravenous central lines. The term *neonatal sepsis* is generally used to describe a systemic infection of bacterial, viral, or fungal origin, with associated clinical manifestations. This definition includes the isolation of a pathogen from a usually sterile body fluid (e.g., blood, cerebrospinal fluid, trachea, or urine); however, the clinical features can be present without identification of an organism, because small volume collections of body fluids often fail to identify the organism responsible. This is called *culture-negative sepsis* or *suspected sepsis*.

Neonatal sepsis can be classified as either early or late-onset sepsis depending on the age of onset. Early onset sepsis is an invasive bacterial infection occurring in the first 3 days after birth. It is strongly associated with perinatal risk factors and likely represents vertical mother-to-infant transmission. It almost always is accompanied by clinical symptoms in the first 24 hours after birth. The most common pathogens are *Escherichia coli* in the preterm infant and group B *Streptococcus* in the term infant (Stoll et al. 2011). The frequency of early onset sepsis has changed dramatically with the use of intrapartum prophylaxis for early onset group B streptococcal sepsis (Figure 1–8). The rate of occurrence is 0.98 infections per 1,000 births, with the highest rates found in preterm infants— 10.96 per 1,000 live births.

Late-onset sepsis is defined as a positive blood culture occurring after 3 days of age and is known to be associated with increased morbidity and mortality in the NICU. Among ELBW survivors, 65% have at least one suspected infection and 35% have culture-proven sepsis (Stoll et al. 2004). ELBW infants with late-onset sepsis have a mortality rate of 18%, prolonged hospital stays, and significantly increased rates of NDI compared with noninfected ELBW infants. For this reason, significant efforts have focused on strategies to reduce the rate of nosocomial infection in NICUs. Quality improvement efforts include hand hygiene procedures, central line care bundles, antifungal prophylaxis, and improvements in NICU design and staffing. An observational study documented a significant improvement in the overall incidence of late-onset sepsis between two eras in the NICHD NRN; however, not all NICUs showed improvement (Greenberg et al. 2017). The 7% decrease likely represents efforts by individual NICUs to reduce infection, but data on which specific interventions were most successful were not studied.

GROWTH AND NUTRITION

Premature infants are born at a point in development at which their nutrient needs are extremely high. Growth failure is a major problem for premature infants during their NICU stay. The goal for these infants is to achieve appropriate increases in weight, length, and head circumference as would be seen in the developing fetus. In addition, premature infants often have other diagnoses that increase their energy expenditure further, increasing the caloric intake needed to achieve adequate growth. Growth is monitored by serial measurements of weight, length, and head circumference and compared with premature growth charts. Targets are weight gain of 15–20 g/day, length increase of 1 cm/week, and head circumfer-

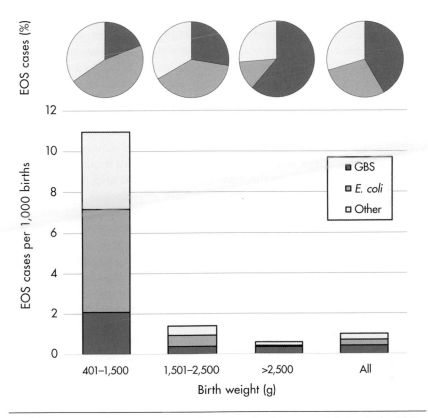

FIGURE 1–8. **Incidence and organisms involved in neonatal sepsis by birthweight.**

E. coli=*Escherichia coli*; EOS=early onset sepsis; GBS=group B *Streptococcus*.
Source. Stoll et al. 2011.

ence increase of 1 cm/week. If the rate of growth is insuficient, nutrient targets are adjusted. The goal is to keep infants growing at rates above the 10th percentile. Dieticians assist NICU medical providers in making needed adjustments to optimize nutrition and growth. The nutritional status of premature infants is also monitored by serial laboratory evaluations.

Early initiation of enteral feedings has been shown to be beneficial; however, due to the immaturity of the gastrointestinal tract, including decreased motility and reduced intestinal enzyme activity, enteral feedings cannot be rapidly advanced. Rapid increases in feeding volumes may result in feeding intolerance or NEC. Feeding protocols guide feeding initiation and advancement. Typically, all infants receive colostrum swabbed on the buccal mucosa every 3 hours beginning in the first day of life. Infants weighing <1,500 g or those unable to take enteral feeds receive parenteral nutrition containing glucose, amino acids, calcium, and lipids within several hours after birth to supply a portion of their nutrient needs. All infants also receive small-volume "trophic" feeds if they are medically stable and have a functional gastrointestinal tract.

Enteral feedings are generally given via tube in babies born earlier than 32–34 weeks' gestation due to their inability to suck or coordinate suck and swallow with breathing. Feeds are delivered via orogastric or nasogastric tube. Ideally, the mother's milk is used; if not available, pasteurized donor human milk is preferred for infants weighing <1,500 g, continued up until approximately 34 weeks' gestation. Feedings are advanced gradually, and parenteral nutrition is tapered slowly. As feedings are increased, fortifier is used to augment the nutrient intake. The rate of advancement depends on the infant's birth weight and feeding tolerance. Feeding tolerance should be routinely assessed; symptoms suggesting feeding intolerance include emesis, abdominal symptoms (e.g., distension, tenderness, or absent bowel sounds), green or red gastric residuals, and presence of blood in stools.

Oral feeding should be started as soon as the infant shows signs of readiness. Some preterm infants born later than 34 weeks can be orally fed from birth; others require periods of tube feeding. Premature infants approach discharge criteria when they are able to maintain their body temperature in an open crib and are feeding by mouth with a good growth rate. Some infants may be discharged to home on tube feedings if they are otherwise stable and a longer period of tube feedings will be needed.

Gastroesophageal Reflux

Gastroesophageal reflux is the transient relaxation of the lower esophageal sphincter, often accompanied by poor coordination of esophageal motility, allowing reflux of gastric contents into the esophagus. The premature infant may also have delayed gastric emptying. Reflux is common and physiological in all newborns in the first few months of life and causes few symptoms. It is seen more frequently in premature infants and may be associated with feeding problems, such as frequent emesis, feeding aversion, poor weight gain, grimacing, aspiration, and exacerbation of chronic lung disease. Numerous studies have failed to demonstrate a temporal association of gastroesophageal reflux and apnea in preterm infants or a worsening of apnea when reflux is present (Peter et al. 2002). Nonpharmacological treatment consists of elevating the head of the bed and positioning the infant left side down so that the lower esophageal sphincter is in a higher position. The most common pharmacological intervention is a histamine H_2 blocker or proton pump inhibitor to decrease gastric acidity.

Necrotizing Enterocolitis

NEC is one of the most common gastrointestinal emergencies in newborn infants. Diagnosis is typically made radiographically by identifying air in the bowel wall, pneumatosis intestinalis, free air in the abdomen, pneumoperitoneum, or portal venous air. A classification system was suggested by Bell that differentiated suspected (Stage I), proven (Stage II), and advanced (Stage III) NEC (Table 1–2) (Bell et al. 1978). Most affected infants are premature, with an increasing incidence as gestational age decreases. The exact etiology is unknown; however, important risk factors include prematurity, intestinal ischemia, enteral feeding, and bacterial colonization. An observational study of preterm infants performed by the NICHD NRN found an overall incidence of 9% (Stoll et al. 2015). The incidence seems to be declining, likely related to quality improvement efforts aimed at reducing risk, including use of antenatal steroids, human milk feedings, and avoiding prolonged antibiotic use. Classic NEC in preterm infants occurs from 10 to 25 days of age, with a peak at 32 weeks' gestation. Clinical presentation can vary from slowly increasing feeding intolerance or bloody stools without other signs of illness to fulminant disease with a shock-like picture.

Treatment of NEC is supportive and includes fluid resuscitation, withholding feedings with gastric decompression via nasogastric tube, and antibiotics to cover enteric pathogens. Management of acidosis, thrombocytopenia, coagulopathy, and shock is needed in patients with more fulminant presentations. Approximately 30% have mild disease and require bowel rest and antibiotics but do not require surgical intervention, whereas another 15%–30% die from NEC. Surgical interventions include peritoneal drain placement or exploratory laparotomy. Prior studies have compared the outcomes of these two approaches but have failed to demonstrate any differences in mortality or time on total parenteral nutrition (Moss et al. 2006; Rees et al. 2008). Several additional interventions show promise for further decreasing rates of NEC, including lactoferrin and probiotics, but data around their impact on outcomes are limited (Barbian et al. 2019; Sari et al. 2012).

An RCT is being performed by the NICHD NRN, and the primary outcome is mortality without NDI at 18–22 months' adjusted age. Recruitment has been completed, and follow-up results are anticipated in the near future. Survivors of surgical NEC may have long-term complications, including prolonged dependence on total parenteral nutrition, short bowel syndrome, failure to thrive, and neurodevelopmental delay (Hintz et al. 2005).

NEUROLOGICAL SYSTEM

Intraventricular Hemorrhage

IVH is the most common type of intracranial pathology seen in the premature infant. Preterm infants are at risk for impaired autoregulation, which results in increases in cerebral blood flow leading to rupture of the fragile blood vessels in the germinal matrix. The germinal matrix, a

Table 1–2.　Modified Bell's staging criteria for necrotizing enterocolitis (NEC)

Stage	NEC classification	Systemic signs	Abdominal signs	Radiographic signs
IA	Suspected	Temperature instability, apnea, bradycardia, lethargy	Gastric retention, abdominal distention, emesis, heme-positive stool	Normal or mild intestinal dilation, mild ileus
IB	Suspected	Same as IA	Grossly bloody stool	Same as IA
IIA	Definite, mildly ill	Same as IA	Same as IB, plus absent bowel sounds with or without abdominal tenderness	Intestinal dilation, ileus, pneumatosis intestinalis
IIB	Definite, moderately ill	Same as IIA, plus mild metabolic acidosis and thrombocytopenia	Same as IIA, plus absent bowel sounds and definite tenderness, with or without abdominal cellulitis or right lower quadrant mass	Same as IIA, plus ascites
IIIA	Advanced, severely ill, intact bowel	Same as IIB, plus hypotension, bradycardia, severe apnea, combined respiratory and metabolic acidosis, disseminated intravascular coagulation, and neutropenia	Same as IIA, plus signs of peritonitis, marked tenderness, and abdominal distention	Same as IIA, plus ascites
IIIB	Advanced, severely ill, perforated bowel	Same as IIIA	Same as IIIA	Same as IIIA, plus pneumoperitoneum

Source.　Reprinted from *Pediatric Clinics*, Vol. 43, Issue 2, Joseph Neu, "Necrotizing Enterocolitis: The Search for a Unifying Pathogenic Theory Leading to Prevention," 409–432, Copyright © 1996, with permission from Elsevier.

periventricular structure between the caudate nucleus and the thalamus, progressively decreases in size as gestational age advances, with nearly complete involution by 36 weeks of gestation. In the premature newborn, the germinal matrix contains a fine vascular network without supportive stroma. The risk of IVH increases with decreasing maturity; it is more common in EPT infants born earlier than 28 weeks' gestation and is rare after 32 weeks. Most hemorrhages occur in the first 48 hours and almost all in the first week of life. IVH is often asymptomatic, but occasionally it will be accompanied by lethargy, seizures, drop in hematocrit, hypotension, or metabolic acidosis. The Papile grading system (Papile et al. 1978) has been used to classify IVH (Table 1–3). The incidence of IVH declined significantly following the widespread use of antenatal steroids and postnatal surfactant in the 1990s. The percentage of babies with severe IVH, defined as grade 3 or 4, also declined significantly between 1993 and 2012 in infants born at 26–28 weeks' gestation but not in infants born at 22–25 weeks' gestation (Stoll et al. 2015).

Table 1–3.   Papile grading system of intraventricular hemorrhage

Grade	Description
Grade I	Blood in the periventricular germinal matrix regions or germinal matrix hemorrhage
Grade II	Blood within the lateral ventricular system without ventricular dilation
Grade III	Blood distending the lateral ventricles
Grade IV	Blood within the ventricular system and intraparenchymal hemorrhage

Source. Adapted from Papile et al. 1978.

Severe IVH can be complicated by posthemorrhagic hydrocephalus, which is defined as progressive ventricular dilatation. Posthemorrhagic hydrocephalus can be transient or persistent and is caused by obstruction of the cerebrospinal fluid flow within the ventricular system or diffusely by decreased absorption by arachnoid villi. Management involves preventing excessive ventricular distension and increased intracranial pressure using serial lumbar puncture, ventriculostomy, or ultimately by placement of a ventriculoperitoneal shunt.

Periventricular Leukomalacia

PVL is described as multifocal areas of necrosis that form cysts in the deep periventricular white matter, occurring in a specific distribution dorsolateral to the external angles of the adjacent lateral ventricles. Perinatal inflammation and cerebral ischemia are two factors known to contribute to PVL. In a recent study, cystic PVL occurred in 6% of premature infants ≤26 weeks' gestation and was found to be transient in 18%, persistent in 20%, and appearing late in 62%; all were associated with NDI and cerebral palsy (CP) (Sarkar et al. 2018).

Seizures

The incidence of seizures in the term neonatal population had been estimated at 1–5 per 1,000 live births, with higher rates of 9–11 per 1,000 live births among premature newborns. These studies did not account for the low diagnostic accuracy of clinical observation alone. It is now recognized that neonatal seizures are frequently either subtle or often subclinical, and thus the rate of seizures is likely much higher. Both continuous electroencephalography and amplitude-integrated encephalography are being used with more frequency in the NICU, resulting in improved detection of seizure activity. Premature infants with neonatal seizures have been found to have an increased risk of adverse neurodevelopmental outcome, independent of multiple other confounding factors (Davis et al. 2010). The adverse outcome may be related to both the underlying cause of the seizures and the impact of seizure activity on the developing brain.

Retinopathy of Prematurity

ROP is the abnormal growth of blood vessels in the retina of premature infants. It leads to a wide range of outcomes, from normal vision to blindness. A review of interventions and short-term outcomes over a 20-year period by the NRN reported ROP stage 3 or higher in about 15% of infants born ≤28 weeks' gestation, with incidence of ROP and high-grade ROP increasing significantly as gestational age decreased (Stoll et al. 2015). ROP is more common in infants with a longer duration of mechanical ventilation, prolonged oxygen administration, and other indicators of illness severity. Careful monitoring of oxygen saturation reduces but does not eliminate ROP. Restriction of supplemental oxygen has been used to reduce ROP, and clinical trials in the neonatal population have been undertaken to evaluate this approach (discussed later).

ROP is classified based on the staging of the disease (stages 1–5), the location of the retina involved (zone I–III), the extent of retinal involvement (1–12 clock hours), and the presence of plus disease (Table 1–4; Figure 1–9). *Plus disease* is defined as dilated and tortuous blood vessels in the posterior pole of the eye and is indicative of aggressive ROP. All infants born at a weight <1,500 g or a gestational age ≤30 weeks, as well as those with a birth weight between 1,500 and 2,000 g who have an unstable clinical course, should be screened by a retina specialist at either 31 weeks' postmenstrual age or 4 weeks' chronological age, whichever is later, and follow-up eye examinations performed every 1–2 weeks. Moderately severe ROP can be managed effectively in many cases by laser therapy or cryotherapy to ablate the avascular retina. Intravitreal injections of antivascular endothelial growth factor therapy are a more recent treatment modality for ROP. A multicenter trial demonstrated a reduced recurrence of ROP with this method when compared with laser treatment and decreased rates of severe myopia (Mintz-Hittner et al. 2011); however, some concerns have arisen about systemic absorption and harmful effects on developing tissues, specifically the brain.

Table 1–4.   Stages of retinopathy of prematurity

Stage	Description
Stage 1	Demarcation line. This is a whitish line visible between the normally vascularized retina and the peripheral retina in which there are no blood vessels.
Stage 2	Visible ridge. The demarcation line develops into a ridge, with height and width, between the vascular retina and peripheral retina.
Stage 3	Blood vessels in the ridge. Blood vessels grow and multiply and are visible in the ridge.
Stage 4	Subtotal retinal detachment. Vitreoretinal surgery may be indicated.
Stage 5	Total retinal detachment. No treatment is usually possible.

Source.   National Eye Institute: Retinopathy of Prematurity. Bethesda, MD, National Institutes of Health, 2019. Available at: https://www.nei.nih.gov/learn-about-eye-health/eye-conditions-and-diseases/retinopathy-prematurity. Accessed September 1, 2019.

SUMMARY

Preterm birth is one of the five leading causes of infant mortality in the United States; approximately 10% of all births occur prior to 37 weeks' gestation. For this reason, reducing preterm birth is a public health priority. Despite substantial research, the causes of preterm birth are poorly understood. Approximately two-thirds are spontaneous preterm births, whereas one-third are medically induced to avoid or minimize maternal or fetal complications. Advances in medical care have decreased mortality; however, the earlier the baby is born, the higher the risk for mortality or complications related to prematurity. Preterm birth is associated with immaturity of almost every organ system, and each system has specific complications. The most common and significant complications of prematurity are BPD, sepsis, NEC, severe IVH, PVL, and ROP.

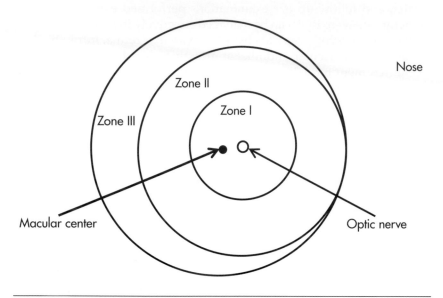

FIGURE 1–9.   Retinopathy of prematurity (ROP) zones.

Neurodevelopmental Outcomes of Extremely Preterm Infants

WHY FOCUS ON THE NEURODEVELOPMENTAL OUTCOMES?

With advances in perinatal and neonatal care and changes in approach to resuscitation, survival for extremely preterm infants has improved significantly in recent decades (Stoll et al. 2015). This survival benefit has extended to the most premature infants born EPT and those with ELBW (<1,000 g). Although some of the most substantial factors contributing to the remarkably improved survival for this vulnerable group have been related to scientific progress leading to new perinatal and neonatal treatments and technologies, the stance toward active antepartum, intrapartum, and neonatal intervention has been increasingly influential (Rysavy et al. 2015). In light of this improved survival for EPT infants, focus has shifted to early childhood neurodevelopmental and other later outcomes. There has subsequently been increasing recognition of the critical significance of understanding postdischarge outcomes, both to evaluate the true impact of interventions and management approaches in the NICU and to inform counseling and direct early detection of neurodevelopmental challenges and intervention.

CHALLENGES TO INTERPRETING NEURODEVELOPMENTAL OUTCOMES AND IMPAIRMENT

Before we a review the neurodevelopmental outcomes literature, we must first consider the challenges to understanding the complexities and limitations of those results. Although predicting survival to NICU discharge been refined beyond the use of gestational age only, there remains substantial variability and lack of precision of predicting even this early endpoint, which is influenced by many variables, including center differences (Lee et al. 2010; Rysavy et al. 2015; Tyson et al. 2008).

The prediction and interpretation of neurodevelopmental outcomes is much more difficult; thus, counseling and education about these outcomes is fraught with tremendous challenges. Medical providers and investigators rely on large studies of children born preterm, which most often report NDI, to direct their understanding of these outcomes. This is a "composite outcome" combining criteria and cut points from several outcome domains, including neuromotor, cognitive, hearing, and vision (Table 1–5). Unfortunately, definitions and levels of severity of NDI differ among studies, which necessarily leads to difficulties in the overall interpretation and to significant challenges in applicability and counseling. This inconsistency was elegantly illustrated by the Canadian Neonatal Follow Up Network, which applied a range of severe NDI definitions to its large database of outcomes at 18–30 months of corrected age among children born EPT (Haslam et al. 2018). The authors found that the *definition* of severe NDI used had a significant influence on its incidence (ranging from 3.5% to 14.9% depending on definition) as well as the associations between risk factors and severe NDI. In addition, significant center variation in neurodevelopmental outcomes among babies of 18–22 months' corrected age has been demonstrated by the NICHD NRN even after adjusting for demographic variables, antenatal interventions, and neonatal clinical factors, thus presenting challenges to accurate counseling from multicenter datasets (Vohr et al. 2004). It may thus seem most appropriate to use data from a local site only in the context of counseling families, but it is unlikely that a single center would have robust and current outcomes data for specific high-risk groups, such as infants born extraordinarily preterm. Furthermore, the largest contributing component to the composite NDI outcome is "cognitive" delay or impairment. Developmental tests performed at 18–30 months are intended to provide some concept of cognitive abilities. However, as we discuss in more detail later, scores on these tests administered in toddler age to children born ELBW and EPT have been shown to be poor predictors of cognitive scores at school age (Hack et al. 2005; Roberts et al. 2010; Schmidt et al. 2012; Spencer-Smith et al. 2015). Early

Table 1–5.   Domains and assessments included in typical definitions of the composite outcome of neurodevelopmental impairment during toddler age among children born preterm

Domain	Evaluations at 18–36 months' corrected age
Motor	Neurological examination for cerebral palsy and GMFCS level; motor composite score on standardized developmental test (i.e., Bayley Scales); cut points based on normed test mean or compared with term-born control group
Cognitive	Cognitive composite score on standardized developmental test (i.e., Bayley Scales); cut points based on normed test mean or compared with term-born control group
Vision	Clinical evaluation of bilateral blindness and ability to perceive light
Hearing	Functional assessment of ability to hear and follow directions with or without aids or cochlear implants
Speech and language*	Determination of ability to follow commands and meaningful words or signs; language composite score on standardized developmental test (i.e., Bayley Scales); cut points based on normed test mean or compared with term-born control group.

*Speech and language assessments have not been included in all definitions of neurodevelopmental impairment in the literature.
GMFCS=Gross Motor Function Classification System.

and especially later cognitive and behavioral outcomes in childhood are extraordinarily complex and greatly impacted by postdischarge environment, relationships, and biological factors (Msall and Park 2008; Treyvaud et al. 2012). Concerns about changes in cognitive, academic, behavioral, motor, and coordination abilities over time underscore the need for later assessment as well as support and interventions that may modify recovery. These issues combine to make attempts at predicting precise individual patient outcomes ill conceived.

It is important to recognize that numerous trials and prospective studies in neonatal medicine, particularly for children born EPT, now have death or NDI at 2–3 years of age as a primary or main secondary outcome. Because death and NDI are competing outcomes, the assumption is often made that these adverse outcomes will not be influenced in the same direction by an intervention. However, this assumption is not always valid. A composite outcome, whether including death or a composite of neurosensory and developmental outcomes only, may also not be the ideal target from a biological, patient-centered, or family-centered perspective (Dahan et al. 2019). Moreover, although neurodevelopmental outcome at 2–3 years of age and beyond is critically important for any prospective observational study or clinical trial that evaluates care and assesses the safety of interventions, it may not be the most appropriate primary outcome for every trial (Marlow 2015).

For families and other medical decision makers, knowing the range of outcomes beyond the neonatal period—and of the limitations in our ability to predict them—is vital to approaching the possible implications and consequences of EPT birth. However, whether information about composite outcomes, either in the prenatal or postnatal setting, is actually meaningful to parents and families remains questionable. Moreover, parents and families of children born preterm may value one outcome or group of outcomes differently than do researchers or others in society. Families may find it hard to understand the information presented on potential outcomes, and statistics are likely to be difficult to grasp (Dupont-Thibodeau et al. 2014; Janvier and Barrington 2012). The value of outcomes also may differ for those who themselves were born preterm (Hack 2009; Hack et al. 2004; Saigal et al. 2006, 2016) and among physicians and other care providers, investigators, educators, and those involved in developing public policy.

Despite these provisos, a large body of literature exists on the early neurodevelopmental outcomes of children born EPT. An understanding of the range of reported outcomes and associated factors described in the literature is important for both the family and the medical care team. In this chapter, we do not attempt to present a comprehensive review of all published neurodevelopmental outcomes studies but concentrate on results from larger cohorts and regional population-based studies. Furthermore, because the substantial majority of studies report early neurodevelopmental outcomes, our focus is on outcomes at ages 18 months to 3 years, although we acknowledge that evaluation at this time point represents only a tiny and incomplete view into the child's future life.

Components of Early Neurodevelopmental Outcomes

MOTOR FUNCTION

Motor impairments, including CP, are among the most frequently reported neurodevelopmental outcomes for EPT and ELBW infants. Motor difficulties may become evident over months or years, but their timely identification may allow for interventions to improve outcomes, thereby reinforcing the critical importance of vigilant long-term follow-up. CP is a disorder of movement and posture that involves abnormalities in tone, reflexes, coordination, and movement as well as delays in motor milestone achievement and aberration in primitive reflexes that is permanent but not unchanging and caused by a nonprogressive interference, lesion, or abnormality in the developing immature brain (Bax et al. 2005; Fawke 2007). CP is also categorized by type (spastic, dyskinetic, or dystonic), topography (limbs involved), and descriptors of the extent and pattern of involvement (monoplegia, diplegia, hemiplegia, and quadriplegia). CP sometimes cannot be diagnosed with confidence until after 18 months of age, although early examinations of general movement assessment and other factors may elevate the risk profile and underscore the need for intervention and follow-up (Kwong et al. 2018; Spittle et al. 2011, 2013).

The five-level Gross Motor Function Classification System (GMFCS) (Palisano et al. 1997, 2007; Rethlefsen et al. 2010) provides a valid and reliable system to classify the extent of activity limitation in CP. Higher levels on the GMFCS are associated with increasing functional difficulty. Importantly for early childhood assessments, distinctions between levels I and II are not as significant as differences between other levels. Nonetheless, the positive predictive value of an early assessment classification of GMFCS level I, II, or III (child will walk with or without aids) compared with level IV or V (child will likely need a wheelchair for mobility) is very high (0.96). The GMFCS provides a sound approximation, rather than a definitive final functional categorization, in this age group (Gorter et al. 2009). Although CP with severe functional limitations is of great concern, it is relatively rare. Children diagnosed with CP may have a spectrum of neurological findings, including a range of motor and coordination deficits, and individualized evaluation and tailored interventions are critical (Vohr et al. 2005).

An Australian CP registry review from the 1970s to 2004 showed an increasing prevalence of CP in the 1970s and 1980s which was attributed to increasing survival of EPT infants; however, CP rates stabilized or decreased between the early 1990s and 2004 (Reid et al. 2011; Spittle and Orton 2014). A recent study over a 4-year period of children born EPT in the NICHD NRN, with assessments at 18–26 months' corrected age, showed that the rate of any level of CP decreased from 16% in 2011 to 12% in 2014. Among those affected, the rate of severe CP decreased over time, while the rate of mild CP increased (Adams-Chapman et al. 2018) (Figure 1–10). A report from a population-based cohort study of nine regions in France found that 6.9% (95% CI 4.7–9.6) of children born at 24 weeks' to 26 weeks, 6 days' gestation were reported to have any CP; however, that study relied on pediatrician questionnaires rather than in-person examinations by certified examiners (Pierrat et al. 2017).

Motor and coordination impairments apart from CP are reported in children born preterm, and some are associated with serious challenges. Even at the relatively early assessment time point of 18–26 months' corrected age, 25%–30% of children born EPT have been reported to have neurological examination results that are "suspect" or abnormal but do

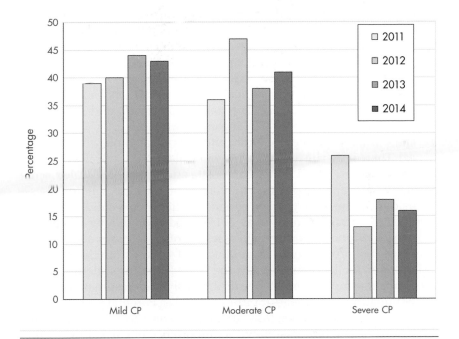

FIGURE 1–10. **Severity of illness among infants with cerebral palsy (CP), 2011–2014.**

Any level of CP decreased from 16% in 2011 to 12% in 2014.

Source. Adams-Chapman et al. 2018.

not meet the criteria for CP, whereas nearly 60% are considered normal on neurological evaluation (Adams-Chapman et al. 2018). Developmental coordination disorder (DCD) is a diagnosis considered best made at 5 years of age or later, but motor performance assessment tools are available from 3 years of age. The criteria for DCD diagnosis include

A. Motor coordination and performance below expected for the child's chronological age and intelligence level (score <15th percentile) on the Movement Assessment Battery for Children (Henderson et al. 2007) or equivalent test such as the Bruininks-Oseretsky Test of Motor Proficiency (Bruininks and Bruininks 2005);
B. Motor disorder interferes with activities of daily living or academic achievement;
C. Motor disorder is not due to a general medical or neurological condition, such as CP; and
D. Motor difficulties are in excess of those associated with any intellectual disability present (Blank et al. 2012; Sugden et al. 2006).

Although the motor difficulties associated with DCD are often considered "minor" motor impairments in comparison with disabling CP, they nonetheless can have a significant impact on the child. These difficulties may include important functional abilities including fine motor skills, speed and accuracy in motor planning, balance, and coordination. Children with DCD or probable DCD have been shown to be at increased risk for reading and attention difficulties, social-emotional and behavior problems, anxiety, speech and language impairment, and other challenges (Kirby and Sugden 2007; Lingam et al. 2012).

The evaluation of neuromotor outcomes throughout childhood is critical. There is debate regarding the value of the Bayley Scales of Infant Development (BSID)-III motor composite and fine motor scaled score normative data and cut points in the context of other gross motor assessments during the early toddler period to determine a child's "impairment" at that time (Duncan et al. 2015). Prediction of later motor and coordination concerns from early assessments also poses a significant dilemma. In a prospective, longitudinal EPT cohort from the 2005 Victorian Infant Collaborative Study, the BSID-III motor scale normative cut points for impairment at 2 years seriously underestimated rates of motor impairment at 4 years (Spittle et al. 2013). Parental perceptions of DCD are also unreliable, yet interventions may ameliorate the functional limitations of DCD, highlighting the importance of clinical evaluation (Roberts et al. 2011). These concerns also extend beyond children born EPT. In a New Zealand cohort at risk for hypoglycemia (i.e., moderately preterm, low birth weight, or large for gestational age), subjects' motor score, fine and gross motor subtest scores, and neurological assessments at 2 years were poorly predictive of motor difficulties at 4.5 years, explaining 0%–7% of variance in MABC-2 scores (Burakevych et al. 2017). There is increasing recognition that physical and environmental effects as well as early intervention approaches may modify recovery of motor delays, which also reinforces the need for serial assessments.

COGNITIVE ASSESSMENT

A central component of the high-risk infant neurodevelopmental follow-up visit has been the administration of a standardized developmental test. These tests are meant to provide a measure of "cognitive" function, although they have widely acknowledged limitations, including 1) the evolution of test versions that make it difficult to compare across cohorts, 2) preclusion of extrapolation of 2- to 3-year results to IQ at later time points, and 3) challenges to interpretation of results in the preterm population using standardized cut points alone and in the absence of a contemporaneous normal birth weight term control group.

With a testing age range of 1–42 months, the BSID is now the most widely used developmental test for high-risk infants across the United

States and Europe. The original version, released in 1969, was revised in 1993 (BSID-II; Bayley 1993). The BSID-II had two developmental scores: the Mental Developmental Index (MDI), a composite of cognitive and language tasks, and the Psychomotor Developmental Index, a composite of fine and gross motor skills. The perceived drawback in combining cognitive and language in a single measure, as well as the drive to revise editions due to the "Flynn effect" (Flynn 1999), contributed to the development of the BSID-III (Bayley 2006). The BSID-III contains a cognitive composite score, a language composite score (with receptive and expressive subscores), and a motor composite score (with gross and fine motor subscores), in addition to social-emotional and adaptive behavior domains. Its goal was to identify delays as well as relative strengths and challenges in specific developmental domains and to target interventions to areas of need. However, in part due to a change in approach to norming the BSID-III and to separation of the cognitive and language scales, cognitive scores on the BSID-III were found to be substantially higher than anticipated among both preterm high-risk children and full-term control groups (Anderson et al. 2010; Vohr et al. 2012).

These findings have led to concern that the BSID-III underestimates developmental delay if normative test means are used alone, which has serious implications for both clinical and research endeavors. Previously, commonly used cut points for the categorization of moderate and severe developmental delay or disability were 2–3 and >3 standard deviations below the normative mean, respectively; thus, for BSID-II, an MDI of 55–70 was considered moderate, whereas an MDI <55 was considered a severe delay (British Association of Perinatal Medicine 2008; Vohr et al. 2012). However, in the era of the BSID-III and in the absence of contemporaneous term-born or normal birth weight control groups, commonly used cut points have shifted. Some have recommended that BSID-III cognitive and language scores <85 or combined BSID-III scores <80 provide the best definition of moderate to severe delay for equivalence with a BSID-II MDI score <70 (Johnson et al. 2014), whereas others have modified the categorization threshold to define moderate delay as 70–84, severe delay as 55–69, and profound delay as <54 (Schmidt et al. 2012; Vohr 2014). The fourth edition of the BSID, Bayley-4, was published in September 2019 (Bayley and Aylward 2019).

Although a full discussion of later childhood assessments is beyond the scope of this chapter, many cognitive development tests are available to provide full-scale IQ or equivalent scores, including the Wechsler Preschool and Primary Scale of Intelligence (age range 2 years, 6 months to 7 years, 7 months), now in its fourth edition (Wechsler 2012); the Differential Ability Scales (age range 2 years, 6 months to 17 years, 11 months), now in its second edition (DAS-II; Elliott et al. 2018), and the Wechsler Intelligence Scale for Children (age range 6 years, 0 months to 16 years, 11 months), now in its fifth edition (Wechsler et al. 2014). The Wechsler

Individual Achievement Test (age range 4 years, 0 months to 50 years, 11 months), now in its third edition (Wechsler 2009), identifies academic strengths and weaknesses and has been used in clinical, research, and educational settings.

Substantial concerns surround the ability of developmental or cognitive test results at toddler ages to predict later cognitive outcomes. Also, some neurocognitive, executive function, and behavioral difficulties may only be detected at later ages. The poor validity of a low Bayley MDI score at 20 months' corrected age to predict cognitive function at school age was highlighted by Hack et al. (2005), although prediction was noted to be better for those with significant neurosensory impairments. In the Caffeine for Apnea of Prematurity international trial cohort (Schmidt et al. 2012), investigators observed a substantial decline in the rate of cognitive impairment as measured by BSID-II MDI scores at 18 months' corrected age compared with Wechsler Preschool and Primary Scale of Intelligence–III full-scale IQ at 5 years. In a single-center longitudinal study from the Netherlands, BSID-II MDI scores at 2 years explained less than half of full-scale IQ at 5 years using predictive modeling, with verbal intelligence more accurately predicted than performance intelligence and processing speed (Potharst et al. 2012). Similarly, although the BSID-III cognitive and language scales at 2 years were associated with cognitive functioning at 4 years as assessed by the DAS-II, developmental delay at 2 years as determined by BSID-III reference data and normative cut points had low sensitivity in predicting future cognitive, verbal, and nonverbal reasoning impairments on the DAS-II at 4 years in a large regional Australian cohort (Spencer-Smith et al. 2015).

These findings have important implications for family and provider education. Given the prognostic uncertainties for individual outcomes prediction and the varying perspectives of the meaning of outcomes to patients and families, neonatologists should be extremely circumspect in attempts to incorporate early cognitive data into counseling strategies that direct delivery-room resuscitation approaches. The findings are also important from the perspective of resource availability and public policy. In countries and regions without specific policies assuring ongoing, longitudinal assessments and services for children born EPT, the 2- or 3-year evaluation may be the final opportunity to identify challenges before these children transition to the school system. If ongoing needs are determined only by scoring below a specific normative cut point on a developmental test, many children at significant risk for future impairments could be left behind. Understanding that later learning and attention problems may occur in children born preterm is a critical step to ensuring adequate support and services for families and teachers to help these children achieve their best possible outcomes and underscores the need to advocate for expanded child- and family-focused policies.

HEARING AND VISION OUTCOMES

Severe neurosensory impairments among preterm infants, including profound hearing and vision impairment, are now low-incidence outcomes but have important long-term consequences. Rates of blindness and significant hearing impairment are inversely related to gestational age (Hintz et al. 2011; Moore et al. 2012). Both moderate to severe vision and hearing impairment are more common among high-risk infants and those with co-occurring characteristics including male sex, multiple birth, CP, hydrocephalus, and seizures (Davis et al. 2010; Hintz et al. 2006; Synnes et al. 2012; Vohr 2014).

Bilateral hearing impairment requiring amplification among preterm cohorts has been reported to range between 1% and 9% depending on risk factors (Vohr 2016). Early detection of hearing impairment leads to optimization of speech and language development, and guidelines and recommendations reflect the importance of recognizing potential problems as early as possible. As stated in the policy statement of the American Academy of Pediatrics (AAP) Joint Committee on Infant Hearing, infants admitted to the NICU for more than 5 days should have auditory brainstem response included as part of their predischarge screening so that neural hearing loss will not be missed; for those who fail this test, referral should be made directly to an audiologist for rescreening and, when indicated, comprehensive evaluation (American Academy of Pediatrics Joint Committee on Infant Hearing 2007). Reevaluation should occur, regardless of initial evaluation results, based on individual risk factors and readmissions. All infants, including healthy infants, should have hearing screening by 1 month of age, with rescreening and referral for audiology evaluation by 3 months of age for those who do not pass the initial screen. In addition, a validated global screening tool is administered to infants at 9, 18, and 24–30 months, or sooner when there is concern about their hearing or language development.

Given that auditory input is crucial for development of the auditory cortex and speech (deRegnier et al. 2002; McMahon et al. 2012), increasing research interest has focused on the NICU setting and interventions to prevent hearing loss and to promote speech and language development in children born EPT. Studies of preterm infants in the NICU have shown that increased exposure to parental talk was a stronger predictor of infant vocalizations at 32 weeks than was exposure to language from other adults, and adult word counts in the NICU were associated with higher BSID-III language and cognitive scores at 18 months' corrected age (Caskey et al. 2011, 2014). Hearing a parent's voice may also have short-term effects in the NICU: parental reading has been shown to decrease desaturation events (Scala et al. 2018). Further research of language interventions that begin in the NICU and continue to home and community will be important in the development of comprehensive and effective approaches for child and family support.

Children born premature have an increased risk of various ophthalmic and visual challenges, especially those with a history of severe or treatment-requiring ROP and those with severe brain injury. Functional visual challenges include strabismus; problems with acuity, convergence, and visual fields; and retinal morphology (Holmstrom and Larsson 2013). However, a short-term outcome of severe ROP in the NICU may not result in the most severe functional vision outcomes in early childhood (SUPPORT Study Group of the Eunice Kennedy Shriver NICHD Neonatal Research Network et al. 2010; Vaucher et al. 2012). Conversely, children born preterm with no history of ROP or only mild ROP may also have an increased risk of visual problems. Neurodevelopmental follow-up studies have demonstrated that ≤50% of infants born VLBW have some visual impairments at later school age and that these problems can be associated with learning and academic challenges (Stephenson et al. 2007). The AAP and the American Association of Pediatric Ophthalmology recommend that ophthalmological follow-up be undertaken in children with a history of ROP within 4–6 months after discharge, regardless of severity or previous need for treatment (Fierson et al. 2018).

For early neurodevelopmental outcomes studies among preterm infants at 18–30 months' corrected age, criteria for profound or severe disability in the hearing domain have generally included some definition of "no useful hearing" even with aids or "some hearing but loss not corrected by aids," whether accompanied by specific decibel hearing loss (dBHL) audiological evaluation cut points (profound, >90 dBHL; severe, 70–90 dBHL) (British Association of Perinatal Medicine 2008) or by examination and observation of bilateral hearing loss not correctable by amplification (Doyle et al. 2010; Serenius et al. 2013; Vohr et al. 2012). Similarly, severe disability in the visual domain has generally been defined as functional bilateral blindness, including visual acuity <20/200, inability to perceive light, ability to perceive only light or reflecting objects (British Association of Perinatal Medicine 2008; Doyle et al. 2010, Vohr et al. 2012), or inability to fixate and follow a light with either eye (Serenius et al. 2013). Definitions of moderate hearing and vision impairment differ among studies.

Overview of Early Outcomes of Selected Extremely Preterm Cohorts

Hundreds of early neurodevelopmental outcomes studies of single- and multicenter, regional, and some population-based cohorts of children born EPT have been reported. An overview of some results from a few selected international cohorts are summarized in Table 1–6. Simple and uniform interpretation of these data is significantly limited; studies vary widely in gestational age inclusion, birth year, age at target follow-up, the personnel and instruments used for neurodevelopmental endpoint evaluation, and patient populations, among both studies and centers in the same cohorts. Crucially, definitions of "impairment" and cut points for levels of impairment severity vary broadly among studies. In part due to these reasons, the reported outcomes differ among studies. However, most importantly, these early reported outcomes do not necessarily predict later outcome or reflect the values and vision of the family and child. Because the various definitions of early NDI have been applied as research tools and may not be of greatest import to parents, investigators must strive to integrate what is truly important to parents as outcomes in future research (Janvier et al. 2019). An example of more detailed NDI information by gestational age from the Canadian Neonatal Follow Up Network for EPT infants born 2009–2011 is shown in Figure 1–11 (Synnes et al. 2017).

Risk Factors for Adverse Outcomes Among Preterm Infants

As described previously, preterm infants are at risk for adverse outcomes throughout childhood. The risks are modified by perinatal, neonatal, and sociodemographic factors and morbidities and complications that occur during the neonatal period. Important neonatal morbidities associated with later outcomes include brain injury, BPD, and ROP. Others include infection, poor growth and nutrition, and NEC. We end this section by addressing the impact of socioeconomic factors on outcomes and touch on the potential and promise of environmental and family interventions.

BRAIN INJURY

Cranial Ultrasound

Cranial ultrasound has been used to image preterm infant brain injury since the late 1970s (Pape et al. 1979; Slovis and Kuhns 1981). With the development of a standardized grading system for ICH, as shown in Table 1–3, cranial ultrasound quickly became and remains the neuroimaging standard for preterm infants (Ment et al. 2002). Although many still seem to rely heavily on simply the presence of grade 3 ICH, intraparenchymal hemorrhage (IPH), or cystic PVL to counsel families about the neurodevelopmental outcomes of their preterm infants, the complexity of interpreting ultrasound findings and the limitations of pre-

Table 1–6. Early neurodevelopmental outcomes of selected extremely preterm cohorts

	CNFUN	NICHD NRN	NSW and ACT	NICHD NRN	EPICure 2
Study	Symnes et al. 2017	Younge et al. 2017	Bolisetty et al. 2018	Rysavy et al. 2015	Moore et al. 2012
Group description	<23 weeks' to 28 weeks + 6 days' GA	22 weeks' to 24 weeks + 6 days' GA	23 weeks' to 28 weeks + 6 days' GA	22 weeks' to 26 weeks + 6 days' GA	22 weeks' to 26 weeks + 6 days' GA
Birth years	2009–2011	2008–2011	2007–2012	2006–2011	2006
Age at follow-up, corrected for prematurity	18–21 months	18–22 months	2–3 years	18–22 months	3 years
Number (% follow-up of eligible survivors)	2,954/3,087 (96%)	487 (98% with BSID-III)	1,514/1,897 (80%)	2,630 (92%)	576 (55%)[a]
Outcomes					
Vision: Blind[a]/Severe impairment	1.6%	0.4%	1.0%	0.4%	1.0%
Hearing: Deaf/Require aids	2.6%	3.0%	Aids: 2% Cochlear implant: 1%	1.4%	Improved by aids: 5% Not improved by aids: 0.2%
Developmental/Cognitive	BSID-III cognitive: <85: 15.7% <70: 3.3%	BSID-III cognitive: <85: 41%	BSID-III used; data not separately reported	BSID-III cognitive: 70–84: 16.5% <70: 9.3%	Predicted MDI[b]: 70–84: 34% <70: 30%

Table 1–6. Early neurodevelopmental outcomes of selected extremely preterm cohorts *(continued)*

	CNFUN	NICHD NRN	NSW and ACT	NICHD NRN	EPICure 2
Outcomes *(continued)*					
CP or motor delay	Any CP: 6.4%	Moderate-severe: 11%	Any CP: 7%	Moderate: 3.4%	Any CP: 14%
	CP with GMFCS level ≥III: 2.2%	Severe: 5%	Quadriplegia: 1%	Severe: 2.5%	Moderate motor: 3% Severe motor: 5%
Disability or impairment	Any NDI: 46% Significant NDI: 16.5%	Any NDI: 43%	Mild: 20% Moderate-severe: 11%	Moderate NDI: 23.5% Severe NDI: 3.6%	None/mild: 75% Moderate: 12% Severe: 13%

Note.   Data regarding CP and ESID-II scores were reported in Schlapbach et al. 2011.
ACT=Australian Capital Territory; BSID=Bayley Scales of Infant Development; CNFUN=Canadian Neonatal Follow-Up Network; CP=cerebral palsy; GA=gestational age; GMFCS=Gross Motor Function Classification System; MDI=mental developmental index; NDI=neurodevelopmental impairment; NICHD NRN=National Institute of Child Health and Human Development Neonatal Research Network; NSW=New South Wales.
[a]Defined as no functional vision in one or both eyes.
[b]For Victorian Infant Collaborative Study: Developmental quotient compared with a contemporaneous normal birth weight control group; for EPICure 2: Predicted MDI BSID-II from BSID-III; for Extremely Preterm Infants in Sweden Study: aggregated BSID-III cognitive and language score information, with mean and standard deviation relative to a contemporaneous 37- to 41-week GA control group.
Source.   Data regarding CP and ESID-II scores were reported in Schlapbach et al. 2011.

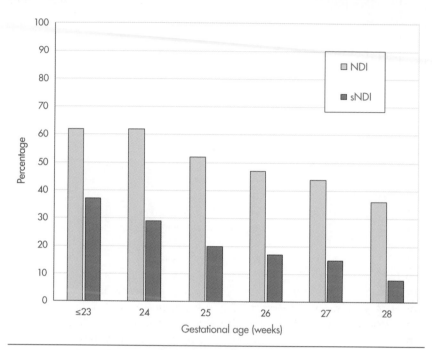

FIGURE 1–11.   Rates of any NDI and significant NDI (sNDI) by gestational age in the Canadian Neonatal Follow-Up Network.

Assessments were performed at 21 months of age corrected for prematurity. Any NDI: Any of CP with GMFCS level I or greater; BSID-III cognitive, language, or motor <85; sensorineural/mixed hearing loss; or unilateral or bilateral visual impairment. sNDI: Any of CP with GMFCS level III, IV, or V; BSID-III cognitive, language, or motor <70; hearing aid or cochlear implant; or bilateral visual impairment.

BSID=Bayley Scales of Infant Development; CP=cerebral palsy; GMFCS=Gross Motor Function Classification System; NDI=neurodevelopmental impairment.

Source.   Synnes A, Luu TM, Moddemann D, et al: "Determinants of Developmental Outcomes in a Very Preterm Canadian Cohort. *"Archives of Disease in Childhood: Fetal and Neonatal Edition* 102:F238, 2017. Copyright © 2017 BMJ. Used with permission.

dicting outcomes with any single neuroimaging or other finding should give clinicians cause for prudence and careful consideration.

Virtually every major study of early neurodevelopmental outcomes among preterm and ELBW infants has confirmed an association between major cranial ultrasound abnormalities and adverse neurological and developmental outcomes. Definitions of ultrasound abnormalities as well as outcomes differ among studies; however, most consider IPH, ventriculomegaly, or cystic changes to be severe abnormalities, regardless of laterality or extent of findings. In some, persistence of periventricular echodensity is included among cranial ultrasound abnormalities (Ancel et al. 2006; de Vries et al. 2004, 2011). The diagnosis reported in studies is frequently based on the results from a single ultrasound, either the "worst" or the "final" imaging study, but some prospective cohorts include serial imaging.

Many studies have focused on exploring the association of major cranial ultrasound findings with CP. The Extremely Low Gestational Age Newborn (ELGAN) study followed infants born <28 weeks' gestation between 2002 and 2004 from 14 institutions across five U.S. states (Kuban et al. 2009; O'Shea et al. 2009). Three sets of ultrasounds were performed during hospitalization and were reviewed by certified study radiologists. BSID-II and standardized neurological examinations for CP were performed at 2 years. The investigators found strong independent associations between ultrasound findings and CP. About half of the children with echolucency or ventriculomegaly developed CP, and late occurrence of ventriculomegaly, bilateral echolucency, and IPH or PVL were strongly predictive of quadriparesis. However, almost half of the children with CP at 2 years had completely normal cranial ultrasounds, and the positive predictive value of ventriculomegaly or echolucency for moderate or severe CP was poor. Isolated IVH was not strongly predictive of CP. In a single center, deVries et al. (2004) reported 76% sensitivity and 95% specificity of ultrasound abnormalities for CP at 2 years for patients younger than 32 weeks' estimated gestational age. Of importance, among those with major cranial ultrasound abnormalities who developed CP, approximately 30% were noted only after 28 days. Major abnormalities were also not strongly associated with cognitive delay at 2 years.

However, cranial ultrasound findings alone have low sensitivity and therefore are poorly predictive of early developmental outcomes or later childhood cognitive and learning outcomes (Hack et al. 2000; Wood et al. 2005). As many as 30%–40% of those with "normal" ultrasounds have neurodevelopmental challenges at 18–30 months (Laptook et al. 2005). The ELGAN study showed that IVH was associated with increased risk for motor or developmental impairment at 2 years *only* when accompanied or followed by white matter lesions, highlighting the limited predictive value of using only early cranial ultrasound findings and IVH (O'Shea et al. 2012). In longer-term follow-up studies of the Etude Epidémiologique sur les Petits Ages Gestationnels cohort born at 24 weeks' to 28 weeks, 6 days' gestation, major cranial ultrasound abnormalities remained strongly associated with CP (Beaino et al. 2010). However, approximately 40% of those with major neonatal ultrasound abnormalities had no significant cognitive or learning challenges identified at 8 years of age, whereas 30%–40% of those with no neonatal abnormalities had moderate to severe challenges (Marret et al. 2013). This underscores the need for long-term surveillance throughout childhood for all children born very preterm. Nevertheless, in skilled hands, with meticulous technical attention and serial cranial ultrasound imaging, much can be seen beyond ICH. In a single center, deVries et al. (2004) reported 76% sensitivity and 95% specificity of ultrasound abnormalities for CP at 2 years for patients born at <32 weeks' estimated gestational age. Of importance, among those with major cranial ultrasound abnormalities who developed CP, approximately 30% were noted only after 28 days. Major abnormalities were also not strongly associated with cognitive delay at 2 years. More recent findings from this group, using MRI at term-equivalent age to refine specific cranial ultrasound findings, has resulted in positive and negative predictive values of 96% and 69%, respectively, for CP at 2 years among preterm infants (de Vries et al. 2011).

Cranial ultrasound is an operator-dependent modality; imaging procedures and views vary among institutions and studies, and no uniform approach to serial imaging protocols exists. Although interrater reliability and accuracy are very good to excellent for severe ICH, agreement is only fair or poor for subtler findings and PVL alone (Hintz et al. 2007). Cerebellar hemorrhage, a finding that could be missed without the appropriate ultrasound views, is increasingly recognized to be associated with neurodevelopmental disabilities in children born preterm (Limperopoulos et al. 2007, 2014). Isolated IPH and of course large IVH can be seen by cranial ultrasound; however, not all "severe" hemorrhages can be considered equivalent in terms of association with early neurodevelopmental outcomes. Characteristics of the hemorrhage, including laterality, midline shift, and extent (Bassan et al. 2007; Davis et al. 2014), as well as the presence or absence of other adverse clinical factors (Merhar et al. 2012), impact prediction of neurodevelopmental outcomes. In light of all these findings, the limitations of cranial ultrasound abnormalities as a single predictive factor for long-term outcomes, particularly developmental and cognitive endpoints, should be recognized.

Brain Magnetic Resonance Imaging

Brain MRI has been used among preterm infants more extensively in recent years, both for research and for clinical indications. MRI generally provides a more comprehensive and detailed picture of the brain, with better delineation of deep structure and cortical injury and improved detection of white matter injury, which is common among preterm infants at term-corrected age. Identification of white matter injury is important for understanding the structure-function relationship of the developing preterm brain, influences on later neuromotor and cognitive outcomes, and developing future neuroprotective strategies (Volpe et al. 2011). Subtle white matter injury seen on MRI has been reported to be associated with reduced total brain and gray matter volumes, reduced cerebellar volume, and reduced basal ganglia and thalamic volumes, which in turn are associated with childhood developmental impairments among preterm infants. These findings and others provide evidence that white matter injury in the preterm is associated with brain maturational disturbances, suggesting an overall link to impaired neural connectivity (Dean et al. 2014). Therefore, clinical investigations have focused on whether MRI may provide enhanced prognostic information.

Following early and small studies that compared cranial ultrasound and MRI, white matter injury scoring approaches were developed, and larger cohort studies have been published. Among the first was a multicenter effort in Australia and New Zealand that compared serial cranial ultrasound with near-term MRI findings and their association with 2-year outcomes in 167 infants born at <30 weeks' estimated gestational age (Woodward et al. 2006). This study showed that moderate-severe white matter injury on near-term MRI was significantly associated with neuromotor delay and CP, independent of ultrasound findings and other risk factors. Increasing severity was also related to lower BSID-II MDI scores, but an independent association of moderate-severe white matter injury with severe cognitive delay was not detected. However, cranial ultrasound was assessed only with regard to early findings, including grade of ICH and periventricular cystic changes. Furthermore, a substantial proportion of infants with moderate to severe white matter injury on MRI did not have adverse 2-year outcomes.

The NICHD Neuroimaging and Neurodevelopmental Outcomes study was a prospective study of early and late cranial ultrasound and near-term MRI in 480 infants born <28 weeks' gestation, with outcomes including BSID-III assessed at 18–22 months (Hintz et al. 2015). In multivariable models, both the late ultrasound findings reflective of white matter injury and the MRI findings of significant cerebellar injury remained independently associated with adverse neurodevelopmental outcomes. In models that did not include late cranial ultrasound, MRI findings of both moderate to severe white matter injury and significant cerebellar lesions were independently associated with adverse outcomes. Early ultrasound findings were not associated with adverse outcomes when late neuroimaging was taken into account. These results demonstrate the need to understand the evolution of brain injury over time rather than rely on early findings.

A prospective study of serial cranial ultrasound and near-term MRIs among infants born at <27 weeks in Sweden showed associations between MRI findings and 30-month outcomes, but the investigators determined that any substantial MRI abnormalities were detected by the late cranial ultrasound done the same day (Skiöld et al. 2012). Follow-up of the NICHD cohort to 6–7 years of age showed that severe late ultrasound findings, which were rare, were most strongly associated with cognitive impairment and disability at school age, and significant cerebellar lesions on MRI were associated with disability; however, near-term MRI did not substantively enhance prediction of significant cognitive disability or impairment at school age (Hintz et al. 2018). Diffuse excessive high signal intensity on near-term MRI has been shown not to be associated with adverse early or later childhood outcomes (Brostrom et al. 2016; Jeon et al. 2012).

In summary, despite what appears to be substantial experience with cranial ultrasound and conventional brain MRI in preterm infants, controversies and questions remain about which studies to perform, when and under what circumstances to perform them, and their relative values in prognosis. These are not simple questions because the value of additional information may vary by clinical circumstances and for individual parents and physicians (Janvier and Barrington 2012). Cerebellar injury seen on MRI but not on cranial ultrasound may be associated with higher risk for neurodevelopmental abnormalities (Hintz et al. 2015; Tam et al. 2011), although the importance of punctate lesions remains unclear (Steggerda et al. 2013). Other studies have shown that MRI may provide additive information to predict neuromotor outcomes (de Vries et al. 2011) complementary to specific findings, such as periventricular echodensities, on cranial ultrasound (Sie et al. 2005) or neurological examination (Skiöld et al. 2013; Spittle et al. 2009). Neonatal sepsis and NEC have been linked with progressive or higher rates of white matter injury on MRI, and adverse 2-year outcomes associated with these morbidities may be mediated by white matter injury (Glass et al. 2008; Shah et al. 2008). Nevertheless, a recent publication has suggested avoiding routine term-equivalent conventional brain MRI for screening purposes due to insufficient evidence that the practice improves long-term outcomes (Ho et al. 2015).

Future studies should focus on identifying specific high-risk groups of preterm infants for whom MRI would definitively improve prediction of neurodevelopmental outcomes and allow risk stratification for neuroprotective or interventional studies. Investigations with advanced techniques, including diffusion tensor imaging, resting-state functional connectivity MRI, surface morphometry, and volumetric methods, hold promise to help explore these questions (Anderson et al. 2015).

BRONCHOPULMONARY DYSPLASIA

BPD is associated with later adverse respiratory, developmental, educational, and health economical outcomes. EPT infants with BPD have greater coughing, respiratory medication use, and hospitalizations and impact of respiratory disease on the family at 18–22 months' corrected age compared with those without BPD (Stevens et al. 2014). A meta-analysis of pulmonary function testing in children born preterm with BPD, preterm without BPD, or at term showed significantly decreased forced expiratory volume in 1 second (FEV1) in those born preterm, with a further decrease in those with BPD (Kotecha et al. 2013). Several investigators have reported poor neurodevelopmental outcomes in infants with BPD compared with preterm infants without BPD (Grégoire et al. 1998; Lodha et al. 2014; Majnemer et al. 2000; Roberts et al. 2009; Schmidt et al. 2015). BPD is a consistent independent predictor of adverse developmental outcomes at 2 and 5 years of age (Schmidt et al. 2012). The adjusted odds of adverse neurodevelopmental outcome at 5 years are 2.3 (95% CI 1.8–3.0) times higher among very preterm born children with BPD than among those without BPD (Schmidt et al. 2015). In addition, the ELGAN investigators evaluated behavioral outcomes at 10 years of age for children whose BPD status prior to discharge was known and found that autism spectrum disorder and communication impairment were more common among children with more severe BPD relative to children with milder or no BPD (Sriram et al. 2018).

Several large randomized trials have studied interventions in the NICU to decrease the rate of BPD in EPT infants and have followed these cohorts beyond discharge. Vitamin A reduces BPD or death in ELBW infants (relative risk 0.89) but does not improve developmental outcomes at 18–22 months (Ambalavanan et al. 2005). A Cochrane review that examined the benefits and risks of late-treatment systemic corticosteroids (>7 days) found short-term benefits of reduced need for assisted ventilation and rate of BPD and perhaps also reduced death during the first 28 days of life (Doyle et al. 2017). However, at higher doses, short-term complications were also recognized. Although a trend toward increased CP or abnormal neurological examination was found in the steroid versus control groups, no significant difference was found between groups in neurosensory disability or the combined rates of either death or CP or of death or major neurosensory disability (Doyle et al. 2017). Caffeine reduces BPD at 36 weeks, CP at 2 years, and motor impairment severity at 5 years (Schmidt et al. 2006, 2007, 2012). Surfactant therapy for RDS reduces both air leak syndromes and mortality (Bahadue and Soll 2012) but does not reduce moderate or severe disability at 1 year or any adverse outcomes at 2 years (Sinn et al. 2002). Another Cochrane review showed that antenatal corticosteroids reduce many complications of prematurity, including mortality, RDS, need for mechanical ventilation, systemic infection in the first 48 hours, and IVH, but do not appear to have a statistically significant effect on BPD or neurodevelopmental outcome (Roberts and Dalziel 2017). However, an overall reduction in rates of cognitive impairment and CP among infants of 22–25 weeks' gestation treated with antenatal steroids has been reported in some large studies (Carlo et al. 2011).

RETINOPATHY OF PREMATURITY

With advances in surveillance and treatment, including laser therapy and bevacizumab, bilateral blindness due to ROP is now rare in the developed world, although globally as many as 20,000 children annually are blind due to ROP (Blencowe et al. 2013). Nevertheless, long-term visual problems related to ROP remain a challenge; more than one-third of a Swedish cohort of children born EPT had at least some ophthalmological abnormality at school age that was strongly associated with ROP treatment and lower gestational age, including blindness, strabismus, and refractive errors (Hellgren et al. 2016). Severe ROP is also associated with important nonvisual disabilities. Severe ROP or treated ROP is a strong independent predictor of poor neurodevelopmental outcome at 5 years of age among children born EPT (Schmidt et al. 2015). These children have more than four times higher odds of motor and cognitive disability than infants without severe ROP (Schmidt et al. 2014) and are more likely to have impairment in multiple domains.

As mentioned earlier, restriction of supplemental oxygen has been used to reduce ROP. In a meta-analysis of five oxygen saturation targeting trials in EPT infants, targeting lower oxygen saturations (85%–89%) compared with higher saturations (91%–95%) was associated with somewhat lower risk of ROP (RR 0.72, 95% CI 0.50–1.04) (Manja et al. 2015). However, the lower versus higher oxygen saturation strategy was also associated with increased risk of death before discharge (RR 1.18, 95% CI 1.03–1.36), but no significant difference in death by 18–24 months. Furthermore, in a meta-analysis of the 18- to 24-months' corrected age outcomes of these trials (Manja et al. 2017), no difference was found in death or NDI between lower and higher oxygen saturation groups, nor did the rates of NDI or severe visual loss differ between the groups. Mortality before 18–24 months' corrected age was higher in the lower saturation group. Therefore, the potential benefit of lower oxygen saturation targeting for ROP appears to be substantially offset by the increased risk of mortality and lack of benefit to neurodevelopmental outcomes.

The effect of ROP treatment may also have implications for both visual and developmental outcomes. Laser therapy is the current standard treatment, but injection of antivascular endothelial growth factor agents such as bevacizumab is increasingly being used to treat acute ROP. In one small randomized trial, an antivascular endothelial growth factor agent appeared to be superior to laser therapy for treatment of zone 1 ROP (Mintz-Hittner et al. 2011). However, due to concerns about systemic absorption of the drug, late proliferative vascular changes that lead to retinal detachment, and only minimal differences in refractive outcomes at 2.5 years in the trial (Mintz-Hittner et al. 2011), concerns have been raised regarding this approach (Darlow 2015). A retrospective analysis of infants born at <27 weeks' gestation in the NICHD NRN compared 18- to 26-month corrected age outcomes of those who underwent bevacizumab with those who had surgery for ROP (Natarajan et al. 2019). Perinatal and neonatal factors between the groups differed, including that infants treated with bevacizumab had lower median birth weight, longer duration of ventilation and supplemental oxygen, and lower rates of maternal Medicaid insurance. In adjusted multivariable analyses, death or severe NDI and severe NDI at 18–26 months did not differ between groups. However, adjusted odds of BSID-III cognitive scores <85 and GMFCS levels above level II were both approximately 1.7 times higher in the bevacizumab group compared with the surgery group. In an earlier case series of 2-year outcomes in infants treated with laser, bevacizumab, or both (Lien et al. 2016), infants treated with both therapies had significantly higher rates of mental and psychomotor impairment on the BSID-II than infants treated with laser. No difference was found between the laser- and bevacizumab-treated infants. Further research is needed to identify novel strategies for the prevention of ROP and treatments that are safe and lead to improved visual outcomes without increasing adverse developmental outcomes.

INFECTIONS

Infection is associated with poor growth, and particularly with poor head growth, which is an independent predictor of adverse outcome in preterm infants (Ehrenkranz et al. 2006). Furthermore, infection is associated with increased risk for low cognitive performance, CP, and vision impairment at 18–22 months (Schlapbach et al. 2011; Stoll et al. 2004). When adjusted for multiple factors predictive of CP, 2-year-old children with a history of extreme prematurity and confirmed sepsis have more than three times higher odds of CP (Schlapbach et al. 2011). By 5 years of age, both early and late-onset sepsis in very preterm infants are associated with significantly increased odds of CP but may not be associated with cognitive impairment (Mitha et al. 2013).

Infants with *Candida* sepsis or meningitis and infants with bacterial meningitis experience the most significant increase in risk for poor developmental outcomes in early childhood (Adams-Chapman et al. 2013; Bassler et al. 2009). Ultimately, however, the overall risk for NDI (any one of cognitive impairment, CP, or vision or hearing impairment) associated with neonatal infection is slightly less significant than risks associated with severe IVH, ROP, or BPD (Bassler et al. 2009; Schlapbach et al. 2012).

NECROTIZING ENTEROCOLITIS

Infants with NEC are at greater risk of death, cognitive delay, CP, severe vision or hearing impairment, and the composite outcome of developmental impairment at 18 months (Bassler et al. 2009; Schulzke et al. 2007). In one large observational study, nearly all of this increased risk was associated with NEC requiring surgical intervention (Hintz et al. 2005). Surgical NEC and spontaneous intestinal perforation are associated with more than doubled odds of NDI among survivors (Wadhawan et al. 2014). However, similar to infection, overall risk of adverse outcome associated with NEC is less significant than risks associated with severe IVH, ROP, or BPD (Bassler et al. 2009).

Although antenatal corticosteroid treatment leads to a significant re-duction in NEC (Carlo et al. 2011; Roberts and Dalziel 2017), the impact of antenatal steroids on developmental outcomes remains uncertain. Exclusive maternal milk feeding reduces risk for NEC and improves neu-rodevelopmental outcomes; however, both NEC and developmental out-comes are complex and multifactorial, so direct association and causation are difficult to ascertain (Patel and Kim 2018). Use of pasteurized donor milk compared with formula has been proposed as potentially retaining some outcome benefits for preterm infants when the mother's own milk is unavailable (Section on Breastfeeding 2012; World Health Organiza-tion 2011). A meta-analysis of randomized or quasi-randomized trials of formula compared with pasteurized donor milk showed that formula feeding nearly doubled the risk of NEC (Quigley et al. 2019); however, no difference between groups was found in terms of mortality or early childhood neurodevelopmental outcome from the data available. Several trials are currently ongoing worldwide, including the NICHD NRN milk trial (NCT01534481), which will substantively add to our understanding of longer-term outcomes. Donor milk is currently recommended by the World Health Organization and the AAP as the preferred choice if the mother's own breast milk is not available for low birth weight and pre-term infants, if the donor milk is from a safe and reliable source (Section on Breastfeeding 2012; World Health Organization 2011). Availability of human milk banks and use of donor milk are increasing in NICUs (Wil-liams et al. 2016). Several additional interventions show promise for fur-ther decreasing rates of NEC, including lactoferrin and probiotics, but data are limited around impact on outcomes, and there is complexity around site-specific decisions to implement some treatments (Barbian et al. 2019; Sari et al. 2012).

GROWTH AND NUTRITION

A focus on growth and nutrition both in the NICU and after discharge is increasingly recognized as essential for optimizing longer-term de-velopmental outcomes. In a large cohort study, infants born weighing 501–1,000 g were divided into quartiles of in-hospital growth velocity (Ehrenkranz et al. 2006). Quartile of in-hospital growth velocity was as-sociated with risk for CP and developmental outcomes more than two standard deviations below the mean at 18–22 months' corrected age, even after adjustment for other factors predictive of poor growth and development. Preterm infants who fail to thrive in the first 8 months af-ter discharge have poor developmental outcomes compared with those who demonstrate catch-up growth or maintain an appropriate growth trajectory (Hack et al. 1982).

Substantial focus has been placed on growth failure among preterm infants as measured by weight alone. Despite changes in nutritional practices in NICUs, this weight-based growth failure remains a significant concern. Although the proportion of VLBW infants discharged from NICUs with growth failure as measured by weight in the Vermont Oxford Network has decreased over time, approximately 50% were less than 10th percentile and one in four were less than 3rd percentile as measured on the Fenton weight charge at discharge for birth year 2013 (Horbar et al. 2015). Still, other somatic measures are important components to growth delay and may be more important markers of later neurodevelopmental outcome. Linear growth represents fat free mass or lean body mass and protein accretion, which is more closely linked to organ growth and differentiation (Pfister and Ramel 2014). Poor linear growth is common among preterm infants and is associated with cognitive impairment at 2 years, with a mechanism that may link to the insulin-like growth factor 1/growth hormone axis. In a retrospective study of preterm infants whose growth was appropriate for their gestational age, Ramel et al. (2012) reported that even when controlling for weight and head circumference Z-scores, lower length Z-score at 4 months and 12 months was associated with lower cognitive function scores at 24 months. In a study of participants born preterm in the Infant Health and Development Program, Belfort et al. (2013) demonstrated that more rapid linear growth from term-adjusted age to 4 months was associated with lower odds for cognitive delay at 8 years, but this gain was offset by somewhat by higher odds for obesity. Poor head growth has also been demonstrated to be highly predictive of adverse developmental outcomes through at least 8–9 years (Hack et al. 1991).

Because of the strong association between nutrition and growth during the first year of life and developmental outcomes, multiple strategies to improve growth have been evaluated. Although many strategies used to feed preterm infants in the NICU successfully improve growth, there is currently little evidence that they improve developmental outcomes (Brown et al. 2016; Poindexter et al. 2006). Future interventions that expand focus on optimizing linear growth and fat-free mass gains may lead to benefits. Of importance, the complex interactions of nutritional deficits in the NICU, infection and inflammatory illness, and brain injury and development with respect to impact on cognitive outcomes are likely to be rich and ongoing targets for protective approaches (Ehrenkranz et al. 2011; Pfister and Ramel 2014; Ramel et al. 2012).

SOCIOECONOMIC STATUS AND PSYCHOSOCIAL FACTORS

Socioeconomic and demographic factors have long been seen as critically important to the neurodevelopmental outcomes of children born preterm and high-risk (Hack et al. 1992). Socioeconomic factors that influence cognitive outcomes include parent education, having a two-parent household, neighborhood, and social and racial background (Aylward 2005; Manley et al. 2015). Furthermore, disparities in these areas influence a child's upward or recovering cognitive status in the first years of life (Manley et al. 2015). As preterm children move beyond the early neurodevelopmental assessment period into school age, the association between the clinical events experienced in the NICU and outcomes wanes, whereas socioeconomic factors such as parental education remain influential, particularly on cognitive and behavioral outcomes (Linsell et al. 2015; McGowan and Vohr 2019). In a large prospective cohort of children born preterm in France (Beaino et al. 2011), lower parental education was an independent predictor of both mild and severe cognitive delay at 5 years of age. Among children born moderately preterm in a Dutch population-based cohort, low socioeconomic status as measured by parent education, family income, occupation, and single-parent household was a risk factor for both adverse cognitive and behavioral-emotional outcomes (Potijk et al. 2013, 2015). Decreasing gestational age was also found to be a risk factor, with low socioeconomic status and prematurity multiplying risk for these adverse outcomes. In addition, children with motor, coordination, and functional limitations are more likely to live in families with limited resources and more constrained access to the health care system and therefore potential interventions (Hogan et al. 2000).

Parental mental and emotional stressors can also affect child and family outcomes. Mothers of infants in the NICU have been shown to be at high risk for anxiety, depression, and PTSD (Shaw et al. 2009) and can exhibit dysfunctional coping strategies, which are strongly correlated with increased risk for PTSD (Shaw et al. 2013). Furthermore, mothers who have experienced significant trauma symptoms are more likely to see their children as vulnerable after discharge, display dysfunctional coping styles, and experience low social support (Horwitz et al. 2015a, 2015b). Evidence also suggests that a history of mental health disorders may predispose mothers to feel less ready to care for their child at discharge. Enhanced transition and support services should be deployed in these cases (McGowan et al. 2017). Unfortunately, mental health history may be unknown unless a comprehensive approach to psychological assessment and support is in place for the mother, baby, and family in the NICU. Given the critical relationship between a high-risk infant's postdischarge environment, parental psychosocial challenges, and neurodevelopmental and behavioral outcome in childhood, interventions that include psychosocial interventions for mothers as well as parental education and transitional support for families are crucial for achieving best possible outcomes for the child and family (Benzies et al. 2013). Early interventions with mothers in the NICU, particularly those that focus on strengthening the parent–infant relationship and coping skills, have been shown to have a positive influence on motor and cognitive outcomes (Colditz et al. 2019). Furthermore, a range of parental interventional components to reduce stress and anxiety have been shown to be effective (Sabnis et al. 2019). Cognitive behavioral–based therapy interventions with mothers of NICU infants have been shown to result in reduced acute trauma symptoms and depression. Benefits of these interventions persisted following discharge with sustained and significantly reduced trauma, anxiety, and depression symptoms (Shaw et al. 2013, 2014).

Long-Term Mental Health Outcomes of Prematurity

It is not surprising that the well-recognized early delays in development and neurocognitive functioning seen in premature infants are reflected in adverse longer-term outcomes in adolescence and early adulthood. Young adults born preterm with VLBW are reported to have more mental health problems than adults born full-term, in particular, an increased prevalence of attention deficits, internalizing symptoms, and social difficulties (Husby et al. 2016). These mental health challenges also have implications for the families of premature infants. Wolke et al. (2017), for example, reported that parental quality of life was also predicted by the offspring's mental health and peer relationships in childhood.

INTERNALIZING AND EXTERNALIZING DISORDERS

Research has shown a high prevalence of behavioral and emotional problems, specifically anxiety and depression, in long-term follow-up studies of premature infants (Hack 2009; Leon Hernandez 2018; Lund et al. 2012). The risk of these adverse outcomes is increased in the presence of cognitive and motor difficulties in the child (Hayes and Sharif 2009). In a sample of 96,677 children ages 2–17 years living in the United States, Singh et al. (2013) found a 28.7% prevalence of parent-reported mental health problems among children born with VLBW compared with 15% in children born full-term. Multiple studies have supported these findings, even after correcting for socioeconomic factors, severe developmental impairment, and other chronic conditions. For example, Johnson et al. (2010), in an 11-year follow-up cohort study of 219 children born at <26 weeks' gestation compared with 153 control subjects born at term, found that premature infants were three times more likely to have a psychiatric disorder, including significantly increased risk of autism, ADHD, and other emotional disorders. Räikkönen et al. (2008) found that low birth weight subjects born small for gestational age had higher scores on the Beck Depression Inventory and were four times more likely to use antidepressants compared with control subjects.

These findings are also confirmed in studies of self-reported mental health in adults with histories of prematurity (Pyhälä et al. 2017). A large meta-analysis from six different study cohorts found that adults born preterm are at a higher risk of internalizing problems and socially avoidant personality traits and have a decreased likelihood of rule breaking, intrusive behavior, antisocial personality problems, and externalizing symptoms. Pyhälä et al. (2017) suggested that there may be a universal phenotype of mental health problems and that adults born with VLBW tend to worry more, be more anxious and withdrawn, and engage in fewer risk-taking behaviors and romantic relationships. Proposed mechanisms include interaction between neurobiological, endocrinological, and psychosocial processes, including disruptions in brain development. Hack (2009) also drew attention to the lower rates of risk-taking and delinquency in VLBW adults, including lower rates of substance abuse, which has been hypothesized to be related to various factors including increased parental monitoring, social isolation, and increased behavioral inhibition. Several large, population-based studies from Scandinavia have examined this issue. Indredavik et al. (2010) looked at perinatal risk and psychiatric outcomes in a sample of 65 adolescents either born preterm with VLBW or born at term but small for gestational age. In the VLBW group, lower birth weight was associated with inattention, psychiatric diagnoses, and reduced psychosocial function. IVH increased the risk for a high inattention score, and lower Apgar scores increased the risk for autism spectrum symptoms and internalizing symptoms.

Not all studies support these findings. Both Darlow et al. (2013) from New Zealand and Gäddlin et al. (2009) from Sweden reported long-term follow-up data suggesting that young adults born with VLBW made a good transition to adulthood and had similar scores across many aspects of health and social functioning as their same-age peers. Similarly, Jaekel et al. (2018) found no persistently increased risk for anxiety or mood disorders in individuals after very preterm birth or those with VLBW and that having a romantic relationship was a protective factor.

AUTISM

Research has shown a higher prevalence of autism spectrum disorder in long-term follow-up studies of infants born premature (Leon Hernandez 2018). As mentioned, Johnson et al. (2010), in their follow-up cohort study of 219 children born at <26 weeks' gestation, found that premature infants were three times more likely than term-born subjects to have a psychiatric disorder, including a significantly increased risk of autism. These findings have been replicated in large registry studies from Scandinavia (Lampi et al. 2012). Pyhälä et al. (2014), in a study of 110 VLBW subjects using the Autism-Spectrum Quotient, found a higher prevalence of autism spectrum traits, in particular traits related to social interaction. These authors suggested that the autism spectrum traits relevant to premature infants were limited to the social interaction deficits.

SOCIAL RELATIONSHIPS

Findings are mixed regarding the question of adult social relationships for those born preterm. Finnish researchers Kajantie et al. (2008) found that a group of young adults born with VLBW had difficulty leaving home and establishing an adult independent life and intimate peer relationships. Pyhälä et al. (2017) reported that adults born with VLBW lack self-confidence in social relationships, while Lund et al. (2012) also reported less social interaction with friends in VLBW subjects. A review by Hack (2009) suggested that adults born with VLBW are less likely to find a romantic partner than are term-born control subjects.

INCREASED RATES OF PSYCHIATRIC HOSPITALIZATION

Norsati et al. (2012) reported data from a historical population-based cohort study from Sweden. They found that preterm birth was significantly associated with increased risk of psychiatric hospitalization in adulthood across a range of psychiatric disorders. Compared with adults born at term (37–41 weeks), those born at 32–36 weeks' gestation were 1.6 times more likely to have nonaffective psychosis, 1.3 times more likely to have depressive disorder, and 2.7 times more likely to have bipolar affective disorder. Those born at <32 weeks' gestation were 2.5 times more likely to have nonaffective psychosis, 2.9 times more likely to have depressive disorder, and 7.4 times more likely to have bipolar affective disorder. Results also showed that nonoptimal fetal growth was significantly associated with drug or alcohol dependence. The authors concluded that vulnerability for hospitalization with a range of psychiatric diagnoses may increase with younger gestational age.

In a Swedish national cohort study of 545,628 individuals born between 1973 and 1979, Lindström et al. (2009) reported on the hazard ratios of hospital admissions for psychiatric disorders and alcohol/illicit drug abuse. Results showed a stepwise increase in psychiatric hospital admissions with an increasing degree of preterm birth. A total of 5.2% of children born at 24–28 weeks' gestation and 3.5% born at 29–32 weeks' gestation had been hospitalized because of a psychiatric disorder.

QUALITY OF LIFE

Most studies assessing the issue of quality of life in low birth weight populations have shown outcomes consistent with those of control groups (Lund et al. 2012). However, one Danish group of researchers found a decrease in objective but not subjective quality of life in VLBW subjects (Dinesen and Greisen 2001). Lund et al. (2012), in a sample of 43 VLBW subjects, found lower quality of life in the domain of mental health compared with control subjects, while Saigal et al. (2016) reported that adults born with VLBW are less likely to live independently, more often receive social benefits, and more often have periods of unemployment.

IMPLICATIONS

The large amount of data suggesting potential negative outcomes with respect to psychopathology among young adults born with low birth weight raises important public health questions. The presence of significant internalizing and externalizing symptoms in these at-risk youth has the potential for long-term impact on their overall health and well-being. The situation is compounded by findings indicating that only a very small percentage of these individuals are referred for psychiatric consultation, suggesting that these problems are often underrecognized (Hayes and Sharif 2009). It will be important to look at whether findings in young adults are predictive of future outcomes.

In addition, these data suggest the importance of understanding the mechanisms by which these psychological outcomes evolve. Pesonen et al. (2008) suggested that one mechanism to consider is that of parental concerns related to child vulnerability. These concerns may create a family environment that reinforces certain behaviors and personality qualities in the child, such as obedience, cautiousness, and low impulsiveness. Parents of premature infants tend to be more directive and intrusive and to show less dyadic reciprocity compared with parents of term infants (Feldman 2007). In fact, findings that prenatal and neonatal variables are not necessarily predictive of later psychological issues suggest that environment, including parent–child relational issues, may play a large role in the genesis of these difficulties (Hayes and Sharif 2009). However, Pesonen et al. (2008) also drew attention to the importance of considering biological mechanisms that may influence behavior and personality development, including findings that lower gestational age and lower birth weight are associated with altered functioning in the hypothalamic-pituitary-adrenal axis and with increased cortisol levels. Cortisol levels in particular have been associated with extroversion, warmth, and social anxiety (Oswald et al. 2007). These hypotheses suggest the need to develop and validate early interventions that target the infant, the parent–infant relationship, and parenting approaches. Pyhälä et al. (2014), in the study cited earlier describing the relationship between autism and prematurity, found that faster growth of premature infants from birth to term may ameliorate these effects, suggesting that targeted interventions could aid long-term neural development.

Summary

Multiple adverse events during the neonatal course can impact biological, developmental, and behavioral risk for children born preterm. Each

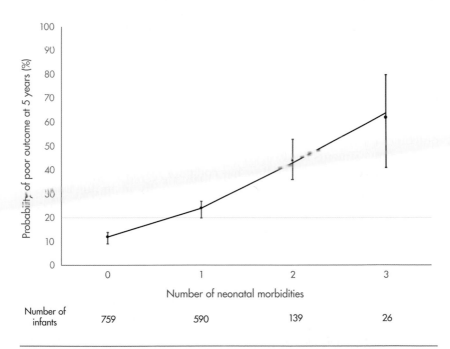

FIGURE 1–12. **Probability of death or disability at 5 years among very low birth weight (VLBW) infants surviving to 36 weeks' postmenstrual age.**

Cumulative effect of three neonatal morbidities (N=1,514) with none, one, two, and all three neonatal morbidities; 95% CI indicated by *error bars*. *Sloping solid line* indicates predictions based on the fitted morbidity count model; *horizontal gray line* indicates the overall probability of a poor 5-year outcome. Morbidities were bronchopulmonary dysplasia (need for supplemental oxygen at 36 weeks' postmenstrual age), serious brain injury (grade 3 or 4 hemorrhage, cystic periventricular leukomalacia, porencephalic cyst, ventriculomegaly with or without hemorrhage); and severe retinopathy of prematurity (unilateral or bilateral disease of stage 4 or 5 or receipt of retinal therapy in at least one eye).

Source. Schmidt B, Roberts RS, Davis PG, et al.: "Prediction of Late Death or Disability at Age 5 Years Using a Count of 3 Neonatal Morbidities in Very Low Birth Weight Infants." *Journal of Pediatrics* 167(5):984, 2015. Copyright © 2015 Elsevier. Used with permission.

of these peri- and neonatal factors may impact physical development and neurodevelopment in unique ways. Furthermore, these morbidities may combine to additionally increase risk. Three of the most substantial neonatal risk factors associated with NDI at toddler age and through at least early school age are severe ICH, ROP, and BPD; the count of these morbidities has been shown to strongly predict risk for later neurodevelopmental disability (Figure 1–12) (Schmidt et al. 2003, 2015). These morbidities are associated with a linear, additive increase in risk for adverse developmental outcome, although the 95% confidence intervals are wide with increasing number of morbidities, particularly at later age.

Neonatal infection (particularly fungal infection and meningitis) and NEC (particularly surgical NEC) add to the prediction of poor outcome. Other neonatal risk factors independently associated with adverse developmental outcomes have also been noted. Thus, these findings present crucial opportunities for continued quality improvement in the NICU. Socioeconomic disparities represent substantial risk factors for developmental and behavioral difficulties among children born preterm, particularly with longer-term endpoints into school age. This represents perhaps the most important challenge to supporting optimal long-term outcomes for our patients and their families. Given the substantial and ongoing investments made to ensure survival of even the smallest and most premature infants, the time has come for neonatology to focus efforts toward the transition to home and community, including interventions to support the mother and family as well as the infant and advocacy to ensure truly long-term follow-up through school age.

References

Adams-Chapman I, Bann CM, Das A, et al: Neurodevelopmental outcome of extremely low birth weight infants with Candida infection. J Pediatr 163(4):961–967, 2013

Adams-Chapman I, Heyne RJ, DeMauro SB, et al: Neurodevelopmental impairment among extremely preterm infants in the Neonatal Research Network. Pediatrics 141(5), 2018

Ambalavanan N, Tyson JE, Kennedy KA, et al: Vitamin A supplementation for extremely low birth weight infants: outcome at 18 to 22 months. Pediatrics 115(3):249–254, 2005

American Academy of Pediatrics Joint Committee on Infant Hearing: Year 2007 position statement: principles and guidelines for early hearing detection and intervention programs. Pediatrics 120(4):898–921, 2007

American College of Obstetricians and Gynecologists, Society for Maternal-Fetal Medicine: Obstetric care consensus No. 6: periviable birth. Obstet Gynecol 130(4):e187–e199, 2017

Ancel PY, Livinec F, Larroque B, et al: Cerebral palsy among very preterm children in relation to gestational age and neonatal ultrasound abnormalities: the EPIPAGE Cohort Study. Pediatrics 117(3):828–835, 2006

Anderson PJ, De Luca CR, Hutchinson E, Roberts G, et al: Underestimation of developmental delay by the new Bayley-III scale. Arch Pediatr Adolesc Med 164(4):352–356, 2010

Anderson PJ, Cheong JL, Thompson DK: The predictive validity of neonatal MRI for neurodevelopmental outcome in very preterm children. Semin Perinatol 39(2):147–158, 2015

Aylward GP: Neurodevelopmental outcomes of infants born prematurely. J Dev Behav Pediatr 26(6):427–440, 2005

Bahadue FL, Soll R: Early versus delayed selective surfactant treatment for neonatal respiratory distress syndrome. Cochrane Database Syst Rev 11:CD001456, 2012

Barbian ME, Buckle R, Denning PW, Patel RM: To start or not: factors to consider when implementing routine probiotic use in the NICU. Early Hum Dev 135:66–71, 2019

Bassan H, Limperopoulos C, Visconti K, et al: Neurodevelopmental outcome in survivors of periventricular hemorrhagic infarction. Pediatrics 120(4):785–792, 2007

Bassler D, Stoll BJ, Schmidt B, et al: Using a count of neonatal morbidities to predict poor outcome in extremely low birth weight infants: added role of neonatal infection. Pediatrics 123(1):313–318, 2009

Batton B, Li L, Newman NS, et al: Use of antihypotensive therapies in extremely preterm infants. Pediatrics 131(6):e1865–e1873, 2013

Batton B, Li L, Newman NS, et al: Early blood pressure, antihypotensive therapy and outcomes at 18–22 months' corrected age in extremely preterm infants. Arch Dis Child Fetal Neonatal Ed 101(3):F201–F206, 2016

Bax M, Goldstein M, Rosenbaum P, et al: Proposed definition and classification of cerebral palsy, April 2005. Dev Med Child Neurol 47(8):571–576, 2005

Bayley N: Bayley Scales of Infant Development, 2nd Edition. San Antonio, TX, The Psychological Corporation, 1993

Bayley N: Bayley Scales of Infant Development, 3rd Edition. San Antonio, TX, The Psychological Corporation, 2006

Bayley N, Aylward GP: Bayley Scales of Infant and Toddler Development, 4th Edition. San Antonio, TX, The Psychological Corporation, 2019

Beaino G, Khoshnood B, Kaminski M, et al: Predictors of cerebral palsy in very preterm infants: the EPIPAGE prospective population-based cohort study. Dev Med Child Neurol 52(6):e119–e125, 2010

Beaino G, Khoshnood B, Kaminski M, et al: Predictors of the risk of cognitive deficiency in very preterm infants: the EPIPAGE prospective cohort. Acta Paediatr 100(3):370–378, 2011

Behrman RE: Preterm Birth: Causes, Consequences, and Prevention. The National Academies Collection. Washington, DC, National Academies Press, 2007

Belfort MB, Gillman MW, Buka SL, et al: Preterm infant linear growth and adiposity gain: trade-offs for later weight status and intelligence quotient. J Pediatr 163(6):1564–1569, 2013

Bell MJ, Ternberg JL, Feigin RD, et al: Neonatal necrotizing enterocolitis: therapeutic decisions based upon clinical staging. Ann Surg 187(1):1–7, 1978

Benitz WE: Treatment of persistent patent ductus arteriosus in preterm infants: time to accept the null hypothesis? J Perinatol 30(4):241–252, 2010

Benitz WE: Learning to live with patency of the ductus arteriosus in preterm infants. J Perinatol 31(suppl 1):S42–S48, 2011

Benzies KM, Magill-Evans JE, Hayden KA, Ballantyne M: Key components of early intervention programs for preterm infants and their parents: a systematic review and meta-analysis. BMC Pregnancy Childbirth 13(suppl 1):S10, 2013

Blank R, Smits-Engelsman B, Polatajko H, et al: European Academy for Childhood Disability (EACD): recommendations on the definition, diagnosis and intervention of developmental coordination disorder (long version). Dev Med Child Neurol 54(1):54–93, 2012

Blencowe H, Lawn JE, Vazquez T, et al: Preterm-associated visual impairment and estimates of retinopathy of prematurity at regional and global levels for 2010. Pediatr Res 74(suppl 1):35–49, 2013

Bolisetty S, Tiwari M1, Sutton L, et al: Neurodevelopmental outcomes of ex-
    tremely preterm infants in New South Wales and the Australian Capital
    Territory. J Paediatr Child Health 55(8):956–961, 2018
British Association of Perinatal Medicine: Report of a BAPM/RCPCH Working
    Group: Classification of Health Status at 2 Years as a Perinatal Outcome. Ver-
    sion 1.0, January 8, 2008. Available at: https://www.networks.nhs.uk/nhs-
    networks/staffordshire-shropshire-and-black-country-newborn/documents/
    2_year_Outcome_BAPM_WG_report_v6_Jan08.pdf. Accessed September 1,
    2019.
Brostrom L, Bolk J, Padilla N, et al: Clinical implications of diffuse excessive
    high signal intensity (DEHSI) on neonatal MRI in school age children born
    extremely preterm. PLoS ONE 11(2):e0149578, 2016
Brown JV, Embleton ND, Harding JE, McGuire W: Multi-nutrient fortification of
    human milk for preterm infants. Cochrane Database Syst Rev (5):CD000343,
    2016
Bruininks R, Bruininks B: Bruininks-Oseretsky Test of Motor Proficiency, 2nd
    Edition. Minneapolis, MN, NCS Pearson, 2005
Burakevych N, Mckinlay CJ, Alsweiler JM: Bayley-III motor scale and neurolog-
    ical examination at 2 years do not predict motor skills at 4.5 years. Dev
    Medicine and Child Neurol 59(2):216–223, 2017
Carlo WA, McDonald SA, Fanaroff AA, et al: Association of antenatal cortico-
    steroids with mortality and neurodevelopmental outcomes among infants
    born at 22 to 25 weeks' gestation. JAMA 306(21):2348–2358, 2011
Caskey M, Stephens B, Tucker R, Vohr B: Importance of parent talk on the de-
    velopment of preterm infant vocalizations. Pediatrics 128(5):910–916, 2011
Caskey M, Stephens B, Tucker R, Vohr B: Adult talk in the NICU with preterm
    infants and developmental outcomes. Pediatrics 133(3):e578–e584, 2014
Colditz PB, Boyd RN, Winter L, et al: A randomized trial of baby Triple P for pre-
    term infants: child outcomes at 2 years of corrected age. J Pediatr 210:48–54,
    2019
Cummings J, Committee on Fetus and Newborn: Antenatal counseling regard-
    ing resuscitation and intensive care before 25 weeks of gestation. Pediatrics
    136:588, 2015
Dahan S, Bourque CJ, Reichherzer M, et al: Beyond a seat at the table: the added
    value of family stakeholders to improve care, research, and education in
    neonatology. J Pediatr 207:123–129, 2019
Darlow BA: Retinopathy of prematurity: new developments bring concern and
    hope. J Paediatr Child Health 51(8):765–770, 2015
Darlow BA, Horwood LJ, Pere-Bracken HM, Woodward LJ: Psychosocial outcomes
    of young adults born very low birth weight. Pediatrics 132(6):e1521–e1528, 2013
Davis AS, Hintz SR, Van Meurs KP, et al: Seizures in extremely low birth weight
    infants are associated with adverse outcome. J Pediatr 157(5):720–725, 2010
Davis AS, Hintz SR, Goldstein RF, et al: Outcomes of extremely preterm infants
    following severe intracranial hemorrhage. J Perinatol 34(3):203–208, 2014
de Vries LS, Van Haastert IC, Rademaker KJ, et al: Ultrasound abnormalities preced-
    ing cerebral palsy in high-risk preterm infants. J Pediatr 144(6):815–820, 2004
de Vries LS, Van Haastert IC, Benders MJ, Groenendaal F: Myth: cerebral palsy
    cannot be predicted by neonatal brain imaging. Semin Fetal Neonatal Med
    16(5):279–287, 2011

Dean JM, Bennet L, Back SA, et al: What brakes the preterm brain? An arresting story. Pediatric Research 75(1–2):227–233, 2014

deRegnier RA, Wewerka S, Georgieff MK, et al: Influences of post-conceptional age and postnatal experience on the development of auditory recognition memory in the newborn infant. Dev Psychobiol 41(3):216–225, 2002

Dinesen SJ, Greisen G: Quality of life in young adults with very low birth weight. Arch Dis Child Fetal Neonatal Ed 85(3):F165–F169, 2001

Doyle LW, Roberts G, Anderson PJ, et al: Outcomes at age 2 years of infants <28 weeks' gestational age born in Victoria in 2005. J Pediatr 156(1):49–53, 2010

Doyle LW, Cheong JL, Ehrenkranz RA, Halliday HL: Late (>7 days) systemic postnatal corticosteroids for prevention of bronchopulmonary dysplasia in preterm infants. Cochrane Database Syst Rev (10):CD001145, 2017

Duncan AF, Bann C, Boatman C, et al: Do currently recommended Bayley-III cutoffs overestimate motor impairment in infants born <27 weeks gestation? J Perinatol 35(7):516–521, 2015

Dupont-Thibodeau A, Barrington KJ, Farlow B, Janvier A: End-of-life decisions for extremely low-gestational-age infants: why simple rules for complicated decisions should be avoided. Semin Perinatol 38(1):31–37, 2014

Ehrenkranz RA, Dusick AM, Vohr BR, et al: Growth in the neonatal intensive care unit influences neurodevelopmental and growth outcomes of extremely low birth weight infants. Pediatrics 117(4):1253–1261, 2006

Ehrenkranz RA, Das A, Wrage LA, et al: Early nutrition mediates the influence of severity of illness on extremely LBW infants. Pediatr Res 69(6):522–529, 2011

Eichenwald EC, Aina A, Stark AR: Apnea frequently persists beyond term gestation in infants delivered at 24 to 28 weeks. Pediatrics 100(3 pt 1):354–359, 1997

Elliott CD, Salerno JD, Dumont R, Willis JO: The differential ability scales—second edition, in Contemporary Intellectual Assessment: Theories, Tests, and Issues, 4th Edition. Edited by Flanagan DP, McDonough EM. New York, Guilford, 2018, pp 360–382

Engle WA, American Academy of Pediatrics Committee on Fetus and Newborn: Surfactant-replacement therapy for respiratory distress in the preterm and term neonate. Pediatrics 121(2):419–432, 2008

Fawke J: Neurological outcomes following preterm birth. Semin Fetal Neonatal Med 12(5):374–382, 2007

Feldman R: Maternal versus child risk and the development of parent–child and family relationships in five high-risk populations. Dev Psychopathol 19(2):293–312, 2007

Ferrero DM, Larson J, Jacobsson B, et al: Cross-country individual participant analysis of 4.1 million singleton births in 5 countries with very high human development index confirms known associations but provides no biologic explanation for 2/3 of all preterm births. PLoS One 11(9):e0162506, 2016

Fierson WM, American Academy of Pediatrics Section on Ophthalmology, American Academy of Ophthalmology, et al: Screening examination of premature infants for retinopathy of prematurity. Pediatrics 142(6):e20183061, 2018

Finer NN, Carlo WA, Walsh MC, et al: Early CPAP versus surfactant in extremely preterm infants. N Engl J Med 362(21):1970–1979, 2010

Flynn J: Searching for justice: the discovery of IQ gains over time. Am Psychol 54(1):5–20, 1999

Gäddlin PO, Finnström O, Sydsjö G, Leijon I: Most very low birth weight sub-
    jects do well as adults. Acta Paediatr 98(9):1513–1520, 2009

Glass HC, Bonifacio SL, Chau V, et al: Recurrent postnatal infections are associ-
    ated with progressive white matter injury in premature infants. Pediatrics
    122(2):299–305, 2008

Gorter JW, Ketellar M, Rosenbaum P, et al: Use of the GMFCS in infants with CP:
    the need for reclassification at age 2 years or older. Dev Med Child Neurol
    51(1):46–52, 2009

Green NS, Damus K, Simpson JL, et al: Research agenda for preterm birth: recom-
    mendations from the March of Dimes. Am J Obstet Gynecol 193(3 pt 1):626–
    635, 2005

Greenberg RG, Kandefer S, Do BT, et al: Late-onset sepsis in extremely prema-
    ture infants: 2000–2011. Pediatr Infect Dis J 36(8):774–779, 2017

Grégoire MC, Lefebvre F, Glorieux J: Health and developmental outcomes at 18
    months in very preterm infants with bronchopulmonary dysplasia. Pediatrics
    101(5):856–860, 1998

Gyamfi-Bannerman C, Thom EA, Blackwell SC, et al: Antenatal betamethasone for
    women at risk for late preterm delivery. N Engl J Med 374(14):1311–1320,
    2016

Hack M: Adult outcomes of preterm children. J Dev Behav Pediatr 30(5):460–470,
    2009

Hack M, Merkatz IR, Gordon D, et al: The prognostic significance of postnatal
    growth in very low-birth weight infants. Am J Obstet Gynecol 143(6):693–
    699, 1982

Hack M, Breslau N, Weissman B, et al: Effect of very low birth weight and subnor-
    mal head size on cognitive abilities at school age. N Engl J Med 325(4):231–237,
    1991

Hack M, Breslau N, Aram D, et al: The effect of very low birth weight and social
    risk on neurocognitive abilities at school age. J Dev Behav Pediatr
    13(6):412–420, 1992

Hack M, Wilson-Costello D, Friedman H, et al: Neurodevelopment and predic-
    tors of outcomes of children with birth weights of less than 1000 g: 1992–
    1995. Arch Pediatr Adolesc Med 154(7):725–731, 2000

Hack M, Youngstrom EA, Cartar L, et al: Behavioral outcomes and evidence of
    psychopathology among very low birth weight infants at age 20 years. Pe-
    diatrics 114(4):932–940, 2004

Hack M, Taylor HG, Drotar D, et al: Poor predictive validity of the Bayley Scales
    of Infant Development for cognitive function of extremely low birth weight
    children at school age. Pediatrics 116(2):333–341, 2005

Haslam MD, Lisonkova S, Creighton D, et al: Severe neurodevelopmental im-
    pairment in neonates born preterm: impact of varying definitions in a Ca-
    nadian cohort. J Pediatr 197:75–81, 2018

Hayes B, Sharif F: Behavioural and emotional outcome of very low birth weight
    infants—literature review. J Matern Fetal Neonatal Med 22(10):849–856, 2009

Hellgren KM, Tornqvist K, Jakobsson PG, et al: Ophthalmologic outcome of ex-
    tremely preterm infants at 6.5 years of age: Extremely Preterm Infants in
    Sweden Study (EXPRESS). JAMA Ophthalmol 134(5):555–562, 2016

Henderson SE, Sugden D, Barnett A: Movement Assessment Battery for Children,
    2nd Edition. San Antonio, TX, Pearson Clinical Assessment Group, 2007

Henderson-Smart DJ: The effect of gestational age on the incidence and duration of recurrent apnea in newborn babies. Aust Paediatr J 17(4):273–276, 1981

Higgins RD, Jobe AH, Koso-Thomas M, et al: Bronchopulmonary dysplasia: executive summary of a workshop. J Pediatr 197:300–308, 2018

Hintz SR, Hendrick DE, Stoll BJ, et al: Neurodevelopmental and growth outcomes of extremely low birth weight infants after necrotizing enterocolitis. Pediatrics 115(3):696–703, 2005

Hintz SR, Kendrick DE, Vohr BR, et al: Gender differences in neurodevelopmental outcomes among extremely preterm, extremely-low-birthweight infants. Acta Paediatr 95(10):1239–1248, 2006

Hintz SR, Slovis T, Bulas D, et al: Interobserver reliability and accuracy of cranial ultrasound scanning in premature infants. J Pediatr 150(6):592–596, 2007

Hintz SR, Kendrick DE, Wilson-Costello D, et al: Neurodevelopmental outcomes are not improving for infants born at <25 weeks' gestational age. Pediatrics 127(1):62–70, 2011

Hintz SR, Barnes PD, Bulas D, et al: Neuroimaging and neurodevelopmental outcome in extremely preterm infants. Pediatrics 135(1):e32–e42, 2015

Hintz SR, Vohr BR, Bann CM, et al: Preterm neuroimaging and school-age cognitive outcomes. Pediatrics 142(1), 2018

Ho T, Dukhovny D, Zupancic JAF, et al: Choosing wisely in newborn medicine: five opportunities to increase value. Pediatrics 136(2):e482–e489, 2015

Hogan DP, Rogers ML, Msall ME: Functional limitations and key indicators of well-being in children with disability. Arch Pediatr Adolesc Med 154(10):1042–1048, 2000

Holmstrom G, Larsson E: Outcome of retinopathy of prematurity. Clin Perinatol 40(2):311–321, 2013

Horbar JD, Ehrenkranz RA, Badger GJ, et al: Weight growth velocity and postnatal growth failure in infants 501 to 1500 grams: 2000–2013. Pediatrics 136(1):e84–e92, 2015

Horwitz SM, Leibovitz A, Lilo E, et al: Does an intervention to reduce maternal anxiety, depression and trauma also improve mothers' perceptions of their preterm infants' vulnerability? Infant Ment Health J 36(1):42–52, 2015a

Horwitz SM, Storfer-Isser A, Kerker BD, et al: A model for the development of mothers' perceived vulnerability of preterm infants. J Dev Behav Pediatr 36(5):371–380, 2015b

Husby IM, Stray KM, Olsen A, et al: Long-term follow-up of mental health, health-related quality of life and associations with motor skills in young adults born preterm with very low birth weight. Health Qual Life Outcomes 14:56, 2016

Indredavik MS, Vik T, Evensen KA, et al: Perinatal risk and psychiatric outcome in adolescents born preterm with very low birth weight or term small for gestational age. J Dev Behav Pediatr 31(4):286–294, 2010

Jaekel J, Baumann N, Bartmann P, Wolke D: Mood and anxiety disorders in very preterm/very low-birth weight individuals from 6 to 26 years. J Child Psychol Psychiatry 59(1):88–95, 2018

Janvier A, Barrington K: Trying to predict the future of ex-preterm infants: who benefits from a brain MRI at term? Acta Paediatr 101(10):1016–1017, 2012

Janvier A, Bourque CJ, Dahan S, et al: Integrating parents in neonatal and pediatric research. Neonatology 115(4):283–291, 2019

Jeon TY, Kim JH, Yoo SY, et al: Neurodevelopmental outcomes in preterm infants: comparison of infants with and without diffuse excessive high signal intensity on MR images at near-term-equivalent age. Radiology 263(2):518–526, 2012

Johnson S, Hollis C, Kochhar P, et al: Psychiatric disorders in extremely preterm children: longitudinal finding at age 11 years in the EPICure study. J Am Acad Child Adolesc Psychiatry 49(5):453–463, 2010

Johnson S, Moore T, Marlow N: Using the Bayley-III to assess neurodevelopmental delay: which cut-off should be used? Pediatr Res 75(5):670–674, 2014

Kajantie E, Hovi P, Raikkonen K, et al: Young adults with very low birth weight: leaving the parental home and sexual relationships—Helsinki study of very low birth weight adults. Pediatrics 122(1):e62–e72, 2008

Kirby A, Sugden DA: Children with developmental coordination disorders. J R Soc Med 100(4):182–186, 2007

Kotecha SJ, Edwards MO, Watkins WJ, et al: Effect of preterm birth on later FEV1: a systematic review and meta-analysis. Thorax 68(8):760–766, 2013

Kuban KCK, Allred EN, O'Shea TM, et al: Cranial ultrasound lesions in the NICU predict cerebral palsy at age 2 years in children born at extremely low gestational age. J Child Neurol 24(1):63–72, 2009

Kwong AKL, Fitzgerald TL, Doyle LW, et al: Predictive validity of spontaneous early infant movement for later cerebral palsy: a systematic review. Dev Med Child Neurol 60(5):480–489, 2018

Lampi KM, Lehtonen L, Tran PL, et al: Risk of autism spectrum disorders in low birth weight and small for gestational age infants. J Pediatr 161(5):830–836, 2012

Laptook AR, O'Shea RM, Shankaran S, et al: Adverse neurodevelopmental outcomes among extremely low birth weight infants with a normal head ultrasound: prevalence and antecedents. Pediatrics 115(3):673–680, 2005

Laughon M, Bose C, Allred E, et al: Factors associated with treatment for hypotension in extremely low gestational age newborns during the first postnatal week. Pediatrics 119(2):273–280, 2007

Laughon M, Allred EN, Bose C, et al: Patterns of respiratory disease during the first 2 postnatal weeks in extremely premature infants. Pediatrics 123(4):1124–1131, 2009

Lee HC, Green C, Hintz SR, et al: Prediction of death for extremely premature infants in a population-based cohort. Pediatrics 126(3):e644–e650, 2010

Leon Hernandez A: The impact of prematurity on social and emotional development. Clin Perinatol 45(3):547–555, 2018

Lien R, Yu MH, Hsu KH, et al: Neurodevelopmental outcomes in infants with retinopathy of prematurity and bevacizumab treatment. PLoS ONE 11(1):e0148019, 2016

Limperopoulos C, Bassan H, Gauvreau K, et al: Does cerebellar injury in premature infants contribute to the high prevalence of long-term cognitive, learning, and behavioral disability in survivors? Pediatrics 120(3):584–593, 2007

Limperopoulos C, Chilingaryan G, Sullivan N, et al: Injury to the premature cerebellum: outcome is related to remote cortical development. Cereb Cortex 24(3):728–736, 2014

Lindström K, Lindblad F, Hjern A: Psychiatric morbidity in adolescents and young adults born preterm: a Swedish national cohort study. Pediatrics 123(1):e47–53, 2009

Lingam R, Jongmans MJ, Ellis M, et al: Mental health difficulties in children with developmental coordination disorder. Pediatrics 129(4):e882–e889, 2012

Linsell L, Malouf R, Morris J, et al: Prognostic factors for poor cognitive development in children born very preterm or with very low birth weight: a systematic review. JAMA Pediatr 169(12):1162–1172, 2015

Lodha A, Sauvé R, Bhandari V, et al: Need for supplemental oxygen at discharge in infants with bronchopulmonary dysplasia is not associated with worse neurodevelopmental outcomes at 3 years corrected age. PLoS ONE 9(3):e90843, 2014

Lund LK, Vik T, Lydersen S, et al: Mental health, quality of life and social relations in young adults born with low birth weight. Health Qual Life Outcomes 10:146, 2012

Majnemer A, Riley P, Shevell M, et al: Severe bronchopulmonary dysplasia increases risk for later neurological and motor sequelae in preterm survivors. Dev Med Child Neurol 42(1):53–60, 2000

Malviya MN, Ohlsson A, Shah SS: Surgical versus medical treatment with cyclooxygenase inhibitors for symptomatic patent ductus arteriosus in preterm infants. Cochrane Database Syst Rev (3):CD003951, 2013

Manja V, Lakshminrusimha S, Cook DJ: Oxygen saturation target range for extremely preterm infants: a systematic review and meta-analysis. JAMA Pediatr 169(4):332–340, 2015

Manja V, Saugstad OD, Lakshminrusimha S: Oxygen saturation targets in preterm infants and outcomes at 18–24 months: a systematic review. Pediatrics 139(1), 2017

Manley BJ, Roberts RS, Doyle LW, et al: Social variables predict gains in cognitive scores across the preschool years in children with birth weights 500 to 1250 grams. J Pediatr 166(4):870–876, 2015

Marlow N: Is survival and neurodevelopmental impairment at 2 years of age the gold standard outcome for neonatal studies? Arch Dis Child Fetal Neonatal Ed 100(1):F82–F84, 2015

Marret S, Marchand-Martin L, Picaud JC, et al: Brain injury in very preterm children and neurosensory and cognitive disabilities during childhood: the EPIPAGE cohort study. PLoS ONE 8(5):e62683, 2013

McGowan EC, Vohr BR: Neurodevelopmental follow-up of preterm infants what is new? Pediatr Clin N Am 66(2):509–523, 2019

McGowan EC, Du N, Hawes K, et al: Maternal mental health and neonatal intensive care unit discharge readiness in mothers of preterm infants. J Pediatr 184:68–74, 2017

McMahon E, Wintermark P, Lahav A: Auditory brain development in premature infants: the importance of early experience. Ann NY Acad Sci 1252:17–24, 2012

Ment LR, Bada HS, Barnes P, et al: Practice parameter: neuroimaging of the neonate. Report of the Quality Standards Subcommittee of the American Academy of Neurology and the Practice Committee of the Child Neurology Society. Neurology 58(12):1726–1738, 2002

Merhar SL, Tabangin ME, Meinzen-Derr J, Schibler KR: Grade and laterality of intraventricular haemorrhage to predict 18–22 month neurodevelopmental outcomes in extremely low birthweight infants. Acta Paediatr 101(4):414–418, 2012

Mintz-Hittner HA, Kennedy KA, Chuang AZ, et al: Efficacy of intravitreal bev-
    acizumab for stage 3+ retinopathy of prematurity. N Engl J Med 364(7):603–
    615, 2011

Mitha A, Foix-L'Hélias L, Arnaud C, et al: Neonatal infection and 5-year neuro-
    developmental outcome of very preterm infants. Pediatrics 132(2):e372–
    e380, 2013

Moore T, Hennessy EM, Myles J, et al: Neurological and developmental out-
    come in extremely preterm children born in England in 1995 and 2006: the
    EPICure studies. BMJ 345:e7961, 2012

Moss RL, Dimmitt RA, Barnhart DC, et al: Laparotomy versus peritoneal drain-
    age for necrotizing enterocolitis and perforation. N Engl J Med
    354(21):2225–2234, 2006

Msall ME, Park JJ: The spectrum of behavioral outcomes after extreme prema-
    turity? Regulatory, attention, social, and adaptive dimensions. Semin Peri-
    natol 32(1):42–50, 2008

Natarajan G, Shankaran S, Nolen TL, et al: Neurodevelopmental outcomes of
    preterm infants with retinopathy of prematurity by treatment. Pediatrics
    144(2), 2019

NIH Consensus Development Panel on the Effect of Corticosteroids for Fetal
    Maturation on Perinatal Outcomes: Effect of corticosteroids for fetal matu-
    ration on perinatal outcomes. JAMA 273(5):413–418, 1995

Nosarti C, Reichenberg A, Murray RM, et al: Preterm birth and psychiatric dis-
    orders in young adult life. Arch Gen Psychiatry 69(6):E1–E18, 2012

O'Shea TM, Allred EN, Dammann O, et al: The ELGAN study of the brain and
    related disorders in extremely low gestational age newborns. Early Hum
    Dev 85(11):719–725, 2009

O'Shea TM, Allred EN, Kuban KCK, et al: Intraventricular hemorrhage and de-
    velopmental outcomes at 24 months of age in extremely preterm infants.
    J Child Neurol 27(1):22–29, 2012

Oswald LM, Zandi P, Nestadt G, et al: Relationship between cortisol responses
    to stress and personality. Neuropsychopharmacology 31(7):1583–1591,
    2007

Palisano R, Rosenbaum P, Walter S, et al: Development and reliability of a sys-
    tem to classify gross motor function in children with cerebral palsy. Dev
    Med Child Neurol 39(4):214–223, 1997

Palisano R, Rosenbaum P, Bartlett D, et al: Gross Motor Function Classification
    System: Expanded and Revised (GMFCS–E&R). Hamilton, ON, CanChild
    Centre for Childhood Disability Research, McMaster University, 2007. Avail-
    able at: https://canchild.ca/system/tenon/assets/attachments/000/000/
    058/original/GMFCS-ER_English.pdf. Accessed October 7, 2019.

Pape KE, Blackwell RJ, Cusick G, et al: Ultrasound detection of brain damage in
    preterm infants. Lancet 1(8129):1261–1264, 1979

Papile LA, Burstein J, Burstein R, et al: Incidence and evolution of subependy-
    mal and intraventricular hemorrhage: a study of infants with birth weight
    less than 1,500 gm. J Pediatr 92(4):529–534, 1978

Patel AK, Kim JH: Human milk and necrotizing enterocolitis. Semin Pediatric
    Surg 27(1):34–38, 2018

Patel RM, Kandefer S, Walsh MC, et al: Causes and timing of death in extremely pre-
    mature infants from 2000 through 2011. N Engl J Med 372(4):331–340, 2015

Pesonen AK, Räikkönen K, Heinonen K, et al: Personality of young adults born prematurely: the Helsinki study of very low birth weight adults. J Child Psychol Psychiatry 49(6):609–617, 2008

Peter CS, Sprodowski N, Bohnhorst B, et al: Gastroesophageal reflux and apnea of prematurity: no temporal relationship. Pediatrics 109(1):8–11, 2002

Pfister KM, Ramel SE: Linear growth and neurodevelopmental outcomes. Clin Perinatol 41(2):309–321, 2014

Pierrat V, Marchand-Martin L, Arnaud C, et al: Neurodevelopmental outcome at 2 years for preterm children born at 22 to 34 weeks' gestation in France in 2011: EPIPAGE-2 cohort study. BMJ 358:j3448, 2017

Poindexter BB, Langer JC, Dusick AM, et al: Early provision of parenteral amino acids in extremely low birth weight infants: relation to growth and neurodevelopmental outcome. J Pediatr 148(3):300–305, 2006

Potharst ES, Houtzager BA, Van Sonderen L, et al: Prediction of cognitive abilities at the age of 5 years using developmental follow-up assessments at the age of 2 and 3 years in very preterm children. Dev Med Child Neurol 54(3):240–246, 2012

Potijk MR, Kerstjens JM, Bos AF, et al: Developmental delay in moderately preterm-born children with low socioeconomic status: risks multiply. J Pediatr 163(5):1289–1295, 2013

Potijk MR, de Winter AF, Bos AF, et al: Behavioural and emotional problems in moderately preterm children with low socioeconomic status: a population-based study. Eur Child Adolesc Psychiatry 24(7):787–795, 2015

Pyhälä R, Hovi P, Lahti M, et al: Very low birth weight, infant growth, and autism-spectrum traits in adulthood. Pediatrics 134(6):1075–1083, 2014

Pyhälä R, Wolford E, Kautiainen H, et al: Self-reported mental health problems among adults born preterm: a meta-analysis. Pediatrics 9(4), 2017

Quigley M, Embleton ND, McGuire W: Formula versus donor breast milk for feeding preterm or low birth weight infants. Cochrane Database Syst Rev (7):CD002971, 2019

Räikkönen K, Pesonen AK, Heinonen K, et al: Depression in young adults with very low birth weight: the Helsinki study of very low-birth-weight adults. Arch Gen Psychiatry 65(3):290–296, 2008

Ramanathan R, Corwin MJ, Hunt CE, et al: Cardiorespiratory events recorded on home monitors: comparison of healthy infants with those at increased risk for SIDS. JAMA 285(17):2199–2207, 2001

Ramel SE, Demerath EW, Gray HL, et al: The relationship of poor linear growth velocity with neonatal illness and two-year neurodevelopment in preterm infants. Neonatology 102(1):19–24, 2012

Rees CM, Eaton S, Kiely EM, et al: Peritoneal drainage or laparotomy for neonatal bowel perforation. Ann Surg 248:44–51, 2008

Reid SM, Carlin JB, Reddihough DS: Rates of cerebral palsy in Victoria, Australia, 1970 to 2004: has there been a change? Dev Med Child Neurol 53(10):907–912, 2011

Rethlefsen SA, Ryan DD, Kay RM: Classification systems in cerebral palsy. Orthop Clin North Am 41(4):457–467, 2010

Roberts D, Dalziel SR: Antenatal corticosteroids for accelerating fetal lung maturation for women at risk of preterm birth. Cochrane Database Syst Rev (3):CD004454, 2017

Roberts G, Anderson PJ, Doyle LW, et al: Neurosensory disabilities at school age in geographic cohorts of extremely low birth weight children born between the 1970s and the 1990s. J Pediatr 154(6):829–834, 2009

Roberts G, Anderson PJ, Doyle LW: The stability of the diagnosis of developmental disability between ages 2 and 8 in a geographic cohort of very preterm children born in 1997. Arch Dis Child 95:786–790, 2010

Roberts G, Anderson PJ, Davis N, et al: Developmental coordination disorder in geographic cohorts of 8-year-old children born extremely preterm or extremely low birthweight in the 1990s. Dev Med Child Neurol 53(1):55–60, 2011

Rojas-Reyes MX, Morley CJ, Soll R: Prophylactic versus selective use of surfactant in preventing morbidity and mortality in preterm infants. Cochrane Database Syst Rev (3):CD000510, 2012

Rysavy MA, Li L, Bell EF, et al: Between-hospital variation in treatment and outcomes in extremely preterm infants. N Engl J Med 372:1801–1811, 2015

Sabnis A, Fojo S, Nayak SS, et al: Reducing parental trauma and stress in neonatal intensive care: systematic review and meta-analysis of hospital interventions. J Perinatol 9(3):375–386, 2019

Saigal S, Stoskopf B, Pinelli J, et al: Self-perceived health-related quality of life of former extremely low birth weight infants at young adulthood. Pediatrics 118(3):1140–1148, 2006

Saigal S, Day KL, Van Lieshout RJ, et al: Health, wealth, social integration, and sexuality of extremely low birth weight prematurely born adults in the fourth decade of life. JAMA Pediatr 170(7):678–686, 2016

Sari FN, Akdag A, Dizdar EA, et al: Antioxidant capacity of fresh and stored breast milk: is −80°C optimal temperature for freeze storage? J Matern Fetal Neonatal Med 25(6):777–782, 2012

Sarkar S, Shankaran S, Barks J, et al: Outcome of preterm infants with transient cystic periventricular leukomalacia on serial imaging up to term equivalent age. J Pediatr 195:59–65, 2018

Scala M, Seo S, Lee-Park J, et al: Effect of reading to preterm infants on measures of cardiorespiratory stability in the neonatal intensive care unit. J Perinatol 38(11):1536–1541, 2018

Schlapbach LJ, Aebischer M, Adams M, et al: Impact of sepsis on neurodevelopmental outcome in a Swiss National Cohort of extremely premature infants. Pediatrics 128:e348–e357, 2011

Schlapbach LJ, Adams M, Prioletti E, et al: Outcome at two years of age in a Swiss national cohort of extremely preterm infants born between 2000 and 2008. BMC Pediatr 12:198, 2012

Schmidt B, Davis P, Moddermann D, et al: Long-term effects of indomethacin prophylaxis in extremely low-birth-weight infants. N Eng J Med 344:1966–1972, 2001

Schmidt B, Asztalos EV, Roberts RS, et al: Impact of bronchopulmonary dysplasia, brain injury, and severe retinopathy on the outcome of extremely low-birth-weight infants at 18 months: results from the trial of indomethacin prophylaxis in preterms. JAMA289(9):1124–1129, 2003

Schmidt B, Roberts RS, Davis P, et al: Caffeine for apnea of prematurity trial group. Caffeine therapy for apnea of prematurity. N Engl J Med 354(20):2112–2121, 2006

Schmidt B, Roberts RS, Davis P, et al: Long-term effects of caffeine therapy for apnea of prematurity. N Engl J Med 357(19):1893–1902, 2007

Schmidt B, Anderson PJ, Doyle LW, et al: Survival without disability to age 5 years after neonatal caffeine therapy for apnea of prematurity. JAMA 307(3):275–282, 2012

Schmidt B, Davis PG, Asztalos EV, et al: Association between severe retinopathy of prematurity and nonvisual disabilities at age 5 years. JAMA 311(5):523–525, 2014

Schmidt B, Roberts RS, Davis PG, et al: Prediction of late death or disability at age 5 years using a count of 3 neonatal morbidities in very low birth weight infants. J Pediatr 167(5):982–986, 2015

Schulzke SM, Deshpande GC, Patole SK: Neurodevelopmental outcomes of very low-birth weight infants with necrotizing enterocolitis: a systematic review of observational studies. Arch Pediatr Adolesc Med 161(6):583–590, 2007

Section on Breastfeeding: Breastfeeding and the use of human milk. Pediatrics 129(3):e827–e841, 2012

Serenius F, Källén K, Blennow M, et al: Neurodevelopmental outcome in extremely preterm infants at 2.5 years after active perinatal care in Sweden. JAMA 309(17):1810–1820, 2013

Shah DK, Doyle LW, Anderson PJ, et al: Adverse neurodevelopment in preterm infants with postnatal sepsis or necrotizing enterocolitis is mediated by white matter abnormalities on magnetic resonance imaging at term. J Pediatr 153:170–175, 2008

Shaw RJ, Bernard RS, Deblois T, et al: The relationship between acute stress disorder and posttraumatic stress disorder in the neonatal intensive care unit. Psychosomatics 50(2):131–137, 2009

Shaw RJ, Bernard RS, Storfer-Isser A, et al: Parental coping in the neonatal intensive care unit. J Clin Psychol Med Settings 20(2):135–142, 2013

Shaw RJ, St John N, Lilo E, et al: Prevention of traumatic stress in mothers of preterms: 6-month outcomes. Pediatrics 134(2):e481–e488, 2014

Sie LTL, Hart AAM, van Hof J, et al: Predictive value of neonatal MRI with respect to late MRI findings and clinical outcome. A study in infants with periventricular densities on neonatal ultrasound. NeuroPediatrics 36(2):78–89, 2005

Singh GK, Kenney MK, Ghandour RM, et al: Mental health outcomes in US children and adolescents born prematurely or with low birthweight. Depress Res Treat 570743, 2013

Sinn JK, Ward MC, Henderson-Smart DJ: Developmental outcome of preterm infants after surfactant therapy: systematic review of randomized controlled trials. J Paediatr Child Health 38(6):597–600, 2002

Skiöld B, Vollmer B, Böhm B, et al: Neonatal magnetic resonance imaging and outcome at age 30 months in extremely preterm infants. J Pediatr 160(4):559–566, 2012

Skiöld B, Eriksson C, Eliasson AC, et al: General movements and magnetic resonance imaging in the prediction of neuromotor outcome in children born extremely preterm. Early Hum Dev 89(7):467–472, 2013

Slovis TL, Kuhns LR: Real-time sonography of the brain through the anterior fontanelle. AJR Am J Roentgenol 136(2):277–286, 1981

Spencer-Smith MM, Spittle AJ, Lee KJ, et al: Bayley-III cognitive and language scales in preterm children. Pediatrics 135(5):e1258–e1265, 2015

Spittle AJ, Orton J: Cerebral palsy and developmental coordination disorder in children born preterm. Semin Fetal Neonatal Med 19(2):84–89, 2014

Spittle AJ, Boyd RN, Inder TE, Doyle LW: Predicting motor development in very preterm infants at 12 months' corrected age: the role of qualitative magnetic resonance imaging and general movements assessments. Pediatrics 123(2):512–517, 2009

Spittle AJ, Cheong J, Doyle LW, et al: Neonatal white matter abnormality predicts childhood motor impairment in very preterm children. Dev Med Child Neurol 53:1000–1006, 2011

Spittle AJ, Spencer-Smith MM, Cheong JL, et al: General movements in very preterm children and neurodevelopment at 2 and 4 years. Pediatrics 132:e452–e458, 2013

Sriram S, Schreiber MD, Msall ME, et al: Cognitive development and quality of life associated with BPD in 10-year-olds born preterm. Pediatrics 141, 2018

Steggerda SJ, de Bruine FT, van den Berg-Huysmans AA, et al: Small cerebellar hemorrhage in preterm infants: perinatal and postnatal factors and outcome. Cerebellum 12(6):794–801, 2013

Stephenson T, Wright S, O'Connor A, et al: Children born weighing less than 1701 g: visual and cognitive outcomes at 11–14 years. Arch Dis Child Fetal Neonatal Ed 92(4):F265–F270, 2007

Stevens TP, Finer NN, Carlo WA, et al: Respiratory outcomes of the Surfactant Positive Pressure and Oximetry Randomized Trial (SUPPORT). J Pediatr 165(2):240–244, 2014

Stoll BJ, Hansen NI, Adams-Chapman I, et al: Neurodevelopmental and growth impairment among extremely low-birth-weight infants with neonatal infection. JAMA 292(19):2357–2365, 2004

Stoll BJ, Hansen NI, Bell EF, et al: Neonatal outcomes of extremely preterm infants from the NICHD Neonatal Research Network. Pediatrics 126(3):443–456, 2010

Stoll BJ, Hansen NI, Sanchez PJ, et al: Early onset sepsis: the burden of group B streptococcal and *E. coli* disease continues. Pediatrics 127:817–826, 2011

Stoll BJ, Hansen NI, Bell EF, et al: Trends in care practices, morbidity, and mortality of extremely preterm neonates, 1993–2012. JAMA 314(10):1039–1051, 2015

Sugden D, Chambers M, Utley A: Leeds Consensus Statement 2006: Developmental Coordination Disorder as a Specific Learning Difficulty. ESRC Research Seminar Series, 2004–2005. Leeds, UK, Dyscovery Centre, 2006. Available at: https://www.pearsonclinical.co.uk/Psychology/ChildCognitionNeuropsychology andLanguage/ChildPerceptionandVisuomotorAbilities/MABC-2/Resources/LeedsConsensus06.pdf. Accessed October 7, 2019.

SUPPORT Study Group of the Eunice Kennedy Shriver NICHD Neonatal Research Network, Carlo WA, Finer NN, et al: Target ranges of oxygen saturation in extremely preterm infants. N Engl J Med 362(21):1959–1969, 2010

Suresh GK, Soll RF: Overview of surfactant replacement trials. J Perinatol 25(suppl 2):S40–S44, 2005

Synnes A, Anson S, Baum J, et al: Incidence and pattern of hearing impairment in children with ≤ 5 800 g birth weight in British Columbia, Canada. Acta Paediatr 101(2):e48–e54, 2012

Synnes A, Luu TM, Moddemann D, et al: Determinants of developmental outcomes in a very preterm Canadian cohort. Arch Dis Child Fetal Neonatal Ed 102:F235–F243, 2017

Tam EW, Rosenbluth G, Rogers EE, et al: Cerebellar hemorrhage on magnetic resonance imaging in preterm newborns associated with abnormal neurologic outcome. J Pediatr 158(2):245–250, 2011

Treyvaud K, Inder TE, Lee KJ, et al: Can the home environment promote resilience for children born very preterm in the context of social and medical risk? J Exp Child Psychol 112:326–337, 2012

Tyson JE, Parikh NA, Langer J, et al: Intensive care for extreme prematurity— moving beyond gestational age. N Engl J Med 358(16):1672–1681, 2008

Vaucher YE, Peralta-Carcelen M, Finer NN, et al: Neurodevelopmental outcomes in the early CPAP and pulse oximetry trial. N Engl J Med 367(26):2495–2504, 2012

Vohr BR: Neurodevelopmental outcomes of extremely preterm infants. Clin Perinatol 41:241–255, 2014

Vohr BR: Language and hearing outcomes of preterm infants. Semin Perinatol 40:510–519, 2016

Vohr BR, Wright LL, Dusick AM, et al: Center differences and outcomes of extremely low birth weight infants. Pediatrics 113:781–789, 2004

Vohr BR, Msall ME, Wilson D, et al: Spectrum of gross motor function in extremely low birth weight children with cerebral palsy at 18 months of age. Pediatrics 116:123–129, 2005

Vohr BR, Stephens BE, Higgins RD, et al: Are outcomes of extremely preterm infants improving? Impact of Bayley assessment on outcomes. J Pediatr 161(2):222–228, 2012

Volpe JJ, Kinney HC, Jensen FE, et al: The developing oligodendrocyte: key cellular target in brain injury in the premature infant. Int J Dev Neurosci 29:423–440, 2011

Wadhawan R, Oh W, Hintz SR, et al: Neurodevelopmental outcomes of extremely low birth weight infants with spontaneous intestinal perforation or surgical necrotizing enterocolitis. J Perinatol 34(1):64–70, 2014

Wechsler D: The Wechsler Individual Achievement Test, 3rd Edition. San Antonio, TX, The Psychological Corporation, 2009

Wechsler D: Wechsler Preschool and Primary Scale of Intelligence, 4th Edition. San Antonio, TX, The Psychological Corporation, 2012

Wechsler D, Raiford SE, Holdnack JA: Wechsler Intelligence Scale for Children, 5th Edition. San Antonio, TX, The Psychological Corporation, 2014

Williams T, Nair H, Simpson J, Embleton N: Use of donor human milk and maternal breastfeeding rates: a systematic review. J Hum Lact 32(2):212–220, 2016

Wolke D, Baumann N, Busch B, Bartmann P: Very preterm birth and parents' quality of life 27 years later. Pediatrics 140(3), 2017

Wood NS, Costeloe K, Gibson AT, et al: The EPICure study: associations and antecedents of neurological and developmental disability at 30 months of age following extremely preterm birth. Arch Dis Child Fetal Neonatal Ed 90(2):F134–F140, 2005

Woodward LJ, Anderson PJ, Austin NC, et al: Neonatal MRI to predict neurodevelopmental outcomes in preterm infants. N Engl J Med 355(7):685–694, 2006

World Health Organization: Feeding of Low-Birthweight Infants in Low- and Middle-Income Countries. Geneva, World Health Organization, 2011. Available at: http://www.who.int/elena/titles/full_recommendations/feeding_lbw/en. Accessed June 1, 2019.

Younge N, Goldstein RF, Bann CM, et al: Survival and neurodevelopmental outcomes among periviable infants. N Engl J Med 376(7):617–662, 2017

CHAPTER 2

Psychological Adjustment in Mothers of Premature Infants

Richard J. Shaw, M.D.

Angelica Moreyra, Psy.D.

LaTrice L. Dowtin, Ph.D., LCPC, NCSP, RPT

Sarah M. Horwitz, Ph.D.

Difficulties with psychological adjustment are common in postpartum mothers, with estimates of postpartum depression ranging from 13% to 19% (O'Hara and McCabe 2013), postpartum anxiety ranging from 8% to 10% (Woolhouse et al. 2009), and traumatic stress reactions related to pregnancy or childbirth complications ranging from 3.1% to 15.7% (Grekin and O'Hara 2014). In mothers of preterm infants, the prevalence is even higher, with rates of postpartum depression as high as 40% and rates of postpartum anxiety and PTSD up to 23% (Feeley et al. 2011; Lefkowitz et al. 2010; Vigod et al. 2010). Prevalence rates are further increased in high-risk women, for example, those who have had a cesarean section or stillbirth and a prior history of mental health problems and stressful life events. Yildiz et al. (2017) suggested that documented rates of PTSD likely underestimate the true prevalence of the problem.

The NICU as a Traumatic Experience

Having a newborn infant hospitalized in the NICU is typically an unexpected and traumatic event. Negative responses of parents whose infant is in the NICU are well documented. Their reactions are complex and include feelings of guilt, helplessness, sadness over the loss of the "perfect" child, stress, and symptoms of anxiety and depression (Hagan et al. 2004; Kersting et al. 2004; Miles 1989). Parents who experience psychological distress following the birth of a preterm infant have also been found to be at increased risk for later problems with parent–infant relationships (Macey et al. 1987). These reactions are not surprising given the uncertainty about the potential loss of their child, concerns about the current physical condition and likely future impacts to the infant's health and functioning, and the sustained physical separation from their infant in the NICU. Some notable stressors associated with the NICU include financial strain (not able to return to work, cost of transportation to and from hospital, costs of care), physical barriers to bonding with their infant (the isolette, lack of space at bedside, needing to provide care for other children), and the displacement many families may experience if the NICU is located far from their home.

Miles (1989) categorized some specific domains of stress that occur in the NICU. In particular, she emphasized the importance of the alteration in the expected parental role that encompasses parents' experience of not being able to hold or handle their baby or participate in the anticipated experiences of feeding or breastfeeding and caring for their child. The Parental Stressor Scale: NICU (PSS:NICU) she developed quantifies specific stressful NICU experiences into four subscales: infant appearance and behaviors, parental relationship and communication with staff, parental role alteration, and sights and sounds in the NICU (Table 2–1). Several studies have shown a correlation between the scores on the PSS:NICU, particularly the total score that provides a global measure of stress, and symptoms of depression, anxiety, and PTSD (Shaw et al. 2006). Vinall et al. (2018), for example, found that mothers exposed to more invasive medical procedures for their infants had increased symptoms of posttraumatic stress, and those who reported greater anxiety about these procedures were more likely to have symptoms of reexperiencing and avoidance following their discharge from the NICU.

Psychological Distress in Parents of Premature Infants

The reactions of mothers of preterm infants in the NICU environment are complex and include feelings of sadness, guilt, fear, and insecurity about their child's health and development. Guilt is a particularly common and strong emotion associated with the maternal perception of being responsible for their child's premature birth. Symptoms of anxiety and depression, commonly referred to as the "baby blues," are generally elevated in the first 2 weeks following the birth but in many cases resolve within a few weeks without intervention, particularly in families that have strong social support (Cheon 2012). However, the stressors as-

Table 2–1. Parental Stressor Scale: NICU

Infant appearance and behavior

   Tubes and equipment

   Intravenous feeding

   Bruises, cuts, and incisions

   Abnormal breathing patterns

   Infant size and appearance

   Infant pain and distress

Sights and sounds in the NICU

   Monitors and equipment

   Sick babies

   Number of people

   Presence of a respirator

Parental role alteration

   Separation from the infant

   Inability to feed infant

   Inability to hold infant

   Inability to provide care

   Feelings of helplessness

   Inability to share infant with family members

   Concern about staff closeness with infant

Source.   Miles and Funk 1987.

sociated with the NICU environment may complicate the mother's adjustment and lead to more significant clinical symptoms.

Roque et al. (2017) reported that rates of depression were elevated in parents of infants hospitalized in the NICU compared with parents whose infants were not in the NICU. Risk factors for depression include perceived lack of support from the nursing staff, younger gestational age, prolonged hospitalization, and the severity of the infant's medical status (Table 2–2) (Davis et al. 2004; De Magistris et al. 2010; Segre et al. 2014). Risk factors specific to mothers include a prior history of depression, antepartum depression, maternal substance abuse, and perinatal complications (Segre et al. 2014; Vasa et al. 2014). Ukpong et al. (2004) similarly found that mothers of preterm infants had higher rates of both distress (27.3% vs. 3.7%) and depression (15.1% vs. 3.7%) compared with mothers of healthy, full-term infants. These findings have also been replicated at 6-month follow-up visits with mothers of moderate- to late-term infants hospitalized in the NICU (Lotterman et al. 2019). However, some studies have found no difference in prevalence rates of depression in parents following NICU admission when compared with the general population.

Table 2–2.   Risk factors for parental psychological distress in the neonatal intensive care unit

Maternal	Infant	Family/Social
Prior obstetrical complications	Emergency cesarean section	Perceived lack of staff support
Prior mental health history	Younger gestational age	Lack of partner and/or social support
Maternal substance abuse	Perinatal complications	Changes in marital status
Younger maternal age	Need for ventilator support	Lack of family cohesion
Maternal education	Medical severity	Lack of religious/ community support
Prior or current exposure to other traumatic events	Length of hospital stay	
Stressful birth experience		
Maternal coping style		
Maternal guilt		

Nagata et al. (2004) found no difference in symptoms of depression between a sample of NICU mothers compared with control subjects, although they sampled the mothers just 1 week postpartum, which may be too early in the process for the full expression of these symptoms. Other researchers have documented that mothers of preterm infants also report feelings of confidence, joy, and hope for their infants and pleasure in being able to provide care (de Carvalho et al. 2009, 2012; Padovani et al. 2008). Although some discrepancies can be found across the literature regarding the psychological distress reported in parents of preterm infants, overwhelming evidence both in the literature and from clinical observations supports the notion that having a preterm infant can and often does influence a family's psychological functioning both while in the NICU and beyond.

Posttraumatic Stress in the NICU

Although early research focused on symptoms of anxiety and depression in the parents of medically fragile infants, the presence of trauma symptoms in both children and parents following diagnosis of a severe illness is now widely recognized (Shaw and Bernard 2006). Researchers have identified acute stress disorder and PTSD as a model to describe and explain the psychological reaction of parents to their NICU experience (DeMeir et al. 1996; Holditch-Davis et al. 2003; Peebles-Kleiger

2000; Pierrehumbert et al. 2003; Shaw et al. 2006). The model of NICU hospitalization as a traumatic event has many parallels with literature describing PTSD in parents of children with cancer and other pediatric medical conditions, including solid organ transplant recipients (Stuber and Shemesh 2006).

MEDICAL PTSD

Although historically, the parents of children with severe medical illness have often been diagnosed with adjustment disorders, psychological symptoms can be conceptualized using a trauma model (Tedstone and Tarrier 2003). DSM-5 (American Psychiatric Association 2013) recognizes "being diagnosed with a life-threatening illness" as one example of a traumatic stress that may lead to PTSD. Parents' experience of their child being diagnosed with a serious medical condition, including a premature birth, also can lead to trauma symptoms. Typically, medical PTSD reactions occur in response to the news of a serious medical diagnosis, sometimes referred to as the *information stressor*, but they can also arise in response to acute or chronic traumatic aspects of the child's medical treatment (Green et al. 1997). Psychological reactions to the diagnosis of a child's medical illness may include high levels of fear, realistic anxiety about the future, feelings of helplessness, and loss of control.

There are several differences between medical and nonmedical PTSD (Table 2–3). Life-threatening illness differs from the stress encountered in the military setting or in the context of abuse or other types of trauma because the threat to the individual is located within the body of the parent's child and cannot easily be avoided or ignored. Intrusive symptoms typically take the form of recurrent recollections about the diagnosis and anxieties about future treatment or the child's prognosis. Alterations in arousal and reactivity often take the form of hypervigilance to the infant's physical condition or to changes in the infant's appearance that, in many cases, are within the normal expected range. Medical anxiety may lead to difficulties for the parent to leave the infant or, conversely, to the parent avoiding the infant; in other parents, this anxiety may lead to substance abuse. Additionally, persistent pessimistic expectations about the child's future may lead some parents to feel detached and have difficulty developing a healthy attachment. Irrational feelings of guilt and self-blame commonly characterize medical PTSD.

ACUTE STRESS DISORDER

Introduction of acute stress disorder into DSM-IV in 1994 identified individuals with posttraumatic stress reactions occurring between 2 days and 4 weeks following a traumatic event (American Psychiatric Association 1994). Although conceptually similar to PTSD in that it includes reexperiencing, avoidance, and arousal symptoms, acute stress disorder

Table 2–3.   Medical PTSD

Intrusion symptoms	Persistence avoidance
Recurrent recollections about diagnosis and treatment	External avoidance (i.e., hospital settings)
Ruminative, future-oriented fears about treatment, prognosis, relapse, or death	Internal avoidance* (i.e., thoughts and memories related to medical events)
Panic attacks	
Negative cognitions and mood	**Alterations in arousal and reactivity**
Irrational feelings of guilt and blame	Hypervigilance to medical/physical cues or changes in the infant
Negative expectations about the future	Hypervigilance to somatic symptoms in the infant that may indicate recurrence of disease
Detachment from the infant	Excessive medical anxiety
	Irritability
	Sleep disturbance

*Avoidance of aspects of medical trauma may be difficult and complicated by the cues being internal (thoughts, memories, nightmares) or in the child (i.e., required medical equipment, breathing patterns, skin coloring).

differs from PTSD because of its stronger emphasis on dissociative symptoms (Bryant and Harvey 1997). A major rationale for this diagnosis was to identify individuals thought to be at greater risk of developing more chronic symptoms of PTSD (Koopman et al. 1994). Harvey and Bryant (1998), for example, showed that 78% of motor vehicle accident victims who initially satisfied criteria for acute stress disorder had PTSD 6 months after the trauma, whereas only 4% of those with no acute stress disorder subsequently met criteria for PTSD. Acute stress disorder has been demonstrated in multiple studies of children and parents in the medical setting, including the intensive care unit (Balluffi et al. 2004). It has also been described in the context of the NICU, with prevalence rates ranging between 23% and 28% (Jubinville et al. 2012; Lefkowitz et al. 2010; Shaw et al. 2006; Vanderbilt et al. 2009). Associations between acute stress disorder symptoms and several individual and environmental factors have been reported, including stress of parents, female sex, alteration in parental role and family cohesiveness, and parental coping style (Roque et al. 2017; Shaw et al. 2006).

POSTTRAUMATIC STRESS DISORDER

Early research has documented the presence of PTSD in parents of premature infants, with prevalence rates as high as 41%; in some studies, the PTSD has been shown to persist for as long as 14 months after the infant's birth (Holditch-Davis et al. 2003; Kersting et al. 2004; Pierrehumbert et al. 2003). Shaw et al. (2006) showed a correlation between acute stress disorder and later development of PTSD, with rates consistent with findings from previous studies of PTSD in parents of premature infants (Kersting et al. 2004) as well as data from parents of children with cancer (Kazak et al. 2004). The few studies assessing postpartum posttraumatic stress in the parents of premature infants generally report higher levels in mothers than in fathers (Ionio et al. 2016), although Shaw et al. (2006) found that fathers of premature infants had a delayed onset in their PTSD symptoms and by 4 months were at even greater risk than mothers.

Gondwe and Holditch-Davis (2015) conducted a systematic review of 23 studies of posttraumatic stress symptoms in mothers of premature infants and found a range of elevations in symptoms between 18% and 77.8%. Mothers who reported at least one posttraumatic stress symptom had an increased risk of posttraumatic stress compared with mothers of healthy, full-term infants. In this review, increased posttraumatic stress was also associated with less positive mother–infant interactions. However, variations in the times that data collection occurred and the different instruments used to measure posttraumatic stress limited the ability to make firm conclusions about the prevalence of PTSD in the NICU setting (Beck and Woynar 2017). A more recent review by Beck and Harrison (2017) reported prevalence rates of PTSD varying between 14% and 79%.

Risk Factors for Traumatic Stress Reactions

MATERNAL RISK FACTORS

Roque et al. (2017), in their review of 66 studies, reported that sociodemographic characteristics, including being unmarried, having a low family income, and younger age, contribute to increased levels of maternal stress. Prior history of mental health problems in the mother, father, or extended family was also associated with the development of PTSD symptoms (Olde et al. 2006). Similarly, feelings of a lack of control, changes in living arrangements, and legal issues appear to increase the risk of PTSD (Lefkowitz et al. 2010). Chang et al. (2016) reported an association between previous obstetrical problems, including hemorrhage, preeclampsia, preterm premature rupture of membranes, and uterine rupture, and the development of PTSD (Engelhard et al. 2001; Furuta et al. 2012; Seng et al. 2001; Stramrood et al. 2011; Waldenstrom et al. 2004). Previous miscarriage and the presence of chronic disease in the mother were also found to be risk factors for PTSD (Aftyka et al. 2017b).

Alteration in the Parental Role

Building on the work of Miles (1989), many researchers have established that alterations in the expected parental role are stressful and commonly associated with an increased risk of PTSD (Lasiuk et al. 2013; Roque et al. 2017; Shaw et al. 2006, 2009). Severity of acute stress disorder symptoms, in particular being unable to help, hold, or care for the infant, protect the infant from pain, or share the infant with other family members, is significantly related to the parent's stress when assessed using the PSS:NICU. These findings suggest it is also important to try to prepare parents, whenever possible, for the expected psychological reactions that may occur in the event of a NICU hospitalization and, wherever possible, to find ways to involve them in concrete aspects of their infants' care.

Coping Style

An individual's coping style has been associated with PTSD. Problem-solving coping strategies focused on ensuring that the infant receives the best care were associated with more positive coping (Lavoie 2013), whereas escape-avoidant strategies were associated with increased psychological distress (Reichman et al. 2000). For example, mothers who relied on denial and total control over their infants' care reported feelings of rage, guilt, helplessness, and fear (Bronzo 2012). Shaw et al. (2013), in a study of 56 mothers of premature infants who participated in a treatment intervention study to reduce symptoms of PTSD, found that dysfunctional coping measured by the Brief COPE (Coping Orientation to Problems Experienced), a self-report inventory of coping mechanisms, was positively associated with an elevated risk of PTSD. Theories of coping postulate that the expression of emotions allows individuals to release psychological stress, while techniques of cognitive restructuring may allow individuals to reframe their cognitions to reduce their perceptions of threat. By contrast, coping styles that interfere with stress reduction, for example, avoidant coping, have been associated with adverse psychological outcomes, including PTSD, in parents of pediatric cancer patients (Greening and Stoppelbein 2007). Bronner et al. (2009) reported that peritraumatic dissociation following a stressful event and an avoidant coping style were associated with PTSD in a study of Dutch parents 3 months after their child's admission to the ICU.

Data from studies on parents of children with cancer have found that open styles of communication and optimism are associated with positive outcomes, in contrast with coping styles that rely on disengagement (Grootenhuis and Last 1997). Coping strategies that focus on managing emotions and appraisal of the stress may be more adaptive than problem-focused coping in a medical situation in which events are less under the control of parents (Felton and Revenson 1984). For example, mothers of children who received bone marrow transplants were more likely to have symptoms of depression after the transplant if they resorted to active, problem-focused, or avoidant coping than were mothers who had used a coping style that facilitated emotional regulation (Manne et al. 2003). Amir et al. (1999) proposed that the use of suppression in women with breast cancer strengthens avoidance and does not allow the traumatic events to be adequately processed.

Maternal Education

Shaw et al. (2013) also reported that maternal education, which tends to be associated with problem-focused coping, was related to PTSD, with each year's increase in education associated with an 18% increase in the relative risk of PTSD at 1-month follow-up. This is consistent with previous studies that have examined the relationship between coping and educational level. Dasch et al. (2011) found that parents of youth with spinal injury who also had some college education were less likely to use denial as a coping strategy, while Liu et al. (2007) noted that education was associated with "active forms of coping" in parents of children with psychiatric illness. However, this relationship of greater education with PTSD is contrary to data from combat-related PTSD that found a lack of education or lower levels of education and lower IQ to be risk factors (Zohar et al. 2009).

One explanation for these findings may relate to parents' appraisal of the seriousness of their infant's health. Studies have consistently supported the finding that *appraisal* of the traumatic medical event is more strongly associated with PTSD development than the *actual* medical variables (Tedstone and Tarrier 2003). Highly educated mothers not only may have more knowledge about developmental issues related to prematurity but also may place greater weight on future academic aspirations for their children. As a result, they have a more negative appraisal of the personal implications of prematurity for their children. One important implication of these findings is that cognitive behavioral interventions that target maladaptive cognitions and coping strategies may influence the development of trauma symptoms in the NICU situation.

Another possible explanation for these findings may be the aspects of the trauma that are specific to the NICU situation. The "goodness of fit" model of coping suggests that problem-focused coping is less adaptive in the medical setting, where events are not usually under the control of the parent (Felton and Revenson 1984). Highly educated women may, through their life experiences, have found problem-focused coping to be an effective strategy and habituated to this approach. However, the relative failure of this approach in the NICU setting, where very little is under her control, may be particularly stressful for mothers who are less able to resort to emotion-focused coping and, as a result, produce poor psychological outcomes.

INFANT RISK FACTORS

Data on the relationship between infant medical risk factors and parental PTSD are mixed. For example, acute stress disorder symptoms have not been found to be related to any characteristics that directly pertain to the infant's medical status, including length of stay in the NICU, birth weight, gestational age, and Apgar scores. This pattern is consistent with previous findings on PTSD in parents of cancer survivors (Kazak et al. 1998). Shaw et al. (2006, 2009) found that the presence of posttraumatic stress symptoms was not associated with these infant medical variables and suggested that the parents' subjective appraisal of the seriousness of their child's illness, rather than the objective disease characteristics, predicted psychological outcome. Based on this, it was hypothesized that treatment interventions targeting parental psychological variables may limit the development of future trauma symptoms, whereas medical and infant variables may be less relevant. Consistent with these findings, Roque et al. (2017) also found that characteristics directly pertaining to an infant's health status were not related to acute stress disorder.

Holditch-Davis et al. (2003) surveyed 30 mothers of high-risk premature infants and found that infant medical variables were unrelated to maternal PTSD symptoms. However, a discrepancy was found between the mothers' appraisal of the severity of their infants' condition and the real severity of illness as judged by clinical staff, which was thought to explain this finding. By contrast, Gangi et al. (2013) and Jubinville et al. (2012) found that birth weight and gestational age were linked to an increased risk of both acute stress disorder and PTSD, and Roque et al. (2017), in their review of 66 studies, reported that characteristics of the infant, including a diagnosis of cardiovascular disease, were associated with increased levels of maternal stress.

FAMILY/SOCIAL RISK FACTORS

Roque et al. (2017) found that staff, family, friends, and others in the NICU were all cited as potential sources of social support and reduced levels of stress (Grosik et al. 2013; Montirosso et al. 2012; Younger et al. 1997). Mothers have been found to seek emotional support from their spouses, whereas fathers have reported that information from health care providers was supportive (Hughes and McCollum 1994). Goutaudier et al. (2011) reported that, in the absence of psychological support from preexisting networks, mothers drew support from other NICU parents. In addition, mothers who had previous NICU experiences were better able to cope than first-time NICU mothers (Spear et al. 2002). Shaw et al. (2006) reported that family cohesion and expressiveness were associated with less psychological distress in parents, which was consistent with findings from studies of PTSD in other trauma survivors, including families of cancer survivors. More positive outcomes have also been reported by parents who rely on their religious faith to cope and by those who seek out social and spiritual support and engage family resources (Doering et al. 1999; Hughes and McCollum 1994). Overall, increased sources of support, whether family, peers, or religious beliefs, act as protective factors related to a reduction of levels of reported stress for parents in the NICU.

Parental Posttraumatic Stress and Maternal Outcomes

DEPRESSION AND ANXIETY

Parental PTSD is thought to be relevant in the context of parent psychological adjustment. Affleck et al. (1989) reported that mothers who experienced intrusive symptoms of PTSD 6–18 months after their infant's birth were more likely to report symptoms of depression and distress, and those with more avoidant symptoms of PTSD rated themselves as less competent caregivers. Data from epidemiological surveys indicate that the vast majority of individuals with PTSD meet criteria for at least one other psychiatric disorder, and a substantial percentage have three or more other psychiatric diagnoses (Brady et al. 2000). In a military setting, among people with PTSD, 83.3% had a comorbid mental health disorder (Walter et al. 2018), the most common of which were depressive disorder (49.0%), adjustment disorder (37.0%), generalized anxiety disorder (36.1%), and alcohol use disorder (26.9%). These disorders were also much more likely to be diagnosed in those who served in the military and had PTSD than in those without PTSD (OR range 1.52–29.63). These and other studies suggest that comorbid mental health disorders with PTSD, in particular depression and anxiety, should be considered the rule rather than the exception.

SUBSTANCE ABUSE

It has long been recognized that a strong relationship exists between PTSD and later development of alcohol and substance abuse disorders (Taylor et al. 2017). In fact, among men with PTSD, both veterans and civilians, alcohol use disorder is the most commonly co-occurring disorder, with a prevalence of 50% (Kulka et al. 1990). Treatment outcomes in those with comorbid alcohol use disorder and PTSD are worse than outcomes associated with each disorder without comorbidity (McCarthy and Petrakis 2010). Research has also shown that women with PTSD are approximately 4.5 times more likely to develop an alcohol use disorder or other substance use disorder than are those without PTSD (Creamer et al. 2001). In the veteran population, 63% of veterans who met criteria for alcohol use disorder or other substance use disorders also met criteria for PTSD, whereas 76% of those who met criteria for PTSD also met criteria for substance use disorders (Seal et al. 2011). These data, along with the statistics on psychiatric comorbidity, emphasize the importance of early recognition, prevention, and treatment of PTSD in parents of premature infants to prevent future comorbid mental health and substance abuse problems that can negatively impact parent–infant outcomes.

Parental Posttraumatic Stress and Infant Outcomes

A growing body of evidence suggests that PTSD in parents of premature infants may have a significant impact on the parent–infant relationship as well as on infant behavior, social-emotional and cognitive development, and longer-term health outcomes (Table 2–4) (Cook et al. 2018).

Table 2–4.   Complications of parental posttraumatic stress disorder

Parental effects	Parent–infant interaction	Infant/Child development
Depression	Breastfeeding	Motor development
Anxiety	Parental bonding	Sleep
Alcohol abuse	Attachment	Feeding issues
Substance abuse		Cognitive development
Marital conflict		Social-emotional development
		Vulnerable child syndrome

BREASTFEEDING

Research has suggested that postpartum depression can interfere with the ability of mothers to breastfeed their infants and is associated with a shorter duration of breastfeeding (Cook et al. 2018; Dias and Figueiredo 2015). Mothers with postpartum PTSD stop breastfeeding earlier, often contrary to their wishes. Increased rates of maternal emotional distress associated with premature birth, in particular maternal depression and anxiety, have been linked with poor breastfeeding outcomes (Tully and Sullivan 2018; Zanardo et al. 2011). McDonald et al. (2011) reported that premature infants were less likely to be breastfed within 24 hours of birth and that their first breastfeeding attempts were unsuccessful.

Postpartum anxiety has also been associated with reduced duration of breastfeeding (Paul et al. 2013). Challenges with breastfeeding may have a reciprocal effect on maternal well-being, with findings indicating that supplementing with infant formula is associated with increased rates of maternal anxiety and depression (Tully and Sullivan 2018;

Ystrom 2012). Another potentially relevant issue to consider is the dysphoric milk ejection reflex (D-MER), described as a negative emotional reaction to the milk ejection reflex that, in some mothers, may produce a temporary hollow or churning feeling in the stomach associated with feelings of anxiety, panic, and sadness (Ureño et al. 2019; Watkinson et al. 2016). The prevalence of D-MER has been found to be increased in mothers with a history of anxiety or depression and is exacerbated by stress or a lack of sleep (Harris et al. 1994). Given that D-MER is associated with earlier cessation of breastfeeding, interventions that reduce postpartum depression and anxiety may have additional benefits for the infant in terms of breastfeeding and attachment

MATERNAL–INFANT INTERACTION

The relationship between maternal postpartum distress and infant development has been largely attributed to disturbances in the emotional and behavioral exchanges between the mother and her infant (Giallo et al. 2014). Mothers with postpartum depressive or anxiety disorders may present as being withdrawn or passive in interactions with their infants or, conversely, engage in intrusive, controlling, or hostile parent–infant interactions. However, data on the relationship between postpartum PTSD and maternal–infant interaction are mixed (Anderson and Cacola 2017; Cook et al. 2018). Muller-Nix et al. (2004), for example, found no relationship between maternal PTSD and infant behavior at 6 months, whereas Bosquet Enlow et al. (2011) found that infants of mothers with increased symptoms of PTSD displayed more disorganized and avoidance behaviors at 2 months postpartum. Forcada-Guex et al. (2006), in a study of infant behavior problems with personal-social development at 18 months of age, noted a controlling dyadic interaction pattern among mothers with PTSD. Infants with controlling dyadic interactions tended to have fewer positive outcomes, including eating problems and poor personal-social development, than those who had cooperative dyadic interaction patterns with their mothers (Forcada-Guex et al. 2006). Similarly, mothers with a high number of PTSD symptoms were prone to be more intrusive during interactions with their child (Ionio and Di Blasio 2014). Feeley et al. (2011) reported that mothers with more PTSD symptoms were less sensitive and less effective at structuring mother–infant interaction.

ATTACHMENT AND BONDING

Psychological distress has been shown to interfere with mothers' ability to form positive expectations and attachment representations of their infant. In particular, they may develop representations characterized by insensitivity and incoherent, contradictory descriptions of their child

(Cook et al. 2018; Vreeswijk et al. 2012). Davies et al. (2008) found that mothers with partial or full PTSD symptoms viewed their infants as being less warm, more invasive, and having a more difficult temperament and problematic attachment. Other researchers have shown associations with parental posttraumatic stress and impaired bonding in mothers and problems in the parent–child relationship (Parfitt and Ayers 2009; Seng et al. 2013) as well as unbalanced attachment representations and a lower quality of maternal interactive behaviors (Forcada-Guex et al. 2011; Muller-Nix et al. 2004). By contrast, Borghini et al. (2006) found that emotionally distressed parents were able to develop strong bonds with their infants and, in fact, linked high maternal arousal with greater levels of maternal engagement. However, although emotional distress, which is a normative experience of parents in the NICU setting, may provide opportunities for increased engagement and bonding, symptoms of PTSD, which extends beyond the normative emotional distress experienced by parents in the NICU into a pathological cluster of symptoms, not only disrupts but also in many cases inhibits attachment and bonding.

INFANT DEVELOPMENT

In addition to its relationship with attachment and bonding, maternal posttraumatic stress has been associated with effects on social-emotional and cognitive development in the infant (Cook et al. 2018). Although the mechanisms for these effects are not well established, they are likely related to aspects of the parent–child relationship affected by maternal psychological distress.

Social-Emotional Development

A large longitudinal study found that maternal postpartum PTSD symptoms 8 weeks after delivery were associated with poor social-emotional development in the child at 2 years, particularly in boys and in children with difficult temperaments (Garthus-Niegel et al. 2017). One study demonstrated increased salivary cortisol levels in infants of mothers with maternal PTSD (Yehuda et al. 2005), whereas another reported increased sleep and eating difficulties in young children whose mothers had symptoms of PTSD (Pierrehumbert et al. 2003). Kingston et al. (2012) reported a relationship between increased rates of maternal depression and delayed or impaired emotional development in their child.

Cognitive Development

Studies of the relationship between infant cognitive development and symptoms of maternal trauma have shown inconsistent findings. Feeley et al. (2011) found that postpartum PTSD symptoms were not related to infant cognitive development at age 6 months. However, Parfitt et al. (2014) reported an association between maternal postpartum PTSD and delayed cognitive development in the child at age 15 months but no association with language or motor development. These data are in contrast to more robust findings regarding maternal postpartum depression (Anderson and Cacola 2017). Koutra et al. (2013), for example, found postpartum depressive symptoms to be associated with a decrease in cognitive development independent of the presence of antenatal depression. Delays in infant cognitive development have been found to have a reciprocal effect on parents, with increased rates of distress in families whose infants have developmental delays.

Motor Development

Although it is not known whether preterm infants of mothers with symptoms of PTSD at birth are at a higher risk for delays in motor development, preterm infants overall have been recognized to be at increased risk of motor impairment and delayed motor development, with a prevalence of delay three to four times greater than in the general population (Anderson and Cacola 2017; Williams et al. 2010). Among the most frequently occurring problems encountered by preterm children who do not develop cerebral palsy are impaired gross and fine motor skills (Williams et al. 2010). The prevalence of impairments in fine motor skills in preterm infants varies between 40% and 60%, with scores on standardized tests approximately two-thirds of a standard deviation lower than in the general population (Anderson and Cacola 2017). Preterm infants (even those born after 32 weeks' gestation) are at risk for impaired motor development. Koutra et al. (2013) has also reported that postpartum depression is associated with delays in the infant's fine motor development.

VULNERABLE CHILD SYNDROME

The concept of the trauma stress response is useful for explaining many of the clinical phenomena seen in parents of NICU infants. These observations include vulnerable child syndrome, a term describing the tendency seen in parents of premature infants toward being overprotective and having difficulty with setting limits. Ironically, parental hypervigilance, withdrawal, and irritability may lead to poor health care behavior in children with medical illness, and parental perceptions of their child's increased vulnerability may also lead them to limit that child's exposure to new experiences and create difficulties with healthy siblings. Vulnerable child syndrome has also been associated with increased behavior problems as premature infants mature, particularly in the areas of relationships and self-control. Vulnerable child syndrome is covered in more detail in Chapter 8.

NEUROPHYSIOLOGICAL MEASURES

More recent research has focused on finding neurophysiological correlates to help explain some of the findings in infants of parents with posttraumatic stress symptoms (Sanjuan et al. 2016). Perinatal PTSD may affect infant development via mechanisms of impaired parental bonding, disturbed prenatal care, and disruptions in the parent–infant attachment. Perinatal PTSD may also affect the emotional and physiological development of infants, perhaps via maternal corticolimbic dysregulation (Schechter et al. 2015) or impaired responsiveness (Webb and Ayers 2015). Infants born to mothers with perinatal PTSD have been found to have poorer emotional regulation and behavioral reactivity (Bosquet Enlow et al. 2011) and increased symptom severity if they develop PTSD later in life (Bosquet Enlow et al. 2014). Research from infants born to mothers with postpartum depression has shown them to exhibit abnormal frontal electroencephalographic asymmetry (Davis et al. 2004), and infants may have similar reactions in the context of parental trauma.

Sanjuan et al. (2016) used magnetoencephalography to measure resting neural oscillations in the infant brain. These oscillations reflect local and global brain activity and connectivity and serve as an indicator of overall brain health. In infancy, a developmental transition occurs in relative electroencephalographic resting spectral power, with a reduction in low-frequency power (delta and theta bands) and an increase in high-frequency power (alpha, beta, and gamma bands) with increasing age. Evoked theta oscillations emerging in response to stimuli are related to emotional and social processing and internally motivated attention in infants (Michel et al. 2015). Elevated resting theta power in young adults born preterm has been interpreted as indicating delayed maturation (Miskovic et al. 2009). A pilot study of 14 infants age 6 months examined the association between measures of maternal PTSD and infant frontal neural activity measured by magnetoencephalographic theta power (Sanjuan et al. 2016). The authors found a correlation between perinatal PTSD severity and altered infant frontal spectral power, specifically elevated resting theta power, suggesting that maternal symptoms of PTSD were related to delayed infant cortical maturation. Such research provides potential physiological markers in the infant brain that may be directly influenced by maternal psychopathology. However, further work is needed to determine whether theta activity in brain development is associated with the development of anxiety or other poor outcomes, including the intragenerational transmission of PTSD risk.

Posttraumatic Growth

There is increasing interest in the concept of *posttraumatic growth*, defined as a positive change experienced as a result of the struggle with a major life crisis or traumatic event (Aftyka et al. 2017a). In the NICU, posttraumatic growth may be seen in reordered life priorities, stronger connections with family members, or an increased personal resilience (Corcoran 2014). Different models have been developed to explain the relationship between posttraumatic growth and traumatic stress: they 1) are at opposite ends of the continuum and have a negative association with each other; 2) can coexist; and 3) are independent of each other. The Posttraumatic Growth Inventory (Tedeschi and Calhoun 1996) is a 21-item inventory used to measure the five domains of potential growth (Table 2–5). In a study of 106 parents with infants ages 3–12 months requiring NICU care, Aftyka et al. (2017a) used the Posttraumatic Growth Inventory to study the concept of traumatic growth. Their findings indicated that parents of children who survived had significantly higher posttraumatic growth than did the parents of children who died. These authors suggested a model that highlighted the importance of positive reinterpretation, severity of PTSD, and infant survival. Research has also shown that women in general have a greater tendency to experience posttraumatic growth compared with men, particularly greater appreciation of life (Aftyka et al. 2017a; Büchi et al. 2007). Posttraumatic growth has also been positively correlated with an active coping style (Danhauer et al. 2013).

Table 2–5. The Posttraumatic Growth Inventory

Factors	Sample items
Relating to others	I have a greater sense of closeness with others
	I have more compassion for others
New possibilities	I have developed new interests
	I am more likely to change things that need changing
Personal strength	I have a greater feeling of self-reliance
	I know better that I can handle difficulties
Spiritual change	I have a better understanding of spiritual matters
	I have a stronger religious faith
Appreciation of life	I have changed my priorities about what is important in life
	I have a greater appreciation for the value of my own life

Source. Tedeschi and Calhoun 1996.

Conclusions

The premature birth and subsequent hospitalization of an infant in the NICU is a traumatic experience for the family. It is well documented that both parents are at high risk of symptoms of psychological distress, including depression and PTSD. Even parents who do not meet the criteria for PTSD may have troubling symptoms of posttraumatic stress and associated feelings of guilt and blame related to the preterm birth. The consequences for both the infant and the parents are wide reaching, including an increased risk for the parents of other comorbid psychiatric illnesses and alcohol and substance abuse and increased risk for the infant of problems with early cessation of breastfeeding, disruptions to the parent–infant attachment and bonding, and potential longer-term issues related to social-emotional and motor development. An understanding of the specific factors that increase the risk for PTSD is helpful in identifying more at-risk families, although awareness and screening are essential to initiate early intervention and limit long-term effects. Specific interventions to ameliorate parent psychological distress and limit the impact of trauma on the parenting relationship are addressed in subsequent chapters.

References

Affleck G, Tennen H, Rowe J, et al: Effects of formal support on mothers' adaptation to the hospital-to-home transition of high-risk infants: the benefits and costs of helping. Child Dev 60:488–501, 1989

Aftyka A, Rozalska-Walaszek I, Rosa W, et al: Post-traumatic growth in parents after infants' neonatal intensive care unit hospitalisation. J Clin Nurs 26(5–6):727–734, 2017a

Aftyka A, Rybojad B, Rosa W, et al: Risk factors for the development of posttraumatic stress disorder and coping strategies in mothers and fathers following infant hospitalisation in the neonatal intensive care unit. J Clin Nurs 26(23–24):4436–4445, 2017b

American Psychiatric Association: Diagnostic and Statistical Manual of Mental Disorders, 4th Edition. Washington, DC, American Psychiatric Association, 1994

American Psychiatric Association: Diagnostic and Statistical Manual of Mental Disorders, 5th Edition. Arlington, VA, American Psychiatric Association, 2013

Amir M, Kaplan Z, Efroni RMA, et al: Suicide risk and coping styles in posttraumatic stress disorder patients. Psychother Psychosom 68:76–81, 1999

Anderson C, Cacola P: Implications of preterm birth for maternal mental health and infant development. MCN Am J Matern Child Nurs 42(2):108–114, 2017

Balluffi A, Kassam-Adams N, Kazak A, et al: Traumatic stress in parents of children admitted to the pediatric intensive care unit. Pediatr Crit Care Med 5(6):547–553, 2004

Beck CT, Harrison L: Posttraumatic stress in mothers related to giving birth prematurely: a mixed research synthesis. J Am Psychiatr Nurses Assoc 23(4):241–225, 2017

Beck CT, Woynar J: Posttraumatic stress in mothers while their preterm infants are in the newborn intensive care unit: a mixed research synthesis. ANS Adv Nurs Sci 40(4):337–355, 2017

Borghini A, Pierrehumbert B, Miljkovitch R, et al: Mother's attachment representations of their premature infant at 6 and 18 months after birth. Infant
Ment Health J 27:494–508, 2006

Bosquet Enlow M, Kitts RL, Blood E, et al: Maternal posttraumatic stress symptoms and infant emotional reactivity and emotion regulation. Infant Behav
Dev 34:487–503, 2011

Bosquet Enlow M, Egeland B, Carlson E, et al: Mother–infant attachment and
the intergenerational transmission of posttraumatic stress disorder. Dev
Psychopathol 26:41–65, 2014

Brady KT, Killeen TK, Brewerton T, Lucerini S: Comorbidity of psychiatric disorders
and posttraumatic stress disorder. J Clin Psychiatry 61(suppl 7):22–32, 2000

Kronner MB, Kayser AM, Knoester H, et al: A pilot study on peritraumatic dissociation and coping styles as risk factors for posttraumatic stress, anxiety
and depression in parents after their child's unexpected admission to a pediatric intensive care unit. Child Adolesc Psychiatry Ment Health 33(1):3,
2009

Bronzo AM: Narrative Creation as an Aspect of Coping in Response to Preterm
Delivery and Hospitalization (unpublished doctoral dissertation). Berke-
ley, CA, Wright Institute Graduate School of Psychology, 2012

Bryant RA, Harvey AG: Acute stress disorder: a critical review of diagnostic issues. Clin Psychol Rev 17(7):757–757, 1997

Büchi S, Mörgeli H, Schnyder U, Jenewein J, et al: Grief and post-traumatic
growth in parents 2–6 years after the death of their extremely premature
baby. Psychother Psychosom 76:106–114, 2007

Chang HP, Chen JY, Huang YH, et al: Factors associated with post-traumatic symptoms in mothers of preterm infants. Arch Psychiatr Nurs 30(1):96–101, 2016

Cheon K: Psychological Well-Being of Mothers With Preterm Infants (doctoral
dissertation). Los Angeles, CA, UCLA, 2012

Cook N, Ayers S, Horsch A: Maternal posttraumatic stress disorder during the
perinatal period and child outcomes: a systematic review. J Affect Disord
225:18–31, 2018

Corcoran JB: Factors associated with mother's posttraumatic growth following
the birth of a premature infant. Palo Alto University, 2014

Creamer M, Burgess P, McFarlane AC: Post-traumatic stress disorder: findings from
the Australian National Survey of Mental Health and Well-Being. Psychol Med
31:1237–1247, 2001

Danhauer SC, Case LD, Tedeschi R, et al: Predictors of posttraumatic growth in
women with breast cancer. Psychooncology 22:2676–2683, 2013

Dasch KB, Russell HF, Kelly EH, et al: Coping in caregivers of youth with spinal
cord injury. J Clin Psychol Med S 18(4):361–371, 2011

Davies J, Slade P, Wright I, Stewart P: Posttraumatic stress symptoms following
childbirth and mothers' perceptions of their infants. Infant Ment Health J
29:537–554, 2008

Davis EP, Snidman N, Wadhwa PD, et al: Prenatal maternal anxiety and depression predict negative behavioral reactivity in infancy. Infancy 6:319–331,
2004

de Carvalho ALS, dos Reis ACS, Dias FR, et al: Feelings of the mothers with the
babies hospitalized in neonatal intensive care unit. Northeast Network
Nursing Journal 8:26–31, 2012

de Carvalho JBL, Araújo ACPE, Costa, IDCC, et al: Social representation of fathers regarding their premature child in the neonatal intensive care unit. Brazilian Nursing Journal 62(5):734–738, 2009

De Magistris A, Coni E, Puddu M, et al: Screening of postpartum depression: comparison between mothers in the neonatal intensive care unit and in the neonatal section. J Mat-Fetal Neon Med 23(S3):101–103, 2010

DeMeir RL, Hynan MT, Harris HB, et al: Perinatal stressors as predictors of symptoms of posttraumatic stress in mothers of infants at high risk. J Perinatol 16:276–280, 1996

Dias CC, Figueiredo B: Breastfeeding and depression: a systematic review of the literature. J Affect Disord 171:142–154, 2015

Doering LV, Dracup K, Moser D: Comparison of psychosocial adjustment of mothers and fathers of high-risk infants in the neonatal intensive care unit. J Perinatol 19(2):132–137, 1999

Engelhard IM, van den Hout MA, Arntz A: Posttraumatic stress disorder after pregnancy loss. Gen Hosp Psychiatry 23(2):62–66, 2001

Feeley N, Zelkowitz P, Westreich R, Dunkley D: The evidence base for the cues program for mothers of very low birth weight infants: an innovative approach to reduce anxiety and support sensitive interaction. J Perinat Educ 20(3):142–53, 2011

Felton BJ, Revenson TA: Coping with chronic illness: a study of illness controllability and the influence of coping strategies on psychological adjustment. J Consult Clin Psychol 52(3):343–353, 1984

Forcada-Guex M, Pierrehumbert B, Borghini A, et al: Early dyadic patterns of mother–infant interactions and outcomes of prematurity at 18 months. Pediatrics 118(1):e107–e114, 2006

Forcada-Guex M, Borghini A, Pierrehumbert B, et al: Prematurity, maternal posttraumatic stress and consequences on the mother–infant relationship. Early Hum Dev 87:21–26, 2011

Furuta M, Sandall J, Bick D: A systematic review of the relationship between severe maternal morbidity and post-traumatic stress disorder. BMC Pregnancy Childbirth 12:125, 2012

Gangi S, Dente D, Bacchio E, et al: Posttraumatic stress disorder in parents of premature birth neonates. Procedia Soc Behav Sci 82:882–885, 2013

Garthus-Niegel S, Ayers S, Martini J, et al: The impact of postpartum post-traumatic stress disorder symptoms on child development: a population-based, 2-year follow-up study. Psychol Med 47:161–170, 2017

Giallo R, Cooklin A, Wade C, et al: Maternal postnatal mental health and later emotional-behavioural development of children: the mediating role of parenting behaviour. Child Care Health Dev 40(3):327–333, 2014

Gondwe KW, Holditch-Davis D: Posttraumatic stress symptoms in mothers of preterm infants. Int J Afr Nurs Sci 3:8–17, 2015

Goutaudier N, Lopez A, Séjourne N, et al: Premature birth: subjective and psychological experiences in the first weeks following childbirth, a mixed-methods study. J Reprod Infant Psychol 29(4):364–373, 2011

Green BL, Epstein SA, Krupnick JL, et al: Trauma and medical illness: assessing trauma-related disorders in medical settings, in Assessing Psychological Trauma and PTSD. Edited by Wilson JP, Keane TM. New York, Guilford, 1997, pp 160–191

Greening L, Stoppelbein L: Brief report: pediatric cancer, parental coping style, and risk for depressive, posttraumatic stress, and anxiety symptoms. J Pediatr Psychol 32(10).1272–1277, 2007

Grekin R, O'Hara MW: Prevalence and risk factors of postpartum posttraumatic stress disorder: a meta-analysis. Clin Psychol Rev 34(5):389–401, 2014

Grootenhuis MA, Last BF: Adjustment and coping by parents of children with cancer: a review of the literature. Support Care Cancer 5(6):466–484, 1997

Grosik C, Snyder D, Cleary GM, et al: Identification of internal and external stressors in parents of newborns in intensive care. The Permanente Journal 17(3):36, 2013

Hagan R, Evans SF, Pope S: Preventing postnatal depression in mothers of very preterm infants: a randomized controlled trial. BJOG 111(7):641–647, 2004

Harris B, Lovett L, Newcombe RG, et al: Maternity blues and major endocrine changes: Cardiff puerperal mood and hormone study II. BMJ 308:949–953, 1994

Harvey AG, Bryant RA: The relationship between acute stress disorder and posttraumatic stress disorder: a prospective evaluation of motor vehicle accident survivors. J Consult Clin Psychol 66(3):507–501, 1998

Holditch-Davis D, Bartlett TR, Blickman AL, Miles MS: Posttraumatic stress symptoms in mothers of premature infants. J Obstet Gynecol Neonatal Nurs 32:161–171, 2003

Hughes MA, McCollum J: Neonatal intensive care mothers' and fathers' perceptions of what is stressful. J Early Intervent 18(3):258–268, 1994

Ionio C, Di Blasio P: Post-traumatic stress symptoms after childbirth and early mother–child interactions: an exploratory study. J Reprod Infant Psychol 32:163–181, 2014

Ionio C, Colombo C, Brazzoduro V, et al: Mothers and Fathers in NICU: The Impact of Preterm Birth on Parental Distress. Eur J Psychol 12(4):604-621, 2016

Jubinville J, Newburn-Cook C, Hegadoren K, Lacaze-Masmonteil T: Symptoms of acute stress disorder in mothers of premature infants. Adv Neonatal Care (4):246–253, 2012

Kazak AE, Stuber ML, Barakat LP, et al: Predicting posttraumatic stress symptoms in mothers and fathers of survivors of childhood cancers. J Am Acad Child Adolesc Psychiatry 37(8):823–831, 1998

Kazak AE, Alderfer MA, Streisand R, et al: Treatment of posttraumatic stress symptoms in adolescent survivors of childhood cancer and their families: a randomized clinical trial. J Fam Psychol 18(3):493–504, 2004

Kersting A, Dorsch M, Wesselmann U, et al: Maternal posttraumatic stress response after the birth of a very low-birth-weight infant. J Psychosom Res 57:473–476, 2004

Kingston D, Tough S, Whitfield H: Prenatal and postpartum maternal psychological distress and infant development: a systematic review. Child Psychiatry Hum Dev 43(5):683–714, 2012

Koopman C, Classen C, Spiegel D: Predictors of posttraumatic stress symptoms among survivors of the Oakland/Berkeley, California firestorm. Am J Psychiatry 151:888–894, 1994

Koutra K, Chatzi L, Bagkeris M, et al: Antenatal and postnatal maternal mental health as determinants of infant neurodevelopment at 18 months of age in a mother–child cohort (Rhea Study) in Crete, Greece. Soc Psychiatry Psychiatr Epidemiol 48(8):1335–1345, 2013

Kulka RA, Fairbank JA, Jordan BK, et al: Trauma and the Vietnam War Generation: Report of Findings From the National Vietnam Veterans Readjustment Study. New York, Brunner/Mazel, 1990

Lasiuk GC, Comeau T, Newburn-Cook C: Unexpected: an interpretive description of parental traumas' associated with preterm birth. BMC Pregnancy Childbirth 13(suppl 1):S13, 2013

Lavoie JA: Eye of the beholder: perceived stress, coping style, and coping effectiveness among discharged psychiatric patients. Arch Psychiatr Nurs 27(4):185–190, 2013

Lefkowitz DS, Baxt C, Evans JR: Prevalence and correlates of posttraumatic stress and postpartum depression in parents of infants in the neonatal intensive care unit (NICU). J Clin Psychol Med S 17(3):230–237, 2010

Liu M, Lambert CE, Lambert VA: Caregiver burden and coping patterns of Chinese parents of a child with a mental illness. Infant J Ment Health Nurs 16(2):86–95, 2007

Lotterman JH, Lorenz JM, Bonanno GA: You can't take your baby home yet: a longitudinal study of psychological symptoms in mothers of infants hospitalized in the NICU. J Clin Psychol Med S 26(1):116–112, 2019

Macey TJ, Harmon RJ, Easterbrooks MA: Impact of premature birth on the development of the infant in the family. J Consult Clin Psychol 55:846–852, 1987

Manne S, DuHamel K, Winkel G, et al: Perceived partner critical and avoidant behaviors as predictors of anxious and depressive symptoms among mothers of children undergoing hemopaietic stem cell transplantation. J Consult Clin Psychol 71(6):1076–1083, 2003

McCarthy E, Petrakis I: Epidemiology and management of alcohol dependence in individuals with post-traumatic stress disorder. CNS Drugs 24:997–1007, 2010

McDonald S, Slade P, Spiby H, Iles J: Post-traumatic stress symptoms, parenting stress and mother-child relationships following childbirth and at 2 years postpartum. J Psychosom Obstet Gynaecol 32:141–146, 2011

Michel C, Stets M, Parise E, et al: Theta- and alpha-band EEG activity in response to eye gaze cues in early infancy. Neuroimage 118:76–58, 2015

Miles MS: Parents of critically ill premature infants: sources of stress. Crit Care Nurs Q 12:69–74, 1989

Miles MS, Funk SG: Parental Stressor Scale: Neonatal Intensive Care Unit. Manual, School of Nursing, University of North Carolina at Chapel Hill 1987

Miskovic V, Schmidt LA, Boyle M, Saigal S: Regional electroencephalogram (EEG) spectral power and hemispheric coherence in young adults born at extremely low birth weight. Clin Neurophysiol 120:231–223, 2009

Montirosso R, Provenzi L, Calciolari G, et al: Measuring maternal stress and perceived support in 25 Italian NICUs. Acta Paediatrica 101:136–142, 2012

Muller-Nix C, Forcada-Guex M, Pierrehumbert B, et al: Prematurity, maternal stress and mother-child interactions. Early Hum Dev 79:145–158, 2004

Nagata M, Nagai Y, Sobajima H, et al: Depression in the early postpartum period and attachment to children in mothers of NICU infants. Infant Child Dev 13(2):93–110, 2004

O'Hara MW, McCabe JE: Postpartum depression: current status and future directions. Annu Rev Clin Psychol 9:379–407, 2013

Olde E, van der Hart O, Kleber R, van Son M: Posttraumatic stress following childbirth: a review. Clin Psychol Rev 26(1):1–16, 2006

Padovani FHP, Linhares MBM, Pinto ID, et al: Maternal concepts and expectations regarding a preterm infant. Spanish Journal of Psychology 11(2):581–592, 2008

Parfitt YM, Ayers S: The effect of post-natal symptoms of post-traumatic stress and depression on the couple's relationship and parent–baby bond. J Reprod Infant Psychol 27:127–142, 2009

Parfitt Y, Ayers S, Pike A, et al: A prospective study of the parent–baby bond in men and women 15 months after birth. J Reprod Infant Psychol 32:441–456, 2014

Paul IM, Downs DS, Schaefer EW, et al: Postpartum anxiety and maternal–infant health outcomes. Pediatrics 131(4):e1218–e1224, 2013

Peebles-Kleiger MJ: Pediatric and neonatal intensive care hospitalization as traumatic stressor: implications for intervention. Bull Menninger Clin 64:257–280, 2000

Pierrehumbert B, Nicole A, Muller Nix C, et al. Parental post-traumatic reactions after premature birth: implications for sleeping and eating problems in the infant. Arch Dis Child Fetal Neonatal Educ 88: F400–F404, 2003

Reichman SRF, Miller AC, Gordon RM, Hendricks-Munoz KD: Stress appraisal and coping in mothers of NICU infants. Children's Health Care 29(4):279–293, 2000

Roque ATF, Lasiuk GC, Radünz V, Hegadoren K: Scoping review of the mental health of parents of infants in the NICU. J Obstet Gynecol Neonatal Nurs 46(4):576–587, 2017

Sanjuan PM, Poremba C, Flynn LR, et al: Association between theta power in 6-month old infants at rest and maternal PTSD severity: a pilot study. Neurosci Lett 630:120–126, 2016

Schechter DS, Moser DA, Paoloni-Giacobino A, et al: Methylation of NR3C1 is related to maternal PTSD, parenting stress and maternal medial prefrontal cortical activity in response to child separation among mothers with histories of violence exposure. Front Psychol 6:690, 2015

Seal KH, Cohen G, Bertenthal D, et al: Reducing barriers to mental health and social services for Iraq and Afghanistan veterans: outcomes of an integrated primary care clinic. J Gen Intern Med 26:1160–1167, 2011

Segre LS, McCabe JE, Chuffo-Siewertn R, O'Hara MW: Depression and anxiety symptoms in mothers of newborns hospitalized on the neonatal intensive care unit. Nurs Res 63(5):320–332, 2014

Seng JS, Oakley DJ, Sampselle CM, et al: Posttraumatic stress disorder and pregnancy complications. Obstet Gynecol 97(1):17–22, 2001

Seng JS, Sperlich M, Low LK, et al: Childhood abuse history, posttraumatic stress disorder, postpartum mental health, and bonding: a prospective cohort study. J Midwifery Womens Health 58:57–68, 2013

Shaw RJ, Bernard R: Medical posttraumatic stress disorder. Psychiatric Times 23:25–38, 2006

Shaw RJ, Deblois T, Ikuta L, et al: Acute stress disorder among parents of infants in the neonatal intensive care nursery. Psychosomatics 47(3):206–201, 2006

Shaw RJ, Bernard RS, Deblois T, et al: The relationship between acute stress disorder and posttraumatic stress disorder in the neonatal intensive care unit. Psychosomatics 50(2):131–137, 2009

Shaw RJ, Bernard RS, Storfer-Isser A, et al: Parental coping in the neonatal intensive care unit. J Clin Psychol Med S 20(2):135–134, 2013

Spear ML, Leef K, Epps S, Locke R: Family reactions during infants' hospitalization in the neonatal intensive care unit. Am J Perinatol 19(4), 205–213, 2002

Stramrood CA, Wessel I, Doornbos B, et al: Posttraumatic stress disorder follow-
    ing preeclampsia and PPROM: a prospective study with 15 months follow-
    up. Reprod Sci 18(7):645–653, 2011
Stuber ML, Shemesh E: Post-traumatic stress response to life-threatening illnesses
    in children and their parents. Child Adolesc Psychiatr Clin North Am 15:597–
    609, 2006
Taylor M, Petrakis I, Ralevski E: Treatment of alcohol use disorder and co-occurring
    PTSD. Am J Drug Alcohol Abuse 43(4):391–401, 2017
Tedeschi RG, Calhoun LG: The Posttraumatic Growth Inventory: measuring the
    positive legacy of trauma. J Trauma Stress 9(3):455–471, 1996
Tedstone JE, Tarrier N: Posttraumatic stress disorder following medical illness
    and treatment. Clin Psychol Rev 23(3):409–448, 2003
Tully KP, Sullivan CS: Parent–infant room-sharing is complex and important for
    breastfeeding. Evid Based Nurs 21(1):18, 2018
Ukpong DI, Fatoye FO, Oseni SB, Adewuya AO: Postpartum emotional distress
    in mothers of preterm infants: a controlled study. East Afr Med J 80(6):289–
    292, 2004
Ureño TL, Berry-Cabán CS, Adams A, et al: Dysphoric milk ejection reflex: a de-
    scriptive study. Breastfeed Med 14(9):666–673, 2019
Vanderbilt D, Bushley T, Young R, Frank DA: Acute posttraumatic stress symp-
    toms among urban mothers with newborns in the neonatal intensive care
    unit: a preliminary study. J Dev Behav Pediatr 30(1):50–56, 2009
Vasa R, Eldeirawi K, Kuriakose VG, et al: Postpartum depression in mothers of
    infants in neonatal intensive care unit: risk factors and management strat-
    egies. Am J Perinatol 31(5):425–434, 2014
Vigod SN, Villegas L, Dennis CL, Ross LE: Prevalence and risk factors for post-
    partum depression among women with preterm and low-birth-weight in-
    fants: a systematic review. BJOG 117(5):540–550, 2010
Vinall J, Noel M, Disher T, et al: Memories of infant pain in the neonatal inten-
    sive care unit influence posttraumatic stress symptoms in mothers of in-
    fants born preterm. Clin J Pain (10):936–943, 2018
Vreeswijk CMJM, Maas AJBM, van Bakel HJA: Parental representations: a system-
    atic review of the working model of the child interview. Infant Ment Health J
    33:314–328, 2012
Waldenstrom U, Hildingsson I, Rubertsson C, Radestad I: A negative birth experi-
    ence: prevalence and risk factors in a national sample. Birth 31(1):17–27, 2004
Walter KH, Levine JA, Highfill-McRoy RM, et al: Prevalence of posttraumatic
    stress disorder and psychological comorbidities among U.S. active duty ser-
    vice members, 2006–2013. J Trauma Stress 31(6):837–844, 2018
Watkinson M, Murray C, Simpson J: Maternal experiences of embodied emo-
    tional sensations during breast feeding: an interpretative phenomenologi-
    cal analysis. Midwifery 36:53–60, 2016
Webb R, Ayers S: Cognitive biases in processing infant emotion by women with
    depression, anxiety and post-traumatic stress disorder in pregnancy or af-
    ter birth: a systematic review. Cogn Emot 29:1278–1294, 2015
Williams J, Lee KJ, Anderson PJ: Prevalence of motor-skill impairment in
    preterm children who do not develop cerebral palsy: a systematic review.
    Dev Med Child Neurol 52(3):232–237, 2010

Woolhouse H, Brown S, Krastev A, et al: Seeking help for anxiety and depression after childbirth: results of the Maternal Health Study. Arch Womens Ment Health 12(2):75–83, 2009

Yehuda R, Engel SM, Brand SR, et al: Transgenerational effects of posttraumatic stress disorder in babies of mothers exposed to the World Trade Center attacks during pregnancy. J Clin Endocrinol Metab 90:4115–4118, 2005

Yildiz PD, Ayers S, Phillips L: The prevalence of posttraumatic stress disorder in pregnancy and after birth: a systematic review and meta-analysis. J Affect Disord 208:634–645, 2017

Younger JB, Kendell MJ, Pickler RH: Mastery of stress in mothers of preterm infants. Journal for Specialists in Pediatric Nursing 2(1):29–35, 1997

Ystrom E: Breastfeeding cessation and symptoms of anxiety and depression: a longitudinal cohort study. BMC Pregnancy Childbirth 12:3, 2012

Zanardo V, Gambina I, Begley C, et al: Psychological distress and early lactation performance in mothers of late preterm infants. Early Hum Dev 87(4):321–323, 2011

Zohar J, Fostick L, Cohen A, et al: Risk factors for the development of posttraumatic stress disorder following combat trauma: a semiprospective study. J Clin Psychiatry 70(12):1629–1635, 2009

Postpartum Psychological Experiences of Fathers of Premature Infants

LaTrice L. Dowtin, Ph.D., LCPC, NCSP, RPT

Tiffany Willis, Psy.D.

Daniel Singley, Ph.D., ABPP

Although most of the research on parenting infants has focused on maternal psychological processes, including mother–child interactions and maternal well-being, fathers also often experience psychological distress as they embark on parenthood. In a systematic review of 18 studies of fathers in the perinatal period, Philpott et al. (2017) identified significant stress related to negative feelings about the pregnancy, role restrictions related to becoming a father, fear of childbirth, and feelings of incompetence related to infant care. Hollywood and Hollywood (2011) identified several themes specific to the fathers of NICU infants, including anxiety, feelings of helplessness, and fears about the unknown. Fathers commonly report being considered the secondary parent by the NICU team, while constraints of work interfere with their ability to stay involved in their infant's care. Paternal psychological distress is even more likely when maternal psychological distress is high (Kim and Swain 2007). Hugill et al. (2013) also highlighted how fathers struggle to reconcile the tension between what they want to feel and what they believe others expect them to feel.

Good data demonstrate the presence of perinatal mood and anxiety disorders (PMADs) in fathers during the perinatal period that include symptoms of depression, anxiety, OCD, PTSD, and psychosis. Research suggests that 10%–20% of new fathers have a diagnosable PMAD, in particular, depressive and anxiety disorders (Leach et al. 2016). However, despite these data, relatively little attention has been paid to the psychological impact of the NICU experience on fathers, and even less on programs that provide treatment and psychological support. In this chapter, we review risk factors for and symptoms of emotional distress in fathers who have infants in the NICU and outline our psychological consultation approach.

Risk Factors for Paternal Psychological Distress

The combination of hormonal, environmental, and psychological factors has a large impact on the experience of fathers in the NICU setting. These factors often contribute to increased rates of psychological distress and may explain the increased rates of paternal PMADs (Fleming et al. 2002; Kim and Swain 2007).

HORMONAL FACTORS

Testosterone

PMADs in mothers are often attributed to postpartum hormone changes, but it is less widely known that male hormone levels also fluctuate during their partner's pregnancy and postpartum recovery, as well as during interactions with their infants. Kim and Swain (2007) reported that men experience a decrease in their testosterone level throughout their partner's pregnancy, starting a few months prior to delivery and persisting for as long as several months following their infant's birth. Fathers with lower testosterone levels showed greater sympathy and responsiveness to their infants when they cried. The decrease in testosterone has been hypothesized to result in fathers being less aggressive and more focused as the mother approaches her delivery date and to have potential ecological benefits for the family. Results from this study also showed a correlation between lower levels of testosterone and symptoms of depression in fathers ages 45–60 years (Kim and Swain 2007). These findings suggest that the natural and potentially adaptive decrease in testosterone for expectant and new fathers may also be a risk factor for postpartum depression (PPD).

Estrogen and Oxytocin

Kim and Swain (2007) also reported changes in estrogen in fathers during the final stage of the mothers' pregnancy that continued into the early postpartum period. The researchers proposed that increased estrogen levels in fathers promote more nurturing and active parenting practices and, in some cases, may be necessary to facilitate bonding and attachment between the father and infant. These attachment interactions (e.g., holding, talking, singing) are also associated with a surge in oxytocin release. Without routine interactions between the father and his newborn, opportunities for oxytocin release decrease. This finding may have particular relevance for fathers in the NICU environment. Oxytocin, sometimes called the "feel-good" hormone, has been shown in MRI scans to mimic the action of antidepressants (Mottolese et al. 2014). The relative lack of opportunities to hold and engage with their newborn infant may not only result in less frequent oxytocin release but also partly explain the increased rates of PMADs in fathers (Provenzi and Santoro 2015).

Prolactin and Vasopressin

Additional changes in hormone levels in fathers include a rise in prolactin during the pregnancy that continues throughout the first year of the infant's life. Men with high postdelivery levels of prolactin, the hormone responsible for initiation and maintenance of parenting behaviors, were observed to have greater responsiveness to newborn stimuli (Kim and Swain 2007). It has been proposed that fathers with lower prolactin levels may experience a lack of ease with the transition into fatherhood and exhibit more negative emotions, leading to aggression or depression (Cyr-Alves et al. 2018; Kim and Swain 2007). Similarly, vasopressin, another hormone that increases in men after their infant's birth, is thought to play a role in facilitating the paternal–infant bond and other paternal behaviors such as caring for the child and providing shelter and nutrition. However, low levels of this hormone may make bonding and other paternal behaviors more challenging, resulting in another potential risk for the development of a PMAD (Kim and Swain 2007).

Cortisol

The NICU is often a stressful place for fathers (Cyr-Alves et al. 2018). Noergaard et al. (2018) reported higher levels of paternal stress, assessed with the Parental Stressor Scale: NICU (PSS:NICU; Miles et al. 2007), following an intervention to develop a "father-friendly NICU" in which barriers to being present were removed and fathers were encouraged to engage in activities that support bonding and attachment with their infant. This outcome may seem counterintuitive, but it is consistent with other research findings. Although fathers enjoyed the chance to be closer and more connected with their infants, their unfamiliarity and discomfort with novel caregiving tasks increased their stress. This suggests fathers may need more support and encouragement during their initial interactions with their infant. Individuals exposed to stressful environments of any kind may experience a spike in their cortisol levels.

Although the causal relationship between cortisol and depression is still debated, chronic high levels of cortisol have been associated with depression and anxiety (Qin et al. 2016). The role of changes in cortisol may be yet another factor that explains the increased risk for PMADs in fathers.

PATERNAL ROLE

Perhaps now, more than ever before, fathers in the United States are encouraged to be active participants in the childrearing process. This expectation, however, may result in increased levels of emotional distress for men who did not learn caregiving from their own fathers or other male role models (Kim and Swain 2007). The quality of men's relationships with their own parents has a large impact on their psychological experience of being a parent (Cyr-Alves et al. 2018). Men who have not had nurturing relationships with their fathers or were raised in an environment where caretaking was not considered a paternal function may be at increased risk of PMADs during their transition to parenthood (Johnson 2008; Kadivar and Mozafarinia 2013).

Many fathers strongly desire to take on a nurturing parental role and report pleasure and satisfaction when they have positive reciprocal exchanges with their infant (Kim and Swain 2007; Matricardi et al. 2013). However, for the most part, mothers and infants are viewed as the primary dyad, with fathers reporting that they feel invisible in the NICU environment (Cyr-Alves et al. 2018; Helth and Jarden 2013; Logan and Dormire 2018; Mackley et al. 2010). Fathers contribute to this dynamic by allowing mothers to take the primary caregiving role and either are not encouraged or are actively excluded by the mothers or medical staff from engaging in caregiving tasks such as feeding, diapering, holding, bathing, or administering medicine (Logan and Dormire 2018). In a qualitative study that solicited feedback about fathers' experience in the NICU, respondents shared that they often felt unsafe, uncomfortable, or uncertain in caring for their baby due to the infant's size and fragility and the presence of medical equipment, including intravenous lines and leads (Logan and Dormire 2018). Despite systematic efforts to include them in their infant's care, fathers report feeling excluded from receiving medical information regarding their infant from doctors (Arockiasamy et al. 2008; Mackley et al. 2010). As a result of these factors, fathers often find themselves more irritable, less tolerant, and more aggressive to those around them, including their family and friends and the medical staff (Kim and Swain 2007). The exclusion of fathers from their anticipated parental role is a factor found in many studies to be associated with increased rates of depression and anxiety and symptoms of PTSD (Arockiasamy et al. 2008; Kim and Swain 2007; Mackley et al. 2010).

PSYCHOLOGICAL CONTRIBUTIONS

In addition to hormonal and environmental factors, psychological factors can increase the risk of psychological distress for fathers in the NICU.

Parental Couple Relationship

The NICU environment often results in a negative impact on the parents' relationship, with negative repercussions for both the father and mother. In longer-term NICU stays, parents often see less of one another and find that interactions are centered on medical updates and decision making or on logistics related to the care of other children or work and household responsibilities (Logan and Dormire 2018). This transition into the role of being a NICU parent often results in discord in the parents' relationship (Cyr-Alves et al. 2018; Logan and Dormire 2018). If the infant is discharged with ongoing medical supports or needs, this fracture may persist beyond the NICU (Kim and Swain 2007). Fathers also report a decrease in satisfaction in their relationship and sexual intimacy with their partner over time (Kim and Swain 2007). This is often a result of reduced energy, opportunity, and interest from their partner. This lack of physical attention leaves many men feeling abandoned and unfulfilled, contributing to their perception of a low quality of life (Kim and Swain 2007). For some fathers, the foundation of their identity as a parent and partner may be forever changed by the trauma and psychological distress of the NICU experience.

Avoidant Coping

Avoidant coping is one way that fathers commonly react to the stressful experience of the NICU. Many fathers quickly return to work following a NICU admission and see this as a healthy distraction from what is going on in the NICU (Logan and Dormire 2018). Fathers tend to be ambivalent about being present at the bedside (Arockiasamy et al. 2008). They feel pressure to stay emotionally *strong* for the baby and mother and experience a great deal of guilt, wishing they could take the pain away from their child or partner (Logan and Dormire 2018). Avoidant coping may be reinforced in fathers who develop trauma symptoms. In fact, avoidance is a common symptom of PTSD and is one of the mechanisms individuals use to protect themselves from experiences or environments associated with or even similar to the trauma they have experienced. Although avoidance is sometimes an effective coping tool, when avoiding triggers becomes their primary focus, they may fail to process the traumatic event, leading to persistent symptoms of psychological distress. Avoidance may also contribute to fathers feeling isolated from both their infant and partner. When the NICU is not inclusive of fathers, it inadvertently encourages them to actively use avoidance as a coping strategy and may lead to fathers missing out on healthy and reparative interactions with their infant or partner.

Increased Responsibilities

A shift has also occurred in the traditional father role away from an authoritative figure, disciplinarian, and family breadwinner to the more contemporary idea of an involved, nurturing father with an expectation of equal coparenting (Deeney et al. 2012). Having an infant in the NICU can be a pivotal moment for fathers to prioritize parenthood in their lives. However, fathers often assume increased responsibilities outside of the NICU in the immediate aftermath of their child's birth. In many cases, they must return to work to meet financial obligations and maintain health insurance or take on additional responsibilities for the care of older children (Kim and Swain 2007). The father is also often responsible for updating other members of the family on the medical status of the infant and mother, which can be burdensome and time consuming, detracting from time they might otherwise spend with their infant (Arockiasamy et al. 2008; Kim and Swain 2007; Thomson-Salo et al. 2017). The burden of maintaining the expected role of provider, combined with the sanction against expressing feelings, has the potential to increase the father's level of stress and contribute to feelings of burnout and depression (Helth and Jarden 2013).

Perinatal Mood and Anxiety Disorders in Fathers

The diagnosis and recognition of paternal PMADs has been complicated by the bias of classification systems toward maternal health. In DSM-5 (American Psychiatric Association 2013), for example, perinatal depression is coded as a major depressive episode, with the specifier of "with peripartum onset" to signal that it is related to pregnancy or the birth of a child. Similarly, ICD-10 includes the specifier of "with postpartum onset." However, the discussion of PMADs in fathers throughout the literature uses a variety of terminology (e.g., PPD, postpartum/perinatal anxiety [PPA]) that often refers to the same signs and symptoms. Thus, clinicians need to be aware of terminology and symptomatology when considering PMADs in their work with new fathers.

Furthermore, research on paternal PMADs continues to evolve and find its way to the United States. Many current studies either do not explicitly state racial and cultural demographics of their study's sample or include few to no men of color in their research, which means the field knows little about how PMADs may differ in this population. In a study that focused on fathers of color in the United States, the sample was limited to African American fathers who live in low-income communities

(Bamishigbin et al. 2017). Bamishigbin et al. (2017) found that these African American fathers' symptoms of PPD were further complicated by their experiences of racism and potential cultural implications of coping styles. Although this was a crucial step in learning the prevalence and functionality of PMADs in this population, more data need to be gathered to understand paternal PMADs in the heterogeneous group of men of color and across socioeconomic status. Clinicians should also be aware that PMADs in adolescent and young men of color (ages 14–19 years) can also be mitigated by their perceptions of economic stress, racial and social inequities, and their relationship with their own father (Hunt et al. 2015). These findings show that although much of the information discussed about paternal PMADs is helpful, data on paternal PMADs are still largely missing for several populations.

DEPRESSIVE DISORDER

Several meta-analyses have shown that approximately 10% of new fathers experience symptoms of PPD (Cameron et al. 2016; Paulson and Bazemore 2010), yet the field of maternal and even perinatal mental health has almost completely neglected the identification and treatment of mood and anxiety issues that affect new and expectant fathers.

Presentation of Depression

Fathers often manifest symptoms of depression that differ somewhat from the DSM-5 description of major depressive disorder with peripartum onset. Fathers may present with symptoms of anger/irritability, social withdrawal, and somatization and patterns of increased alcohol or substance use (Rabinowitz and Cochran 2008). These differences in presentation compared with women may be explained based on the social and cultural restraints on the expression of feelings in men. Previous research on traditional masculinity has shown *antifemininity* (the belief that specific behaviors and feelings are germane to people who identify as female) to be a common element of a traditional male identity that extolls traits of agency, independence, toughness, and action over caring and openness (Ashmore and Del Boca 1986; David and Brannon 1976). Men also commonly associate depression with femininity (Cole and Davidson 2018). These factors, along with the protector/provider element of the role transition to father, can combine to cause fathers to forgo focusing on their own difficulties in an effort to exude what they believe to be the masculine stance (also referred to as "manning up") to help their partner and infant and make them unwilling to prioritize getting the help they need. Fathers also often have a different timeline for developing PPD; depressive symptoms often spike 3–6 months postpartum, leading many clinicians to fail to connect a father's mental health concerns with their postpartum experience (Paulson and Bazemore 2010).

Implications of Untreated Depression

Depressive symptoms often worsen if left untreated, with detrimental effects on the father, his partner, and their child (Bronte-Tinkew et al. 2007). Among the most common experiences of untreated PPD in fathers are feelings of resentment and a lack of attachment with their newborn (Buist et al. 2003; Lyons-Ruth et al. 2002). This lack of a strong father–infant bond can be associated with a lower sense of confidence and relevance in his child's care. A wealth of research has shown the negative impact of paternal PPD on the children, mothers, and the fathers themselves when the father is not involved with the infant's care in the first year of life (Jacob and Johnson 2001). For example, PMADs in fathers during the pregnancy or at birth are associated with emotional problems in their children at age 3 (Alio et al. 2011). Most research has addressed how the impact of paternal depression on the infant is demonstrated by decreased or problematic patterns of engagement (Yogman et al. 2016). Research has shown that fathers experiencing depression are four times more likely to spank infants than are fathers without depression, and these fathers are also less likely to read to their infants (Davis et al. 2011; Fletcher et al. 2011); this is relevant because reading to young children has been linked to their subsequent cognitive and language outcomes (Duursma et al. 2008), and the impacts of spanking infants may be long term. Longitudinal research has shown that corporal punishment, such as spanking, is associated with increased aggressive behavior in the child (Taylor et al. 2010). In addition, the tendency for men and fathers to show signs of depression characterized by aggression, irritability, and externalizing behaviors can negatively impact their relationship with their partner and result in difficulty coparenting and providing support in the relationship with their child's mother (Bronte-Tinkew et al. 2007). Thus, attending to the specific types of behaviors associated with paternal depression is essential.

Increased knowledge of the relationship between paternal depression and fathers' involvement with their infant has led to development of the Paternal Involvement With Infants Scale (Singley et al. 2018), a self-report measure for assessing fathers' involvement in key aspects of their infant's care. The Frustration subscale of this tool, which measures negative emotional involvement with the infant, has been shown to have a strong relationship with fathers' infant care self-efficacy, the quality of the parental alliance, parenting competence, gender role conflict, and paternal depression (Singley et al. 2018). These findings suggest the need to assess fathers' specific frustrations with their partner and child during the adjustment to parenthood.

Paternal PPD also negatively impacts the couple. Fathers who have symptoms of depression often report feelings of loss or grief at the life they perceive to have given up to become a father, including having their partners' undivided attention. In addition, in couples experiencing birth complications, mothers may engage in a kind of "gatekeeping" in which they control the father's access to the child (Puhlman and Pasley 2013). When a father shows signs of depression, his partner will understandably have concerns about his ability to care for the child independently, and the anxiety about his competence often results in a tendency to restrict or be excessively critical of his care of their child. At the heart of this dynamic are usually unidentified PMAD symptoms in fathers. These can spiral into a feedback loop, with the mother preventing the father from caring for the child, the father feeling resentful of the mother, and opportunities to increase the father's sense of competence as a parent being lost. This can lead to further withdrawal by the father that is interpreted by the mother as disengagement. The mother's resentment and the father's decreased confidence can result in further feelings of estrangement.

Anecdotal evidence suggests that psychoeducation about the nature and role of maternal anxiety and paternal depression may help increase fathers' overall psychosocial functioning during the postpartum period. Couples also benefit from psychoeducation about the potential changes that can happen in their relationship following the birth of their infant and from clarification that fathers tend to parent differently from mothers. For the latter, it is important to highlight for these couples that the although the different parenting approaches between fathers and mothers may have qualitative differences, neither approach is better than the other. Similarly, the couple benefits when mothers are informed that fathers need some encouragement to take incremental or "baby" steps toward caring for his child more independently (Shapiro et al. 2020).

ANXIETY

Although PPD receives moderate attention in the media and academic research, Leach et al. (2016), in a systematic review of 43 papers, found that fathers often experience anxiety disorders at rates exceeding those of depression. Prevalence rates for any anxiety disorder (defined by either diagnostic clinical interviews or above cutoff points on symptom scales) ranged between 4.1% and 16.0% during the prenatal period and between 2.4% and 18.0% during the postnatal period. Prior research has shown that fathers' anxiety is associated with negative outcomes in their child's development, including increased negative affect (Potapova et al. 2014) and internalizing issues (Ramchandani and Psychogiou 2009).

POSTTRAUMATIC STRESS DISORDER

The recognition of symptoms of acute stress disorder and PTSD in the mothers of NICU infants (DeMier et al. 1996; Holditch-Davis et al. 2003) has helped focus attention on the traumatic responses of fathers (Binder

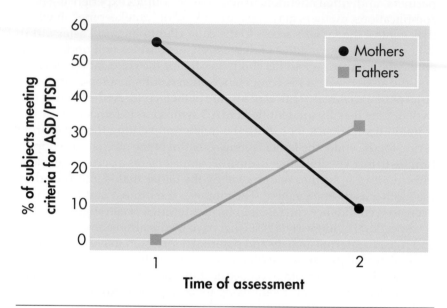

FIGURE 3–1.   Gender differences in proportion of respondents showing post-traumatic stress symptoms.

ASD=acute stress disorder.

Source.   Reprinted from *Psychosomatics*, 50(2), Richard J. Shaw, Rebecca S. Bernard, Thomas DeBlois, et al., "The Relationship Between Acute Stress Disorder and Posttraumatic Stress Disorder in the Neonatal Intensive Care Unit," 131–137, Copyright © 2009, with permission from Elsevier.

et al. 2011). PTSD is common among NICU fathers, with estimates that up to 33% experience PTSD symptoms either while their infant is in the NICU or in the weeks and months following discharge (Hua et al. 2018; Shaw et al. 2006) (Figure 3–1). Research suggests that although NICU fathers often experience PTSD symptoms at a slightly lower rate than do NICU mothers, fathers have been shown to endorse severe PTSD symptoms even at 6 months postdelivery (Binder et al. 2011).

Studies have shown that fathers of premature infants often experience trauma symptoms, including hyperarousal, intrusive thoughts, and increased irritability (Matricardi et al. 2013; Miles et al. 2007). Hypervigilance and avoidance in fathers may trigger behavioral responses ranging from an insistence on being physically near the infant's bedside to avoidant behaviors such as disengagement and finding reasons to stay away from the hospital, such as by working longer hours. The combination of terror, lack of control, and sense of inability to escape the situation may trigger symptoms of acute stress disorder in fathers in response to a completely uncomplicated birth. Premorbid histories of anxiety or trauma exposure may increase the risk of developing trauma symptoms.

Screening for Psychological Distress in Fathers of Premature Infants

Although physicians believe it is their responsibility to recognize postpartum mental health issues, limited time, lack of knowledge and skills, and follow-up care responsibilities often prevent them from detecting such concerns (Leiferman et al. 2008; Singley and Edwards 2015). In addition, barriers arising in the fathers themselves include unwillingness to recognize their own mental health difficulties (Levant et al. 2009) along with a well-documented hesitance to seek help, even when issues are correctly identified by medical providers (Addis 2011, Isacco et al. 2016). However, the growing realization that fathers and their mental health are an essential aspect of a healthy family (especially when a trauma, complicated birth, or a stay in the NICU is involved) is helping draw attention to the needs of this often overlooked population (Garfield et al. 2014; Pleck 2012).

In 2018, the American Psychological Association released *Guidelines for the Psychological Treatment of Boys and Men*, which included consideration of the "generative father" role and the transition to fatherhood. As a broader call for mental health providers to view men as having psychological issues related to their gender, Guideline 1 states that "Psychologists strive to recognize that masculinities are constructed based on social, cultural, and contextual norms" (p. 6). In this way, those providing services to new and expectant fathers can usefully take a multidimensional, intersectional approach to understanding how the mental health challenges that accompany the transition to fatherhood play out psychologically, interpersonally, and culturally.

RECOMMENDATIONS FOR SCREENING

Given that untreated PMADs can have detrimental and long-term impacts for the father and the family, the need for screening both mothers and fathers for symptoms of psychological stress is increasingly evident. However, although at least 10% of fathers in the NICU experience PPD, many go undetected and untreated (Diaz and Plunkett 2018; Fisher et al. 2012; Willis et al. 2018).

In 2018, the National Perinatal Association released a position statement on PMADs that synthesized the literature and recommendations and resulted in a recommendation for screening fathers for PMADs. According to the statement, fathers should be screened for PMADs at least twice during the postpartum year (Willis et al. 2018). Given that the rate of depression for fathers is highest at 3–6 months postdelivery, they recommended that fathers be screened at 2, 4, and 6 months postdelivery. These periods correspond with the infant's routine well-child checks with a pediatrician; therefore, the assessment can be administered to the father in the pediatric office or in the NICU if the baby has not yet been discharged (Willis et al. 2018). The timing of screening is essential, because research suggests that parents are more likely to attend medical appointments for their children than for themselves (Olson et al. 2002). However, many fathers do not accompany their children to well-child visits for various reasons, including work or operating as the secondary parent. In one study, over a 5-year period, 64% of outpatient visits involved exclusively the mother, whereas only 34% included or exclusively involved the father (Fisher et al. 2012). In another a study, when fathers were present at well-child checks and screened for PMADs, 4.4% screened positive for depression, making up 11% of the total positive screens from both mothers and fathers. Given this, the aforementioned protocol increases opportunities to detect PMADs in fathers, but it is only as useful as fathers' attendance at the well-child visits (Cheng et al. 2018). Although adult primary care physicians and mental health clinicians could aid in screening fathers, fathers are less likely to see one of those professionals in time to get appropriate psychological support.

SCREENING MEASURES

When discussing screening for PMADs in fathers, use screening tools that have been validated for fathers (Table 3–1).

Table 3–1. Depression screening tools used for fathers in the NICU*

Screening tool	Number of items	Completion time, *minutes*	Languages available
Edinburgh Postnatal Depression Scale (Cox et al. 1987)	10	<5	18
Postpartum Depression Screening Scale (Beck and Gable 2000)	35	5–10	English, Spanish, Italian
Patient Health Questionnaire–9 (Kroenke and Spitzer 2002)	9	<5	Several
Patient Health Questionnaire–2 (Spitzer et al. 1999)	2	<1	Several
Beck Depression Inventory–II (Beck et al. 1996)	21	5–10	English and Spanish

*All of these tools must be administered by a qualified health care professional.

Edinburgh Postnatal Depression Scale

The Edinburgh Postnatal Depression Scale (EPDS) is the most widely used screener for perinatal depression and has been validated for use with fathers and in 18 different languages (Fisher et al. 2012; Kim and Swain 2007; Willis et al. 2018). It has 10 items and assesses individuals for depression, anxiety, and suicidal ideation (Kim and Swain 2007). The EPDS can be administered by any health care professional and is accessible at no cost online. The cutoff score validated for men is 5/6; this lower clinical cutoff accounts for men's tendency to be less expressive about their feelings (Kim and Swain 2007).

Edinburgh Postnatal Depression Scale–Proxy

The EPDS-Proxy (EPDS-P) was initially designed to be taken by the father or partner to rate the severity of depression in the mother in an attempt to eliminate self-report bias (Cox et al. 1987). However, it is now used as a partner rating scale (Fisher et al. 2012). Mothers can complete the EPDS-P about their partners if the partners are not present to complete the EPDS on their own. Caution should be used with the suicidal ideation item when using the EPDS-P; research suggests that the validity and reliability of this item, as reported by proxy, is low (Fisher et al. 2012). The partner's self-report of depression and suicidal ideation is the most direct and accurate assessment of their experience and should be the goal of paternal depression screening (Fisher et al. 2012). More research is needed on the standardization of tools to assess the unique experience of the NICU as it relates to anxiety and response to trauma.

Fathers Support Scale: NICU

The Fathers' Support Scale: NICU (Mahon et al. 2014) was developed to evaluate the support needs of fathers whose infants are in the NICU (Table 3–2). The authors' goal was to assess some of the more global, experiential stresses reported by fathers, including the ways they preferred to receive information about their infant. Implementation of this tool may be useful in helping the health care team interpret information provided by fathers and be used to help individualize patient care.

Screening at Lucile Packard Children's Hospital

In the NICU at Lucile Packard Children's Hospital (LPCH), screening for select PMADs in fathers is now part of routine care. At 1–2 weeks post admission, NICU social workers make efforts to screen both mothers and fathers for symptoms of acute stress disorder/PTSD, PPA, and PPD. As discussed in Chapter 7, the Perinatal Posttraumatic Stress Questionnaire (PPQ; Quinnell and Hynan 1999) was first used to assess trauma symptoms in both parents. However, our experience has been that the wording in the PPQ makes some fathers feel uncomfortable because some ques-

Table 3–2.   Fathers' Support Scale: NICU

The purpose of this scale is to help us know what fathers need while their baby is in the neonatal intensive care unit (NICU) so that we can provide more support. Please read each question and circle the number that describes best how you feel.

As a father of a baby in NICU, how important are the following things to you?	0 = Not important	1 = A little important	2 = Moderately important	3 = Very important	4 = Extremely important	N/A = Does not apply to me
Section I: Learning about your baby						
1. Getting regular information about your baby's health	0	1	2	3	4	N/A
2. Getting information about your baby in plain, nonmedical language	0	1	2	3	4	N/A
3. Being able to get the information you need about your baby from the NICU doctors	0	1	2	3	4	N/A
4. Being able to understand what you hear about your baby on rounds	0	1	2	3	4	N/A
5. Getting recommendations for your baby's care from one doctor after medical meetings about your baby	0	1	2	3	4	N/A
6. Getting the information you need about your baby from the NICU nurses	0	1	2	3	4	N/A
7. Knowing the roles of staff who care for your baby	0	1	2	3	4	N/A
8. Getting a general idea (rather than a detailed report) about your baby's health daily	0	1	2	3	4	N/A

Table 3–2. Fathers' Support Scale: NICU (*continued*)

As a father of a baby in NICU, how <u>important</u> are the following things <u>to you</u>?	0 = Not important	1 = A little important	2 = Moderately important	3 = Very important	4 = Extremely important	N/A = Does not apply to me
Section I: Learning about your baby (*continued*)						
9. Feeling you are kept as well informed as the baby's mother	0	1	2	3	4	N/A
10. Being able to get information about your baby by phone	0	1	2	3	4	N/A
Section II: Taking care of yourself and your family						
11. Being able to talk with your partner often	0	1	2	3	4	N/A
12. Being able to talk with friends about your baby often	0	1	2	3	4	N/A
13. Being able to go to work	0	1	2	3	4	N/A
14. Being able to take time off work to be with your baby	0	1	2	3	4	N/A
15. Being able to take care of your finances	0	1	2	3	4	N/A
16. Being able to help with the care of your other children	0	1	2	3	4	N/A
17. Being able to talk with other NICU parents	0	1	2	3	4	N/A
18. Being able to talk with your extended family about your baby	0	1	2	3	4	N/A

Table 3–2.   Fathers' Support Scale: NICU (*continued*)

As a father of a baby in NICU, how important are the following things to you?	0=Not important	1=A little important	2=Moderately important	3=Very important	4=Extremely important	N/A=Does not apply to me
Section II: Taking care of yourself and your family (*continued*)						
19. Being able to get away to have some time on your own	0	1	2	3	4	N/A
20. Being able to exercise	0	1	2	3	4	N/A
21. Being able to pray or do other spiritual practices	0	1	2	3	4	N/A
22. Getting away to have some time with your partner	0	1	2	3	4	N/A
23. Being able to talk to an expert about your emotions or feelings	0	1	2	3	4	N/A
Section III: Taking care of your baby						
24. Being able to touch and hold your baby	0	1	2	3	4	N/A
25. Being able to comfort your baby if he/she is in pain or looks upset	0	1	2	3	4	N/A
26. Being able to do routine care for your baby such as feeding and diaper changing	0	1	2	3	4	N/A
27. Being a part of important decisions about your baby's care	0	1	2	3	4	N/A

Table 3–2. Fathers' Support Scale: NICU *(continued)*

As a father of a baby in NICU, how important are the following things to you?	0=Not important	1=A little important	2=Moderately important	3=Very important	4=Extremely important	N/A=Does not apply to me
Section III: Taking care of your baby *(continued)*						
28. Having different doctors' opinions about the best way to treat your baby	0	1	2	3	4	N/A
29. Getting a medical opinion about your baby's care from *one* doctor after a group discussion	0	1	2	3	4	N/A
30. Being able to talk to parents who had a baby in the NICU in the past	0	1	2	3	4	N/A
31. Understanding possible long-term problems your baby might have	0	1	2	3	4	N/A
32. Being able to stay and sleep overnight in the NICU when your baby is sick (even if you live close to the hospital)	0	1	2	3	4	N/A
33. Being able to have your baby take part in research studies	0	1	2	3	4	N/A

Please tell us if there are other things that you or your partner would find helpful in supporting you while your baby is in the NICU.

Source. Reprinted from *Journal of Neonatal Nursing,* 21(2), Paula Mahon, Susan Albersheim, Liisa Holsti, "The Fathers' Support Scale: Neonatal Intensive Care Unit (FSS:NICU): Development and Initial Content Validation," 63–77, Copyright © 2015, with permission from Elsevier.

tions specifically ask about *giving birth*. Although no brief screening measures specifically for paternal traumatic stress are available that can be administered very soon after a traumatic event, one possible, less gender-specific alternative for use with fathers is the Posttraumatic Stress Disorder Checklist–5, Weekly (PCL-5: Weekly; Weathers et al. 2013), a 20-item self-report tool that examines the existence and severity of PTSD symptoms based on criteria from DSM-5. The PCL-5: Weekly can be administered as frequently as every week to monitor symptoms of PTSD.

Preventing Psychological Distress in Fathers of Premature Infants

Although screening fathers for psychological distress is an important first step, a program of psychological consultation in the NICU should include strategies to reduce stress, with measures to address systemic and environmental factors as well as interventions focused on parents.

COMMUNICATION WITH PARENTS

Given that fathers are more likely to use problem-focused coping strategies that rely on information more than on the expression of emotions, NICUs should pay attention to the importance of communicating clearly with parents (Arockiasamy et al. 2008; Ignell Modé et al. 2014; Hugill et al. 2013). Fathers report the value of having medical information about their infant (e.g., saturations, weight, breathing support) and find these numbers both useful and a way to feel more competent as caregivers (Arockiasamy et al. 2008; Logan and Dormire 2018). Fathers have also noted having regularly scheduled meetings with a primary doctor or nurse to be important (Matricardi et al. 2013). Ignell Modé et al. (2014) reported that comprehensible information provided at the onset of the infant's admission increased fathers' sense of security, helped them feel more in control, and facilitated their bonding with their infant and involvement in their infant's care. Regular meetings help fathers feel more included and supported. Fathers also report that having short, written materials that provide information about their infant's medical condition(s) is helpful (Arockiasamy et al. 2008); the more informed and knowledgeable fathers feel about how to care for and interact with their infant, the more empowered they are likely to feel (Kadivar and Mozafarinia 2013).

INVOLVEMENT OF FATHERS WITH NEONATAL CARE

Many fathers avoid physical contact with their infant out of fear of disrupting medical equipment or causing pain or discomfort (Logan and

Dormire 2018). However, the moment at which fathers finally hold their infant is a monumental landmark for them and one that they report helps solidify their connection with their child (Logan and Dormire 2018). A study that examined the impact of skin-to-skin holding between fathers and their infants found that the ability to *act* or to gain an important skill was significant to fathers. They viewed skin-to-skin interaction as something they could actively *do* in an environment where they otherwise often feel helpless (Helth and Jarden 2013). Research has shown that when fathers are more involved with their infant's care, this has positive benefits for the infant's weight and social development during the hospitall zation and at 8 and 18 months following hospital discharge (Noergaard et al. 2018). Olsson et al. (2017) similarly found in a study of 20 fathers of premature infants that those who were encouraged to participate in skin-to-skin contact reported feeling more included in their infant's care and just as important as mothers. Nurses and medical staff should encourage fathers to be active with their infants and to participate in routine care activities, speak gently to their infant, and hold their infant's hand when they are present at the bedside (Johnson 2008; Mackley et al. 2010).

NICU ENVIRONMENTAL CHANGES

To facilitate a healthier experience for fathers in the NICU, large-scale systems changes should be considered. Researchers in Denmark created a model for "father-friendly neonatal units" in which the researchers identify eight basic principles that NICUs should follow (Noergaard et al. 2018)

- Fathers should engage in skin-to-skin holding with their infants upon admission to the NICU when medically appropriate. A fathers' holding and physical touching of the infant is important for the parent–infant bonding, infant healing, and infant development.
- Fathers should receive targeted support and encouragement, especially when the mother has not yet been released from recovery and the infant has not had opportunities to feel parental affection.
- Fathers should be invited to participate in activities such as first baths, holding, diapering, and feeding.
- Medical staff should ensure that fathers are given medical information and guidance directly instead of relying on the mothers to relay information; this makes fathers feel more included in the process.
- Medical teams should make every effort to schedule conferences regarding the infant's care and treatment during times when the father can be present.
- The availability of psychosocial services that address topics such as paternity leave and other issues relevant to fathers can be vital to fathers feeling supported on the unit.
- The NICU should offer fathers' groups in which fathers can talk with one another about their experiences in a safe place.

- Accommodations should be made to lessen the burden placed on fathers when the mother is in the hospital or spending a majority of time with the infant in the NICU. For example, permitting family relatives to stay overnight with the infant so the parents can spend time with older siblings or older siblings to stay overnight in the NICU so the family can be together.

These principles are encouraged for consideration in NICUs to eliminate the numerous barriers associated with fathers' psychological distress (Noergaard et al. 2018).

PATERNITY LEAVE

Many fathers return to work almost immediately after their child is born. For most, this happens out of necessity due to having little or no paternity leave. The United States has no policy for paternity leave, whereas many other countries around the world have paid paternity leave (Kim and Swain 2007). The World Policy Analysis Center (2019) at UCLA's Fielding School of Public Health includes an interactive map denoting which countries around the world offer paternity leave. The map shows regularly updated information of countries that, including but not limited to Canada, Russia, Poland, United Kingdom, and Australia, all allow 14 weeks or more of paternity leave. Nordic countries have been the leaders in paternity leave for the purpose of promoting equality in parent rights. As a standard, Nordic countries started by offering 2 weeks of paternity leave (Haataja 2009), and this has risen to 14 weeks over time (World Policy Analysis Center 2019). Sweden was the first country to offer parental leave without an emphasis on sex, which means a shared amount of time off after delivery can be divided between two caregivers as they see fit (Haataja 2009). Policies focusing on the needs of families give the father equal opportunity to have time off with the infant. These current policies are for standard births and deliveries and often offer extended leave for extenuating circumstances such as NICU admission (World Policy Analysis Center 2019).

Paternity leave would alleviate some of the stressors fathers must manage after their infant is born and is admitted to the NICU. Paternity leave has also been found to have a positive impact on paternal attitudes toward parenting, whereas shorter or lack of paternity leave is associated with lower-quality childcare and less adaptation for men into their new role as fathers (Kim and Swain 2007).

PSYCHOLOGICAL SUPPORT

A deeper exploration into meeting the psychological needs of fathers revealed other core elements that fathers need when seeking support. A recent study by Pilkington et al. (2017) directly assessed fathers' needs for mental health–related support throughout the perinatal period. At the broadest level, they clarified the need to emphasize the importance of fathers getting help for themselves as a way of helping their newborns. In more concrete terms, this study found that new fathers tend to want more informal sources of support, including family and peers, a finding that aligns with using classes or support groups to bring new fathers together with others in a comparable situation. Rominov et al. (2017) also noted a tension between fathers wanting to be more included in perinatal medical and mental health services and their tendency to be reactive rather than proactive by seeking information and support after a crisis has occurred. For this reason, NICU staff members must be familiar with resources specific to fathers' needs and actively promote those supports early and often.

Another recent qualitative study by Eddy et al. (2019) highlighted six themes that are central to understanding the experience of PPD in married men in heterosexual relationships (Figure 3–2). Although these themes can indeed be applied to mothers who experience PPD, Eddy et al.'s (2019) research supports the usefulness of having resources that speak specifically to men's and fathers' most common mental health issues, needs, and options for support throughout the early postpartum period.

Individual and Couples' Therapy

Greater efforts to make interventions and systems both accessible and accommodating for fathers are equally important. Although individual therapy may be helpful for some fathers, Kim and Swain (2007) reported that couples therapy may be more beneficial. Couples therapy allows fathers to express their feelings, receive validation, and have their experience normalized. It also allows the father to express his emotions in a manner that aims to create connection between him and his partner and eliminate stress and tension created or exacerbated by the NICU experience. Fathers tend to be more comfortable with emotional expression for the purpose of accomplishing a task rather than just for the sake of expressing feelings (Helth and Jarden 2013).

Educational Groups

Kaaresen et al. (2006) conducted a randomized controlled trial of 146 premature infants using a modified version of the Mother–Infant Transactional Program and reported data on 112 fathers at 12-month follow up. The intervention comprised a total of eight sessions, including four home visits, with the goal of sensitizing parents to their infant's cues and facilitating parent–infant interactions. Parents in the intervention group reported significantly lower scores of parental stress, with no differences

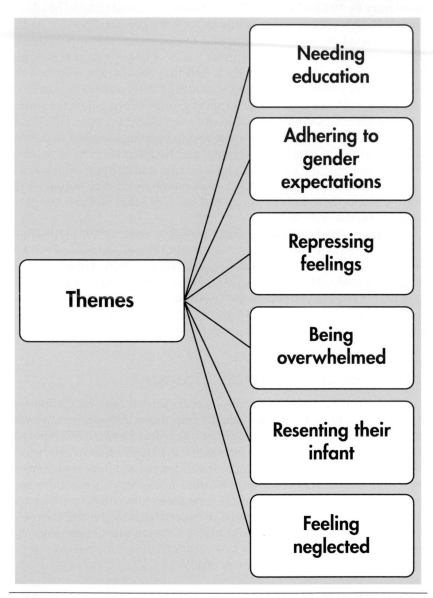

FIGURE 3–2.   Themes found in heterosexual married men with postpartum depression.
Source.   Adapted from Eddy et al. 2019.

in outcome between fathers and mothers. However, Melnyk et al. (2006) reported less robust benefits for fathers compared with mothers participating in an educational-behavioral intervention called Creating Opportunities for Parent Empowerment (COPE), further suggesting that fathers have psychological intervention needs that differ from those of mothers.

Lee et al. (2012) studied an intervention in which 34 fathers received a 25-page booklet during their visits to the NICU. The contents of the booklet had been developed in consultation with neonatal nursing experts and fathers of premature infants and included the following topics: the equipment used by the baby, developmental care in the NICU, baby's nutrition, baby's appearance, what your baby is doing, what you can do with your baby in the NICU, and relaxation tips for fathers. Topics were reviewed with the father by a nurse, who listened to the father's concerns, guided him to focus on the infant, and supported him in the use of relaxation skills. This study, which took place in Taiwan, was developed based on the cultural family postpartum practices in which mothers of newborn infants remain home for the first month following delivery and fathers are the primary visitors to the NICU during this time. The goal of the intervention was to increase fathering ability and reduce paternal stress. Comparison of the intervention group of fathers with historical control subjects showed increased fathering ability, increased perceived nursing support, and reduced parental stress.

Support Groups

There is increasing interest in the use of support groups for new fathers. One such resource is the monthly "Dads Chat" hosted by Postpartum Support International (www.postpartum.net), a monthly telephone call-in group that gives fathers who are experiencing difficulties with early fatherhood the chance to engage in anonymous, on-demand communication with other fathers and receive information and peer support. The group is facilitated by a volunteer member of Postpartum Support International with expertise in paternal perinatal mental health and has been running consecutively for nearly 7 years. Dads Chat is an open, hour-long drop-in format phone call that provides both support and psychoeducational information about common experiences, including relationship changes, conflict, self-care, and mood or anxiety issues. Dads Chat also provides information about relevant resources and, most importantly, creates an environment in which fathers are encouraged to develop a sense of community by directly engaging each other to share reactions and suggestions. Research demonstrates that specific characteristics need to be present for fathers in the NICU to feel supported in group therapy. Fathers often struggle with the public and vulnerable nature of being in the NICU and view group support as emphasizing an already undesired aspect of the NICU experience (Thomson-Salo et al. 2017). In addition, few fathers identify their relationship with other parents in the NICU as a source of support (Arockiasamy et al. 2008). However, when support groups are used as an intervention, fathers find

groups consisting exclusively of fathers and led by men to be most useful. In this context, fathers are better able to experience this time as an
opportunity to debrief about their trauma, share their experience of feeling left out, cry, share negative emotions, and gain a common ground.
Fathers consider the male-only group as a way to provide and receive
mutual support in the context of open and honest discussion (Thomson-
Salo et al. 2017).

Programs for fathers of infants in the NICU are not part of the routine standard of care in the United States. Although some programs may
be geared toward new fathers, data on the efficacy of existing programs
for fathers who have an infant in the NICU are limited to nonexistent.

Interventions for Fathers in the NICU at Lucile Packard Children's Hospital

Since 2017, fathers of NICU infants at LPCH have been able to access
family-based mental health services from an infant mental health perspective, with the goal of improving the outcomes for their infant. Fathers are screened for PMADs and symptoms of posttraumatic stress and
given information about NICU-based mental health support services.
These services include formal psychiatric evaluation by the child psychiatry consult service (including a dedicated NICU psychology fellow), referral for brief trauma-informed treatment (see Chapter 5), parent–infant
psychotherapy, and, more recently, referral to a fathers' support group.
Fathers are also offered joint sessions with their partner to discuss the impact of the NICU admission on both parents and their relationship. All
family constellations are also included in NICU psychological intervention services.

One barrier to engaging fathers in these services is that many already
feel overwhelmed by other responsibilities, such as providing support to
the mother, taking care of older children, and managing general financial
and household responsibilities. The lack of paid paternity leave, as mentioned previously, also results in many fathers returning to work and
having limited time in the NICU. Fathers commonly are less open to ac-
knowledging symptoms of psychological distress or their need for support and prefer to spend their time in the NICU with their infant. Fathers
also have the perception that support services are geared toward mothers rather than fathers.

FATHERS' SUPPORT GROUP IN THE NICU

Currently, we are piloting a novel program to provide support for fathers
in the NICU using an eight-session biweekly curriculum based on the literature of concerns of fathers summarized earlier in this chapter. The con-

cept for and development of this group was led by the NICU psychology fellow. Revision of materials, considerations for session outlines, and inclusion of a session on masculinity culture were all made possible by the dedicated work of our research assistants.[1]

Eligibility

To address anecdotal parent concerns regarding all services being provided to mothers with little to no inclusion of fathers, we are broader in our inclusion criteria for our fathers' group. Different from our group for mothers of premature infants, our fathers' group welcomes fathers of infants in the NICU regardless of their infant's reason for hospitalization. According to information provided by the National Perinatal Association (2019), "Nearly half of all babies in the NICU are born at normal birthweight and are 37-weeks gestation or older." Therefore, support services may be needed for families who have full-term infants who require intensive medical intervention.

Location of Sessions

Currently, we are comparing fathers' groups offered in the NICU with an online format using videoconferencing technology. Benefits of the online format include the potential to improve access for fathers who may have already returned to work or are managing other family responsibilities. This option, which is based on Postpartum Support International's Dads Chat model, may allow underserved families who live far from the hospital or have transportation difficulties to participate. Fathers can attend the group by calling in or using the video chat function on Zoom, which is HIPPA compliant. The facilitator keeps his camera active so participants can make a visual connection with him. However, fathers can choose not to use video or use the Zoom voice calling feature. On-site groups offered in the NICU also have benefits, including the opportunity to recruit fathers who visit the NICU on evenings when the groups are scheduled and the chance to make in-person social connections with other fathers.

Session Format

The proposed telehealth support group consists of eight sessions. Seven 90-minute sessions offer a balance of psychoeducation and opportunities for father-led topics. The eighth session is an open forum in which fathers

---

[1]Pacific Graduate School of Psychology (PGSP)-Stanford Psy.D. Consortium graduate students Maria Ocampo, Jason Tinero, Stephanie Seeman, and Emily Wharton.

are encouraged to discuss concerns relevant to them at the time of the session. We hypothesize that the order of sessions may not be essential; however, we are piloting the sessions starting with Session 1, "Do All New Fathers Feel This: Difficulty Sleeping, Worry, Isolation," which focuses on the initial thoughts and feelings of fathers in the NICU and on psychoeducation about trauma. Session 2, "I Wasn't Ready: Caring for a Premature or Medically Fragile Baby," discusses ways to care for an infant in the NICU. We hypothesized that these two initial sessions can help fathers learn that they are not alone in their feelings and that there are ways that they can interact with their infant.

Session 3, "Protect and Provide: Managing Fatherhood Stress," offers opportunities for fathers to discuss the complexity of additional stressors while balancing the experience of having an infant in the NICU. The session includes psychoeducation about the benefits of rational positive self-statements. In Session 4, "Your Baby Needs You: Advocating for Your Baby in the NICU and Beyond," attention is paid to helping fathers advocate for their infant by talking with hospital staff.

In Session 5, "Manning Up: When It Is Okay for Fathers to Feel Emotions," the facilitator provides a resource that specifically addresses the premise of masculinity culture and fathers' hesitation to express negative emotions. In Session 6, "I'm Not Allowed to Do Anything: Overcoming Gatekeeping to Connect With Your Baby," fathers receive psychoeducation about the rationale for maternal gatekeeping and how they can facilitate father–infant bonding once their baby is discharged from the NICU. Finally, Session 7, "Will I Ever Have Sex Again? Navigating Feelings of Neglect and Resentment," is strategically placed so that if fathers attend all sessions in order, their infant may be home or close to discharge. Families whose infant has been discharged may be settling into a routine at home. This is the time when fathers may begin to feel ready for sexual intimacy with their partners but may have conflicting feelings about resuming their sexual relationships.

The fathers' support group was initially designed to be led by a male clinician experienced in leading parent psychotherapy groups in order to help fathers feel emotionally safe enough to discuss their thoughts and feelings. As discussed, this decision was based on research that found groups for men that are led by men tend to be better received and more effective than those led by women (Thomson-Salo et al. 2017). However, although having a male facilitator is supported in the literature, we believe group facilitators of all sexes and genders could have a positive impact on group members.

Each session in all of the LPCH NICU groups starts with a review of group rules and guidelines, including those for our fathers' group. Included in the handouts and reviewed during the first session is a list of these rules and guidelines, which cover confidentiality; when, where, and how to access the group (e.g., not while driving or in public spaces or while caring for mobile children, avoiding disclosure of what is shared by other members, attendance while in a quiet and private space); and expectations for providing peer support (e.g., not blaming other members or using negatively judgmental language).

At the beginning of each session, the group facilitator introduces himself and asks the first name of each father along with the age of the father's infant and his reason for attending the session. The facilitator then assures each father that he will make time during the session to address the concerns of all participants. To begin the psychoeducation portion of each session, the facilitator leads the group through a brief mindfulness-based stress reduction activity to ground the attendees and set the tone for the group. Likewise, each session concludes by leading the fathers in another mindfulness-based stress reduction technique. Fathers are provided with details regarding these techniques along with session-specific handouts through a shared database.

Conclusions

The limited literature on fathers and interventions during the perinatal and postpartum periods supports that fathers and their mental health needs are often overlooked, especially in the NICU setting. However, considerable research has documented that when fathers are screened, they are often symptomatic for diagnosable PMADs and PTSD related to their child's birth or hospitalization. One problem is that screening for paternal PMADs and PTSD in the NICU is not currently a standard process for most hospitals around the world, and certainly not in the United States, which is further worsened by the fact that few screening tools for paternal psychological distress are available. Although at least one screening tool currently exists for screening PTSD symptoms in the NICU, some fathers report discomfort with the wording of that measure, suggesting it makes them feel it was designed solely for women. Development and validation of screening tools specific to the perinatal mental health needs of fathers are needed. Screening tools for fathers will also need to consider racial and cultural sensitivities because many studies have included few fathers of color, leaving a gap in the field's understanding of the specific needs of these populations. Studies that have included fathers of color, such as African American fathers of various ages, have found experiences of racism to increase a father's likelihood of PPD symptoms and general perceptions of stress.

Research further suggests that infants of parents with unaddressed mental health concerns have poorer outcomes in infancy and throughout childhood. Similarly, when fathers are engaged in romantic relationships with the mother, unmitigated paternal stress has been shown to negatively impact the parental couple relationship. Data from previous studies support that interventions designed to target parental stress in the

NICU have been structured to support the growth and development of the maternal–infant bond and maternal stress rather than being individualized for fathers. Researchers are starting to understand specific components that facilitate a friendly NICU experience for fathers, but the fact remains that many NICUs are mother oriented. Implementing strategies such as psychological intervention and support groups for fathers that decrease paternal barriers and create father inclusion is the next step.

Furthermore, although few interventions exist for new fathers, little data are available on the long-term outcomes on fathers, their infants, and their families resulting from these interventions. Research needs to move in the direction of examining long-term outcomes in these populations. Additionally, future researchers should focus on developing father-specific interventions that use culturally and racially responsive considerations and then test their efficacy for appropriate dissemination. Our proposed consultation method is a data-collecting exploration into learning the needs of new NICU fathers from various backgrounds. We aim to be open and inclusive with efforts to accommodate fathers of various racial, cultural, socioeconomic, and community living arrangements (e.g., fathers living in rural, suburban, and metropolitan areas) by considering when and where services are conducted and how accessible they are to fathers in more rural areas or with restrictive financial resources. By creating evidence-based psychological services designed to address paternal PMADs and PTSD in the NICU and providing a more stable foundation that stimulates the paternal–infant bond that is so advantageous for infant healing and development, clinicians can improve care for infants admitted to the NICU.

References

Addis M: Invisible Men: Men's Inner Lives and the Consequences of Silence. New York, Henry Hold and Company, 2011

Alio AP, Mbah AK, Grunsten RA, Salihu HM: Teenage pregnancy and the influence of paternal involvement on fetal outcomes. J Pediatr Adolesc Gynecol 24(6):404–409, 2011

American Psychiatric Association: Diagnostic and Statistical Manual of Mental Disorders, 5th Edition. Arlington, VA, American Psychiatric Association, 2013

American Psychological Association: Guidelines for the Psychological Treatment of Boys and Men. Washington, DC, American Psychological Association, 2018

Ashmore RD, Del Boca FK: The Social Psychology of Female-Male Relations. London, Academic Press, 1986

Arockiasamy V, Holsti L, Albersheim S: Fathers experiences in the neonatal intensive care unit: a search for control. Pediatr 121(2):215–222, 2008

Bamishigbin ON, Dunkel SC, Guardino CM, et al: Resilience and depressive symptoms in low-income African American fathers. Cultur Divers Ethnic Minor Psychol 23(1):70, 2017

Beck AT, Steer R, Brown G: Beck Depression Inventory Manual, 2nd Edition. The Psychological Corporation, San Antonio, TX, 1996

Beck CT, Gable RK: Postpartum depression screening scale: development and psychometric testing. Nurs Res 49(5):272–282, 2000

Binder WS, Zeltzer LK, Simmons CF, et al: The father in the hallway: posttraumatic stress reactions in fathers of NICU babies. Psychiatr Ann 41(8):396–402, 2011

Bronte-Tinkew J, Moore KA, Matthews G, Carrano J: Symptoms of major depression in a sample of fathers of infants: sociodemographic correlates and links to father involvement. J Fam Issues 28(1):61–99, 2007

Buist A, Morse CA, Durkin S: Men's adjustment to fatherhood: implications for obstetric health care. J Obstet Gynecol Neonatal Nurs 32(2):172–180, 2003

Cameron EE, Sedov ID, Tomfohr-Madsen LM: Prevalence of paternal depression in pregnancy and the postpartum: an updated meta-analysis. J Affect Disord 206:109–203, 2016

Cheng ER, Downs SM, Carroll AE: Prevalence of depression among fathers at the pediatric well-child care visit, JAMA Pediatr 172(9):882–883, 2018

Cole BP, Davidson MM: Exploring men's perceptions about male depression. Psychol Men Masc 20(4):1–8, 2018

Cox J, Holden JM, Sagovsky R: Detection of postnatal depression: development of the 10-item Edinburgh Postnatal Depression Scale. Br J Psychiatry 150(6):782–786, 1987

Cyr-Alves H, Macken L, Hyrkas K: Stress and symptoms of depression in fathers of infants admitted to the NICU. J Obstet Gynecol Neonatal Nurs 47(2):146–157, 2018

David DS, Brannon R: The Forty-Nine Percent Majority: The Male Sex Role. Boston, MA, Addison-Wesley, 1976

Davis RN, Davis MM, Freed GL, Clark SJ: Fathers' depression related to positive and negative parenting behaviors with 1-year-old children. Pediatr 127(4):612–618, 2011

Deeney K, Lohan M, Spence D, Parkes J: Experiences of fathering a baby admitted to neonatal intensive care: a critical gender analysis. Soc Sci Med 75(6):1106–1113, 2012

DeMier RL, Hynan MT, Harris HB, Manniello RL: Perinatal stressors as predictors of symptoms of posttraumatic stress in mothers of infants at high risk. J Perinatol 16(4):276–280, 1996

Diaz NM, Plunkett BA: Universal screening for perinatal depression. NeoReviews 19(3):143–159, 2018

Duursma E, Pan BA, Raikes H: Predictors and outcomes of low-income fathers' reading with their toddlers. Early Child Res Q 23(3):351–365, 2008

Eddy B, Poll V, Whitling J, Clevesy M: Forgotten fathers: postpartum depression in men. J Fam Issues 40(8):1001–1017, 2019

Fisher SD, Kopelman R, O'Hara MW: Partner report of paternal depression using the Edinburgh Postnatal Depression Scale–Partner. Arch Womens Ment Health 15(4):283–288, 2012

Fleming AS, Corter C, Stallings J, Steiner M: Testosterone and prolactin are associated with emotional responses to infant cries in new fathers. Horm Behav 42(4):399–413, 2002

Fletcher RJ, Feeman E, Garfield C, Vimpani G: The effects of early paternal depression on children's development. Med J Aust 195(11–12):685–689, 2011

Garfield CF, Duncan G, Rutsohn R, et al: A longitudinal study of paternal mental health during transition to fatherhood as young adults. Pediatrics 133(5):836–843, 2014

Haataja A: Fathers' Use of Paternity and Parental Leave in the Nordic Countries (Online Working Papers, 2/2009). Kela, Finland, The Social Insurance Institution Research Department, 2009

Helth TD, Jarden M: Fathers experiences with the skin-to-skin method in NICU: competent parenthood and redefined gender roles. J Neonatal Nurs 19(3):114–121, 2013

Holditch-Davis D, Bartlett TR, Blickman AL, Miles MS: Posttraumatic stress symptoms in mothers of premature infants. J Obstet Gynecol Neonatal Nurs 32(2):161–171, 2003

Hollywood M, Hollywood E: The lived experience of fathers of a premature baby on a neonatal intensive care unit. J Neonatal Nurs 17(1):32–40, 2011

Hua A, Pham T, Spinazzola R, Sonnenklar J, et al: PTSD scores among mothers and fathers of NICU graduates aged 1 to 36 months. Pediatr 141(1):551, 2018

Hugill K, Letherby G, Reid T, Lavender T: Experiences of fathers shortly after the birth of their preterm infants. J Ob Gyn Neon Nurs 42(6):655–663, 2013

Hunt TK, Caldwell CH, Assari S: Family economic stress, quality of paternal relationship, and depressive symptoms among African American adolescent fathers. J Child Fam Stud 24(10):3067–3078, 2015

Ignell Modé R, Mard E, Nyqvist KH, Blomqvist YT: Fathers' perception of information received during their infants' stay at a neonatal intensive care unit. Sex Reprod Health 5(3):131–136, 2014

Isacco A, Hofscher R, Molloy S: An examination of fathers' mental health help seeking: a brief report. Am J Mens Health 10(6):NP33–NP38, 2016

Jacob T, Johnson SL: Sequential interactions in the parent–child communications of depressed fathers and depressed mothers. J Fam Psychol 15(1):38–52, 2001

Johnson AN: Engaging fathers in the NICU. J Perinat Neonatal Nurs 22(4):302–306, 2008

Kaaresen PI, Rønning JA, Ulvund SE, Dahl LB: A randomized, controlled trial of the effectiveness of an early intervention program in reducing parenting stress after preterm birth. Pediatrics 118(1):e9–e19, 2006

Kadivar M, Mozafarinia SM: Supporting fathers in a NICU: effects of the hug your baby program on fathers' understanding of preterm infant behavior. J Perinat Educ 22(2):113–119, 2013

Kim P, Swain J: Sad dads. Psychiatry 4(2):36–47, 2007

Kroenke K, Spitzer RL: The PHQ-9: a new depression and diagnostic severity measure. Psychiatr Ann 32:509–521, 2002

Leach S, Poyser C, Cooklin AR, Giallo R: Prevalence and course of anxiety disorders (and symptom levels) in men across the perinatal period: a systematic review. J Affect Disord 190:675–686, 2016

Lee TY, Wang MM, Lin KC, Kao CH: The effectiveness of early intervention on paternal stress for fathers of premature infants admitted to a neonatal intensive care unit. J Adv Nurs 69(5):1085–1095, 2012

Leiferman JA, Dauber SE, Heisler K, Paulson JF: Primary care physicians' beliefs and practices toward maternal depression. J Womens Health 17(7):1143–1150, 2008

Levant RF, Hall RJ, Williams CM, Hasan NT: Gender differences in alexithymia. Psychol Men Masc 10(3):190–203, 2009

Logan RM, Dormire S: Finding my way: a phenomenology of fathering in the NICU. Adv Neonatal Care 18(2):154–162, 2018

Lyons-Ruth K, Lyubchik A, Wolfe R, Bronfman E: Parental depression and child attachment: Hostile and helpless profiles of parent and child behavior among families at risk, in Children of Depressed Parents: Mechanisms of Risk and Implications for Treatment. Washington, DC, American Psychological Association, 2002, pp 89–120

Mackley AB, Locke RG, Spear ML, Joseph R: Forgotten parent. Adv Neonatal Care 10(4):200–203, 2010

Mahon P, Albersheim S, Holsti L: The Fathers' Support Scale: Neonatal Intensive Care Unit (FSS:NICU): development and initial content validation. J Neonatal Nurs 21(2):63–71, 2014

Matricardi S, Agostino R, Fedeli C, Montirosso R: Mothers are not fathers: differences between parents in the reduction of stress levels after a parental intervention in a NICU. Acta Paediatrica 102(1):8–14, 2013

Melnyk BM, Feinstein NF, Alpert-Gillis L, et al: Reducing premature infants' length of stay and improving parents' mental health outcomes with Creating Opportunities for Parent Empowerment (COPE) Neonatal Intensive Care Unit program: a randomized controlled trial. Pediatr 118:1414–1427, 2006

Miles MS, Holditch-Davis D, Schwartz TA, Scher M: Depressive symptoms in mothers of prematurely born infants. J Dev Behav Pediatr 28(1):36–44, 2007

Mottolese R, Redouté J, Costes N, Le Bars D: Switching brain serotonin with oxytocin. Proc Natl Acad Sci 111(23):8637–8642, 2014

National Perinatal Association: NICU Awareness (website). Lonedell, MO, National Perinatal Association, 2019. Available at: http://www.nationalperinatal.org/NICU_Awareness. Accessed December 7, 2019.

Noergaard B, Ammentorp J, Garne E, et al: Fathers' stress in the neonatal intensive care unit. Adv Neonatal Care 18(5):413–422, 2018

Olson AL, Kemper KJ, Kelleher KJ, Hammond CS: Primary care pediatricians' roles and perceived responsibilities in the identification and management of maternal depression. Pediatr Springfield 110(6):1169–1176, 2002

Olsson E, Eriksson M, Anderzén-Carlsson A: Skin-to-skin contact facilitates more equal parenthood: a qualitative study from fathers' perspective. J Pediatr Nurs 34:e2–e9, 2017

Paulson JF, Bazemore SD: Prenatal and postpartum depression in fathers and its association with maternal depression: a meta-analysis. JAMA 303(19):1961–1969, 2010

Philpott LF, Leahy-Warren P, FitzGerald S, Savage E: Stress in the fathers in the perinatal period: a systematic review. Midwifery 55:113–127, 2017

Pilkington PD, Rominov H, Milne LC, Giallo R: Partners to parents: development of an online intervention for enhancing partner support and preventing perinatal depression and anxiety. Advances in Mental Health 15(1):42–57, 2017

Pleck JH: Integrating father involvement in parenting research. Parenting 12(2–3):243–253, 2012

Potapova NV, Gartstein MA, Bridgett DJ: Paternal influences on infant temperament: effects of father internalizing problems, parenting-related stress, and temperament. Infant Behav Dev 37(1):105–110, 2014

Provenzi L, Santoro E: The lived experience of fathers of preterm infants in the neonatal intensive care unit: a systematic review of qualitative studies. J Clin Nurs 24(13–14):1784–1794, 2015

Puhlman DJ, Pasley K: Rethinking maternal gatekeeping. J Fam Theory Rev 5(3):176–193, 2013

Qin D-D, Rizak J, Feng X-L, Yang S-C, et al: Prolonged secretion of cortisol as a possible mechanism underlying stress and depressive behaviour. Sci Rep 6:1–9, 2016

Quinnell FA, Hynan MT: Convergent and discriminant validity of the perinatal PTSD questionnaire (PPQ): a preliminary study. J Trauma Stress 12(1):193–199, 1999

Rabinowitz FE, Cochran SV: Men and therapy: a case of masked male depression. Clin Case Stud 7(6):575–591, 2008

Ramchandani P, Psychogiou L: Paternal psychiatric disorders and children's psychosocial development. Lancet 374(9690):646–653, 2009

Rominov H, Giallo R, Pilkington PD, Whelan TA: Midwives' perceptions and experiences of engaging fathers in perinatal services. Women and Birth 30(4):308–318, 2017

Shapiro AF, Gottman JM, Fink BC: Father's involvement when bringing baby home: efficacy testing of a couple-focused transition to parenthood intervention for promoting father involvement. Psychol Rep 123(3):806–824, 2020

Shaw RJ, Deblois T, Ikuta L, et al: Acute stress disorder among parents of infants in the neonatal intensive care nursery. Psychosomatics 47(3):206–212, 2006

Singley DB, Edwards LM: Men's perinatal mental health in the transition to fatherhood. Professional Psychology: Research and Practice 46(5):309–316, 2015

Singley DB, Cole BP, Hammer JH, et al: Development and psychometric evaluation of the Paternal Involvement With Infants Scale. Psychol Men Masc 19(2):167–183, 2018

Spitzer RL, Kroenke K, Williams JB: Validation and utility of a self-report version of PRIME-MD: the PHQ Primary Care Study. Primary care evaluation of mental disorders. Patient Health Questionnaire. JAMA 282(18):1737–1744, 1999

Taylor CA, Manganello JA, Lee SJ, Rice JC: Mothers' spanking of 3-year-old children and subsequent risk of children's aggressive behavior. Pediatr 125(5):e1057–e1065, 2010

Thomson-Salo F, Kuschel CA, Kamlin OF, Cuzzilla R: A fathers group in NICU: recognising and responding to paternal stress, utilising peer support. J Neonatal Nurs 23(6):294–298, 2017

Weathers FW, Litz BT, Keane TM, et al: PTSD Checklist for DSM-5. Washington, DC, U.S. Department of Veterans Affairs, 2013. Available at: https://www.ptsd.va.gov/professional/assessment/adult-sr/ptsd-checklist.asp. Accessed June 27, 2020.

Willis T, Chavis L, Saxton S, et al: NPA Position Statement 2018: Perinatal Mood and Anxiety Disorders. Lonedell, MO, National Perinatal Association, 2018. Available at: http://www.nationalperinatal.org/resources/Documents/Position Papers/2018 Position Statement PMADs_NPA.pdf. Accessed May 19, 2019.

World Policy Analysis Center: Is paid leave available to mothers and fathers of infants? Los Angeles, CA, World Policy Analysis Center, 2019. Available at: https://www.worldpolicycenter.org/policies/is-paid-leave-available-to-mothers-and-fathers-of-infants/is-paid-leave-available-for-fathers-of-infants. Accessed June 27, 2020.

Yogman M, Garfield CF, Committee on Psychosocial Aspects of Child and Family Health: Fathers' roles in the care and development of their children: the role of pediatricians. Pediatrics 138(1), 2016

CHAPTER 4

Psychological Interventions in the NICU

Melissa Scala, M.D.

Soudabeh Givrad, M.D.

Richard J. Shaw, M.D.

Interventions directed toward the parents of premature infants that are commonly implemented during their child's NICU hospitalization fall broadly into three major categories (Figure 4–1). First is a group of theoretically diverse but commonly available interventions referred to as *developmental care interventions*. Developmental care involves measures that reduce infant pain and stress and provide sensory interventions thought important for the infant's health and development, as well as those that foster engagement and connection between parents and infants. These interventions focus primarily on teaching parents how to recognize their infant's developmental needs and fostering parenting skills believed to promote healthy infant development. Second, the increased awareness of how parents and infants psychologically function as a unit has led to a group of interventions aimed at addressing the evolving relationship between parents and infants, with the goal of improving parental and infant mental health and development. These mental health interventions

Melissa Scala and Soudabeh Givrad contributed equally to this work.

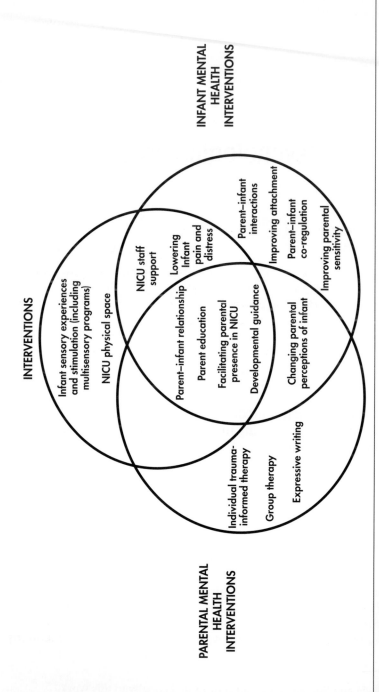

FIGURE 4–1. Psychological interventions in the NICU.

Psychological interventions in the NICU historically have been defined by three broad categories of intervention: developmental care interventions, parental mental health interventions, and infant mental health interventions. In reality, these categories have significant overlap and share many similar interventions. In this image we show some of the components of each category of intervention to demonstrate their overlapping nature.

use parent–infant psychotherapy to facilitate healthy attachment and target relational difficulties in parents and infants in the NICU who might be struggling to establish an optimal bond. Third is a group of interventions that focus primarily on parental distress, with the goal of reducing psychological symptoms of anxiety, depression, and trauma. These categories have some overlap in terms of targets and outcomes; all three can affect both parental mental health and, directly or indirectly, the quality of the relationship between parents and infants and therefore the psychological and developmental outcomes for infants. In this chapter, we review interventions in all of these categories and discuss their integration in the care of both parents and their premature infants.

Developmental Care Interventions

INTRODUCTION

There has been increasing recognition of the close connection between parental and infant mental health, well-being, and how families function as a unit, affecting each other in positive and negative ways. In addition, more and more evidence shows that prematurity, medical illnesses and challenges, and the NICU environment can be a source of vulnerability, stress, trauma, and suboptimal emotional, mental, and physical outcomes for infants. For instance, NICU and premature infants have higher rates of depression and anxiety in childhood, adolescence, and adulthood that are likely to be related, at least in part, to their experiences in the NICU (Burnett et al. 2019; Lund et al. 2012).

Over the past several decades, various interventions have been developed to ameliorate the stressful and traumatic nature of a NICU stay for infants and parents and to move toward creating a more optimal environment that promotes their emotional attachment while addressing the traumas they experience. The field of developmental care is a collaboration of multidisciplinary caregivers and composed of interventions that encourage infants' neurodevelopment and decrease their distress while supporting families (Macho 2017). Concepts from infant mental health, defined as "the developing capacity of the child from birth to age 3 to experience, regulate, and express emotions; form close and secure interpersonal relationships; and explore the environment and learn—all in the context of family, community and cultural expectations for young children" (Zero to Three Infant Mental Health Task Force Steering Committee 2001), have been used in a variety of developmental care programs and models of care. Although most of the work done in the field of infant mental health has focused on healthy-term growing infants, the general framework of infant mental health may be applied to the NICU population.

Family-centered developmental care was initially focused on reducing infant stress; however, the scope has now expanded to include care practices and environments that reduce infant pain and stress, targeted exposures or interventions that promote neuronal connectivity and microbiome assembly, and programs that encourage healthy parent–infant relationships, interactions, and attachments. Many of these components directly impact the psychological health of both infant and parents. Developmental care practices, at their best, can support both parents' and infants' psychological health through individualized care aimed at mitigating the negative effects of the NICU environment.

HISTORY OF DEVELOPMENTAL CARE

Our current mental framework for developmental care owes it roots to Dr. T. Berry Brazelton and Dr. Heidilise Als, who in the 1970s and 1980s began focusing on infants' developmental maturation and emphasized individualized assessment and support. Brazelton (1973) focused on the connection between maternal and infant behavior and developed the Neonatal Behavioral Assessment Scale to assess infant strengths, vulnerabilities, and adaptations. Central to this program was the assertion that infant behavior is a meaningful communication of the infant's wants, needs, and capabilities. Results were used to guide caregiving strategies that supported the parent–infant relationship (Brazelton 1973). The Neonatal Behavioral Assessment Scale was later adapted into the Neonatal Behavioral Observations system for more clinical use (Nugent et al. 2007). Both tools were designed for use in full-term (or term-corrected) infants and parents through the first few months of the child's life, with the goal of improving infant–parent attachment. Some studies reported improvements in caregiver–infant interaction, but a Cochrane review by Barlow et al. (2018) rated the overall quality as weak. One study by Nugent et al. (2014) found decreased postpartum depression among first-time mothers using the Neonatal Behavioral Observations system. Further studies are under way to evaluate the impact of this system on infants, caregivers, and their relationships.

Als (1982) and colleagues developed the Newborn Individualized Developmental Care and Assessment Program (NIDCAP), which emphasized infants' individuality and the evaluation of the regulation and differentiation of five subsets of observable functioning: autonomic, motor, state regulation, attention, and self-regulation systems. NIDCAP's primary intervention involved formalized repetitive observations of infants and emphasized reading infant behavioral cues. Positive sensory input caused infants to move toward the stimulation, and negative input from noxious or overwhelming stimulation created avoidance or stress behaviors. Developmental goals were created based on these observations and modified as the infants matured. Families and medical caregivers were taught to read infants' cues and adjust their interactions with the infants. The NIDCAP construct formalized a communication system in which even very immature infants could effectively respond to their environments and brought emphasis to the parental role in the care of NICU infants (Als 1986).

Infant benefits of NIDCAP include reduced lung disease, shorter hospital stays, improved sleep and reduced pain responses with caregiving, better structural brain development, and improved neurodevelopmental outcomes (Holsti et al. 2004; Ohlsson and Jacobs 2013). Some studies failed to replicate these benefits, but their findings were thought to result from incomplete adoption of the intervention. A Cochrane review by Ohlsson and Jacobs (2013) found no evidence that NIDCAP improved short-term medical or long-term neurodevelopmental outcomes for premature infants. Further concerns about the cost-effectiveness of training, which can take 12 months or longer; the time commitment of multiple infant observations; and changing the nursery to adapt to a NIDCAP model have limited its widespread use, but its theoretical framework forms the base of modern NICU infant developmental care programs worldwide.

Because the work of Brazelton and Als emphasized the importance of parent and caregiver education in the care of NICU infants, numerous programs were developed to meet this need. As our understanding of developmental care has expanded, emphasis on providing specific sensory experiences to NICU infants and interaction opportunities with parents has increased. In the following sections, we describe and summarize various components and targets of developmental care and infant mental health interventions. Several more formalized programs now exist that use these elements in varying degrees based on the focus and orientation of the program. Research on the effectiveness of many of these programs is ongoing.

PARENT EDUCATION INTERVENTIONS

Integration of parents into the NICU care environment led to the creation and evaluation of educational programs designed to teach NICU infant care and cues to parents and caregivers. Programs have been developed in various formats, including written, audio, and video as well as bedside and group classes and simulations. Many of these programs have shown improvements in both parental stress levels and confidence in infant care.

As with many interventions, these programs initially were focused on the family's transition to home and postdischarge periods. The Victorian Infant Brain Studies (VIBeS) is one example of an educational intervention offered following hospital discharge until the infant reaches 1 year's corrected age (Spittle et al. 2010). VIBeS educates parents about key concepts of developmental care, including postural control, behavioral regulation, and mobility in their infants. In a randomized controlled trial (RCT) with 120 participants, the intervention improved both infant dysregulation and externalizing behaviors. Although the intervention did not specifically target parental distress, the study found reduced levels of parental depression and anxiety. Several other programs also showed promise in this intervention (Puthussery et al. 2018), but many included a parent support element and are detailed further in the discussions that follow.

Other programs have focused on parent education and support during the NICU admission. Among those focused on parent education in the inpatient setting, many showed positive impacts on parental mental health. Browne and Talmi (2005) found improvement in maternal knowledge, improved mother–infant interactions, and lower maternal stress scores after maternal education in infant reflexes, attention, motor skills, and sleep-wake states. The HUG Your Baby (Help, Understanding, Guidance for Young Families) program provides digital parent education focused, among other things, on preparation for discharge and has been shown to both decrease maternal stress and increase maternal confidence (Hunter et al. 2019). Another example of a structured parent educational program is the NICU Family Support Core Curriculum, created by the March of Dimes, which teaches parents about NICU infant care, developmental care, infant nutrition, and self-care and prepares parents for discharge. A multisite study of this program showed improved parental knowledge and confidence (Gehl et al. 2020). Beheshtipour et al. (2014) showed lower scores on NICU Parental Stressor Scales (Miles et al. 1993) in parents who were given basic information about the general condition of their infant, the NICU equipment, and partner support. The success of parent educational programs alone has led to their inclusion as part of multicomponent interventions described later in this chapter (see "Multicomponent Interventions").

PAIN REDUCTION

NICU infants may experience up to 17 painful experiences per day with negative neurological consequences due to their developmental immaturity (Porter et al. 1999). Premature infants who experience greater pain exposures in the NICU have been shown to display greater internalizing behaviors (depressive or anxious) at 18 months' and 7 years' corrected age (Vinall and Grunau 2014). Parents can actively help mitigate and reduce infant pain in the NICU using effective nonpharmacological techniques such as parental talking, singing, or playing music (Bergomi et al. 2014; Chen et al. 2019; Shah et al. 2017); kangaroo care/holding/rocking (Chidambaram et al. 2014; Johnston et al. 2008, 2014); infant massage (Chik et al. 2017; Diego et al. 2009); breastfeeding (Erkul and Efe 2017); and administering oral sucrose solution (Shah et al. 2012).

The NICU is a stressful environment for parents and infants. Stress in NICU infants may come from illness, physical discomfort, and noxious stimulation from a bright and often loud environment. D'Agata et al. (2016) used the term *infant medical trauma in the NICU* to capture the traumatic experience of infants in an environment that is neither normal nor nurturing and exposes them to various distressing experiences. Infants are unable to show the same behavioral cues related to experiencing traumas as older infants and children because they are in a preverbal stage of development with immature brain development and ability for sensory integration. Evidence has shown hyperarousal (surges in cortisol, tachycardia, and agitation) in infants and increased medical staff understanding of possible cues of distress at an early age (D'Agata et al. 2016). The mitigation of infant pain and stress is a key component of developmental care and may have a significant impact on infant mental health. Positioning, clustering care times, and making adjustments in lighting and sound are commonly used to help reduce infant stress.

Some mechanisms through which pain and stress can affect infants are epigenetic alterations in hypothalamic-pituitary-adrenal (HPA) axis responsiveness, oxytocin pathways, and structural brain changes (Field 2017; Provenzi et al. 2019; Victoria and Murphy 2016; Walker 2013). Alterations in the HPA axis can have lifelong effects on a person's response to stress. A hyper- or hyporeactive HPA axis, found in many premature infants, may result in long-term negative outcomes such as anxiety, cognitive disorders, metabolic syndrome, and alcohol preference (Huot et al. 2001; Porter et al. 1999). However, oxytocin, a hormone associated with parent–infant bonding, may moderate the effects of pain (Boll et al. 2018). In animal models, degrees of positive care interactions between mothers and their young created lasting epigenetic changes in oxytocin and HPA responsiveness (Champagne et al. 2001).

STRESS REDUCTION

Although painful experiences are a primary source of stress in the NICU, stress may also come from other sources, including environmental factors such as lighting or noise, sleep disruption, and abrupt or nongentle handling. Health care providers should try to reduce stress by keeping noise levels down and lighting conditions low and providing cue-based and two-person care, in which one caregiver calms the infant while the other provides care (e.g., diaper change). However, infant stress can be made worse by the lack of any parental presence; developmental care models facilitate closeness between parents and infants by emphasizing the importance of parental presence in the NICU. This also decreases the stress of separation experienced by parents.

Separation between parents and their infants has been postulated to be the most significant source of trauma and stress for parents and premature infants (Mäkelä et al. 2018; Sanders and Hall 2018). Parents have a strong desire to be close to their infant, but as shown by Mäkelä et al. (2018), NICU parents often experience a roller coaster of closeness and separation while their baby is hospitalized, consisting of moments of bonding followed by disruptions in parent–infant dynamics. The ability to be together as a family in the NICU was cherished by parents of NICU infants and promoted a feeling of normalcy when the usual rhythm and routine of the postpartum period was lost. Mäkelä et al. (2018) further showed that when parents were able to "store closeness," they were able to tolerate the separation and distance better.

For infants, the natural course after birth consists of physical and emotional closeness and connection with caregivers that ideally results in bidirectional regulation and leads to optimal attachment. Historically, the separation of infants and parents in the NICU was seen as inevitable to focus on and deliver medical treatments for infants. However, awareness of the deleterious effects of separation on infants and parents has increased and has led to attempts to make NICUs more family friendly and to provide space for parents to stay by the bedside as much as possible. Beyond the physical presence of parents in the NICU, some interventions now focus on involving parents more in their infant's care, for example, the Family Nurture Intervention (FNI) (Hane et al. 2015).

The relationship between parental and infant stress is not always linear. Although parental presence can mitigate infant distress during upsetting or painful procedures or events and lead to positive results in the parents' role attainment in caregiving after discharge, being present during such painful and difficult procedures does not always lead to decreased stress and may lead to increased rates of PTSD in some parents (Aite et al. 2016; Franck et al. 2011). Therefore, despite an emphasis on family-centered care in NICUs that promotes closeness between parents and infants and facilitates parental presence by the bedside, attention should be paid to parents who may need more emotional and psychological support during this time. Axelin et al. (2010) showed that although being engaged and alleviating their infant's pain and stress was a meaningful and positive experience for parents, they differed on their level of intrinsically motivated engagement in a de-stressing technique (facilitated tucking) based on factors such as level of maternal stress, attachment (including during pregnancy), and adaptation to motherhood. This points to a need for individualizing the level and style of support for parents. Importantly, physical and emotional closeness do not always co-occur, although in many cases physical closeness can facilitate emotional closeness.

SENSORY EXPERIENCES AND STIMULATIONS

Specific sensory experiences may be delivered as part of developmental care, with the primary focus on stress reduction or neural connectivity

(Pineda et al. 2017). Many of these experiences can be provided by the parents, thus allowing them to participate in infant care and supporting healthy parent–infant bonding. Participation in these activities has shown positive benefits for parental mental health as well as improvements in infant outcomes. Specific commonly used sensory experiences and their benefits are discussed and formal programs using these experiences are outlined in the following sections.

Tactile Stimulation

Kangaroo care. Tactile stimulation is the most frequently used and well-studied sensory intervention. In skin-to-skin care, also known as kangaroo care, parents hold their infant, clothed only in a diaper, against their bare chest. The practice began in resource-poor countries where medical equipment to ensure infant temperature control was scarce (Charpak et al. 1994). The rates of infant mortality rise when the infant's temperature drops. This led to using parents and other family members to keep the infant warm. Evidence of its medical benefits brought kangaroo care to resource-rich countries, where it is now a mainstay of infant developmental care in the NICU and universally encouraged, although at times unevenly practiced. Kangaroo care has been shown to benefit both parents and infants. In both term-born and moderately premature infants, kangaroo care reduces salivary cortisol levels and increases oxytocin; other benefits include better cardiorespiratory stability, fewer infections, increased rates of breastfeeding, shorter lengths of stay in the NICU, and positive neurodevelopmental impacts (Boundy et al. 2016). For parents, kangaroo care has been shown to reduce maternal anxiety and depression, and parents who practice it show more attachment behaviors toward their infant (De Alencar et al. 2009; Feldman et al. 2002; Tallandini and Scalembra 2006). However, some studies have failed to demonstrate consistent positive outcomes (Ahn et al. 2010; Chiu and Anderson 2009; Roberts et al. 2000). Kangaroo care has become a common component of multipronged interventions that positively impact parent mental health.

Containment touch. Most research supports gentle touch as an infant calming technique that may reduce stress and improve sleep (Harrison 2010; Im and Kim 2009). Commonly used as an intervention by bedside nurses either during or after infant care times, positive touch, also called *containment touch*, involves placing still hands on the infant's head, abdomen, or limbs and using gentle pressure to mimic the sensation of being in the womb. For parents, this interaction is often among the first offered, particularly for extremely premature or critically ill infants. Research on this simple touch alone is limited, but it may be seen in continuum with kangaroo care as a positive sensory experience linking parents and infants in the NICU.

Simply being held may have positive outcomes for the infant. More hours of parental visitation and holding have been linked with better neurobehavioral measures in premature infants at term equivalence (Reynolds et al. 2013). Surprisingly, some NICU parents may struggle with providing appropriate gentle touch; their fundamental urge for parent–infant interaction often leads to more stimulating touch, including stroking and patting, even when the infant is too immature or medically unstable for this interaction. These parents gain a psychological reward from the response it elicits from their infant, even if it leads to a stress cue or cardiorespiratory change. Unfortunately, medical providers often respond harshly to parent overstimulation in their effort to protect the infant. A construct of the medical provider as parent coach in the care of the infant has been explored as part of the family integrated care model and may be a more effective way to educate and redirect parent–infant interactions in these circumstances.

Infant massage.   Infant massage involves applying systematic tactile stimulation to areas of an infant's body using stroking, stretching, and gentle compression. The goal is to both reduce infant stress and facilitate parent–infant bonding. Although this is seemingly at odds with other developmental goals of reducing stimulation, proponents of infant massage compare the experience with that of the womb, wherein the fetus received constant tactile stimulation from the amniotic fluid and gradual and intermittent pressure from the uterine walls. Infant massage has been shown to improve infant weight gain (Badr et al. 2015) and responses to painful procedures (Chik et al. 2017), shorten lengths of stay when paired with a parent empowerment program (Moradi et al. 2018), and improve time to full feeding and feed tolerance (Choi et al. 2016; Fontana et al. 2018). For parents, infant massage lowers maternal anxiety (Afand et al. 2017) and is associated with a more rapid decline in depressive symptoms and improved parental satisfaction (Holditch-Davis et al. 2013, 2014).

Auditory Stimulation

The normal environment for a healthy-term infant is an auditory-rich home that includes exposure to human speech and, often, music. Prior to birth, fetuses are normally cocooned in a world of sound as the womb supplies a backdrop of voices, digestive noises, and maternal heartbeat (Lahav and Skoe 2014). Both language exposure and music are used as developmental care practices to enrich the auditory experience of infants in the NICU.

Language exposure.   Language exposure is known to be important for speech and language outcomes in infants and children (Gilkerson et al. 2018; Hart and Risley 1992; Rowe 2008). The same has been shown to be true for premature infants in the NICU. A paucity of language exposure from low parent visitation rates and single-patient rooms was found to be associated with poor development of language centers in the brain and lower scores on speech and language outcome measures at 2 years of age in premature infants (Pineda et al. 2014). While recommendations for the quantity and timing of language exposure in the NICU are still being evaluated, soft talking and singing to premature infants have shown benefits at gestational ages as young as 25 weeks, when the infant's sense of hearing is only just developed. Possible auditory exposures include talking, reading, and singing. Exposure to parental reading may improve cardiorespiratory stability (Scala et al. 2018), feed tolerance (Krueger et al. 2010), and neurodevelopmental outcomes (Picciolini et al. 2014) and reduce infant stress. Voice exposure is also used in some multimodal interventions (e.g., FNI). Bedside picture-book reading by parents has shown to improve their feelings of closeness to and intimacy with their infant (Lariviere and Rennick 2011).

Music exposure. Music exposure may involve soft singing by parents or other caregivers and live or recorded music, usually lullabies. Music exposure has been shown to improve infant feeding (Chorna et al. 2014) and cardiorespiratory stability (Arnon et al. 2014) and maternal stress (Loewy 2015) and to reduce infant stress (Picciolini et al. 2014) and responses to pain (Bergomi et al. 2014). Music has also been integrated into multimodal stimulation experiences (e.g., Arnon et al. 2014) in which combined kangaroo care and maternal singing resulted in positive benefits. Although with all sound exposure care must be taken to maintain safe decibel levels, parent involvement in auditory exposure is another mode of parent–infant interaction in the NICU. Evidence is sparse for the impact of music therapy as an interactive experience with infants, although music therapy has been demonstrated to have positive effects on anxiety and stress in parents (Roa and Ettenberger 2018). Two studies compared the impact of combining music plus kangaroo care with kangaroo care alone and found positive effects of music on parental anxiety (Ettenberger et al. 2017; Schlez et al. 2011).

Visual Stimulation

Infants' visual acuity is poor compared with that of older children and adults; full-term infants can focus well only as far as the distance between an adult's lap and that adult's face. Premature infants at the lowest gestations may be born with fused eyelids; however, discriminative visual function has been documented by 31–32 weeks. For these reasons, visual stimulation has not been a prominent part of premature infant developmental care until closer to term gestation and has focused primarily on the infant fixing and following a human face, preferably the parent. There is some concern that visual input before the infant is developmentally ready may alter the normal development of other sensory inputs and integration/processing, prompting low-lit NICU conditions, although many centers use cycled lighting protocols to induce infants' circadian rhythm development and neuroprotective melatonin production and improve weight gain (Vasquez-Ruiz et al. 2014). However, this approach has been reconsidered due to brain impacts from auditory paucity. Animal studies have shown increased development of the visual cortex through visual stimulation (Bourgeois et al. 1989; Volpe 2019), and at least one small study linked exposure to visual patterns with improvements in behavioral organization in premature infants (Marshall-Baker et al. 1998). More research in this area is needed with regard to optimizing infant outcomes; however, more stable and mature infants should be allowed face-to-face stimulation from their parents. Mother–infant bonding also has been related to maternal response to infant facial cues (Dudek et al. 2018).

Olfactory Stimulation

The human sense of smell is often overlooked but is actively engaged in subtle connections between infants and their parents. Maternal skin or breast milk odors can be used to calm infants in the NICU (Maayan-Metzger et al. 2018), may reduce pain scores for mildly painful procedures (Baudesson de Chanville et al. 2017; Zhang et al. 2018), and may promote oral feeding (Davidson et al. 2019). Olfactory signals are important mediators of maternal–infant bonding in mammals; newborn odor triggers dopaminergic responses in the thalami of new mothers but not other women (Lundstrom et al. 2013), suggesting that infant odors may also mediate bonding in humans. Mothers with healthy parent–infant bonds have been shown to prefer their own infant's scent to that of other infants, while mothers with bonding difficulties did not. Mothers with bonding issues could not identify their child's smell over chance (Croy et al. 2019). Use of olfactory cloth scent exchange is part of FNI, a multi-intervention program that has shown positive impacts on the quality of maternal caregiving (Hane et al. 2015; see "Family Nurture Intervention" later in this chapter).

Vestibular Stimulation

Rocking a baby is a normal healthy-term experience that calms the infant by recreating the experience of rocking in the womb. NICU infants often fail to receive stimulation of this kind, and evidence for its individual use is limited. Gentle rocking is a part of several multimodal sensory exposures and has been coupled with many of the experiences already described. The Auditory, Tactile, Visual, and Vestibular (ATVV) intervention, discussed in the following section, includes a vestibular stimulus in its sequence of sensory experiences and is the best-studied multimodal intervention using a vestibular component (White-Traut et al. 2002).

Multimodal Interventions

A number of studies have evaluated the effect of combining multiple sensory activities or exposures either simultaneously or in sequence. Practically, most NICUs have local guidelines regarding any developmental care activities with combined sensory interventions that occur on an unregulated basis. Parents doing skin-to-skin care may decide to read, sing softly, or talk to their infants during massage sessions. Formalized combinations of developmental sensory experiences have shown benefits for infants and parents. Several multimodal studies that combined kangaroo care with music or voice exposure and massage with either olfactory stimulation or kinesthetic stimulation also showed some benefits in maternal stress reduction (Arnon et al. 2014), infant stress reduction (Hernandez-Reif et al. 2007), and infant neurodevelopment (Procianoy et al. 2010).

ATTV is a sequenced sensory approach combining auditory, tactile, visual, and vestibular stimulation (White-Traut et al. 2002). This multimodal intervention was shown to improve developmental outcomes, infant tolerance to handling, and feeding, although other studies that used ATTV failed to replicate these results. Parental benefits include reduced parenting stress and improvement in depressive symptoms (Holditch-Davis et al. 2014). This developmental care sensory construct has been used in multimodal interventions described later in the chapter (see "Multicomponent Interventions").

Other combinations of sensory experiences are currently being studied. Neel et al. (2019) proposed a multisensory intervention for infants starting at 32 weeks' postmenstrual age that included recorded parental voice; kangaroo care plus additional holding; light pressure containment; a parent's voice recorded on a pacifier, which is triggered by infant sucking; parent-scented olfactory stimulation; and vestibular stimulation via therapist chest movements. Primary outcomes are brain-based measures of multisensory processing using time-locked electroencephalography. Secondary outcomes include sensory adaptation, speech sound differentiation, tactile processing, and motor and language function measured at 1 and 2 years' corrected gestational age using Bayley scales and a Infant Toddler Sensory Profile. Published protocols do not include parental responses to this program, and the degree of direct parental involvement in several of these components is unclear.

ROLE OF HEALTH CARE PROVIDERS

Premature birth or birth of a medically ill infant often creates a situation in which parents may not feel competent or confident and struggle to assume their parental role. NICU staff and the infant's health care providers take on a critical role not only in the infant's medical care and survival but also in coaching parents to be active participants in their infant's care. Parents commonly have difficulties understanding their infant's behavioral cues, not knowing how and whether it is safe to touch or hold their infant or to how reduce the infant's stress and pain. NICU staff can be a major source of support and learning for parents so that they can be physically and emotionally close to their infants and mitigate their distress.

Interestingly, and in a somewhat similar fashion, nursing and NICU staff can help mitigate parental stress caused by the inevitable separations and possible disruptions in establishing a parental role. Good relationships between the parents and NICU staff promote parental well-being (Mäkelä et al. 2018), and when parents are able to trust the care their infant is receiving in their absence, it can ameliorate the difficulty and anxiety that separation brings. When the NICU staff is able to use empathy, attunement, and trauma-informed ways of interacting with parents, they will be able to decrease parents' stress, increase their sense of capability, support parent–infant interactions and bonding, and improve outcomes for parents and infants. Therefore, many programs focus both on educating the NICU staff regarding these methods (Hall et al. 2019) and on using them as sources of mentorship and education for parents and for implementing specific interventions.

IMPACT OF THE NICU ENVIRONMENT

Activities in the NICU between parents and their infants to support parental and infant psychological health may only happen if the parents are available and feel welcomed, engaged, and comfortable at the infant's bedside. Shifts in NICU design have improved access to single-family rooms that allow more parental presence (Pineda et al. 2012). Parents may find that the quiet space and more natural lighting afforded in these rooms make the NICU feel more like a "healing environment" (Kotzer et al. 2011). Studies comparing infants who were cared for in open bay units with infants cared for in single-family rooms found improved neurobehavioral and medical outcomes for babies in the latter, including greater weight gain, reduced rates of infection and chronic lung disease, improved attention and muscular tone, higher scores on neurodevelopmental testing at 18–24 months, and shorter lengths of NICU stay (Domanico et al. 2010; Lester et al. 2014, 2016; Ortenstrand et al. 2010; Vohr et al. 2017). Some of the positive differences were mediated by greater developmental support, and some (e.g., signs of stress and pain as well as higher cognitive scores) by more maternal involvement, which has been found to be higher in single-family rooms (Jones et al. 2016; Lester et al. 2016; Raiskila et al. 2017).

Single-family rooms have been associated with more stress in NICU mothers in some studies (Pineda et al. 2012) and in more social isolation from other NICU parents (Domanico et al. 2010). However, most parents expressed improved satisfaction with their infant's care (Stevens et al. 2012), and preference for this room type increased with greater length of stay (Domanico et al. 2010). As more NICUs transition to this model, care should be taken to provide emotional support and opportunities to connect parents with other NICU families.

Some NICUs have taken the single-patient room a step further, integrating parents more fully into the infant's daily care. This has required a frame shift on the part of nurses, who must transition from being the primary caregivers themselves to becoming educators and coaches for parents who are assuming their parental roles in the NICU as well as taking on tasks previously assigned only to nurses. The FiCare system in Canada requires parents to be active participants in infant care for a minimum of 6–8 hours per day. Parents receive education and bedside nursing support that allows them to take a more active role in their infant's care. Outcomes include improved infant weight gain, decreased parental stress and anxiety, and improved rates of breastfeeding (O'Brien et al. 2018). Providing facilities where parents can stay with their infants from admission to discharge takes family integration a step further. In Sweden, providing family areas adjacent to NICU infants shortened lengths of stay (Ortenstrand et al. 2010). A similar program in Italy that supported parental involvement for 8 hours per day reduced parental stress and improved infant weight gain (De Bernardo et al. 2017).

Parental mood may also be negatively affected by the lighting environment of the NICU, which may disrupt their circadian rhythms either through exposure to low lighting conditions or altered rhythms due to artificial lighting. Light exposure has been linked to sleep disturbance and depression in NICU mothers (Lee and Kimble 2009).

Infant Mental Health and Parent–Infant Psychotherapy

The parents' relationship with their infant begins in the prenatal period in the parents' minds. They form thoughts and fantasies about their infant, their own transition to parenthood, and the expansion of their family (referred to as parental representational world or internal working models) (Stern 1998; Zeanah et al. 1985). Parents' perceptions and representations of their infants and their parent–infant interactions are influenced by parental characteristics, including their history of trauma (Chamberlain et al. 2019; Schechter et al. 2006). When infants are born prematurely or ill, these fantasies and images may be disrupted in ways that can affect parental emotional well-being and the way parents see, experience, and interact with the infant. Moreover, having a premature or medically vulnerable infant may create barriers in the parents' psychological transition into parenthood, their role assumption, and feelings of competence. These stressors have consequences for the child's mental health and development as well as parental mental health and the parent–infant relationship (Borghini et al. 2006; González-Serrano et al. 2012; Hall et al. 2015; Korja et al. 2012; Provenzi and Santoro 2015; Spinelli et al. 2016). Premature infants often do not show the same behavior cues as term infants and are less alert. Thus, families in the NICU may struggle to establish an optimal relationship due to their infant's medical vulnerabilities, their own emotional and psychological reactions to the infant's health, the reduced degree of infant engagement, a history of trauma in the family, or parental psychopathology, among others.

The research on relationships between NICU infants and their caregivers has focused on the quality of interactions, maternal sensitivity, parental representational mind, parental attachment representations, and patterns of attachment. Importantly, due to biological and psychological factors, there may be differences among groups of extremely low gestational age (ELGA), very low gestational age (VLGA), and late premature infants and their parents. More studies are needed to investigate these potential differences as they relate to the parent–infant relationship and infant psychological outcomes. Some of the more commonly used terms and concepts in the field of infant mental health are defined in Table 4–1.

Infant illness and immaturity necessitate that much of the infant's care be done by health care providers with specific training in neonatology. This replacement of their role as primary caregiver has been identified as one of the major sources of stress for parents (Woodward et al. 2014) and can impair the developing parent–infant bond and impede or create challenges in the psychological transition of parents into parenthood. Infants admitted to the NICU may be too premature or too ill to give recognizable cues or be engaged in typical interactions with their caregivers in the same way that term infants do. For many parents, this leads to uncertainty as to how to engage with their infant, while the failure to understand the infant's cues may lead to patterns of withdrawal or attempts to engage that result in infant overstimulation. In both scenarios, parents are likely to receive negative feedback from bedside providers that their infant interaction is inappropriate. Although such feedback is well meaning, it tells the parent that the health care provider is more competent in caring for the infant and increases the barriers to parent engagement.

PARENT–INFANT INTERACTIONS AND MATERNAL SENSITIVITY IN THE NICU

The research to date on maternal representations in mothers of premature and medically vulnerable infants has not shown a clear pattern. Al-

---

Table 4–1. Glossary of terms in infant mental health

Parental sensitivity

Parents' ability to be aware of and understand the meaning behind the infant's behavior and to see the infant as a person with autonomous feelings, such as hopes, needs, wishes, and goals (Grossmann et al. 2013). To have a reasonable level of sensitivity, parents must be accessible and have a reasonable threshold for picking up on the infant's communications and responding to them. Parents show a range of thresholds in noticing, understanding, and responding to their infant's cues. To properly understand and make meaning of these communications, parents should be aware of them, not distort them, and have empathy (Leerkes et al. 2004). Maternal sensitivity is one of the main factors in the development of a healthy relationship and a secure attachment between the parent and the child.

Parental representational mind

The parent's mind creates the stage on which the infant's psychological life will begin (Gilmore and Meersand 2014). Parents develop ideas, images, and fantasies in their minds of who their baby is, how the baby will look, what their relationship with the baby will be, and who they are going to be as parents. These fantasies and ideas are called *representations*. For many parents, representations start developing prior to pregnancy and, for most parents, evolve and change throughout their life and pregnancy. Representations are significantly affected by the parents' own history, their major relationships and the quality of these relationships, how they were cared for as children, traumatic or significant incidents in their lives, their beliefs and culture, and their hopes and fears, among other factors (Stern 1998).

Parent–infant interactions

During infancy and early childhood, the interactions and relationship between parents and the infant affect the infant's physical, emotional, and cognitive development. Parent–infant interactions are directly affected by parental sensitivity and responsiveness and are significantly influenced not only by parental emotions and representational mind but also by what the infant brings to the relationship in terms of temperament, cues, needs, and ways of responding to the parent. When assessing parent–infant interactions, some of what is evaluated includes the initiation of physical and emotional contact between the parents and infant; the quality of touch, gaze, and vocalization; synchrony; and mutuality as well as the consistency and contingency of interactions and responses and levels of playfulness, pleasure, hostility, and blame. On the infant's side, it is important to evaluate the infant's ability to communicate, seek comfort, and be soothed. When parents and infants engage in positive, contingent, and sensitive interactions, infants do better in social emotional, language, and cognitive development and tend to form more secure attachments (Wyly 2018).

Table 4–1.	Glossary of terms in infant mental health *(continued)*

Attachment

"Attachment describes the infant's tendency to seek comfort, support and nurturance, and protection, selectively from a small number of caregivers" (Finelli et al. 2019, p. 452). Throughout this process, they become more selective about from whom they seek protection and comfort and form their own "internal working models" of relationships. They also become selective in choosing and attaching salience to incoming information in their social interactions and the way they make meaning of these interactions (Finelli et al. 2019). Attachment patterns are strong predictors of childhood and adulthood mental and emotional health. Using the Strange Situation protocol, during which the parent and infant go through phases of exploration—introduction to a stranger, separations, and reunions—four main attachment classifications have been identified in children (Solomon and George 2016). These consist of

1. Secure attachment (child is able to use parent as a secure base and a reliable source of comfort and protection, explore when the parent is present, and feels upset at separation but is able to reunite with parent and eventually return to exploration)

2. Anxious-avoidant attachment (child is able to explore without using parent as a secure base, is not distressed by the separation, and avoids parent at reunion)

3. Anxious-ambivalent or resistant attachment (child is distressed by the separation but also does not feel comforted or reassured by parent and can give mixed signals of seeking closeness with and rejecting parent)

4. Disorganized attachment (child's behavior does not seem to fit any of the other three attachment patterns)

Ports of entry

Parents and infants their form a unit in which their interactions affect each other. These interactions are, in turn, influenced by aspects of their internal world, including emotions, thoughts, and beliefs. Various considerations determine which are the best targets for intervention for each dyad/triad and at any given point in time. However, no matter what the therapist focuses on in the parent–infant unit, these interventions may result in changes in the entire system (Stern 1998).

Reflective functioning

"Reflective functioning refers to the essential human capacity to understand behavior in the light of underlying mental states and intentions" (Slade 2005, p. 269). Parental capacity to be reflective (parental reflective functioning) is tied to the development of secure attachment and better self and affect regulation (Slade 2005).

though some studies have shown that mothers of very low or extremely low birth weight infants have more negative representations of their infant and see them as weak and fragile, other researchers have found no increased rate of disrupted representations in mothers of premature infants compared with their initial expectation (Cox et al. 2000; González-Serrano et al. 2012; Hall et al. 2015). However, some studies have shown mothers of premature infants to have lower coherence and intensity of involvement; less richness of perceptions, openness to change, and acceptance; and more fear for their infant's safety in their representations (Borghini et al. 2006; Korja et al. 2009). These distortions in the quality of maternal representations of their premature and medically ill infant can have concerning implications for mother–child dynamics and relationship. Notably, most research has been done on maternal characteristics and behaviors, but it is also important to consider fathers and other parenting figures.

Consensus is also lacking about the level of maternal sensitivity and quality of mother–infant interactions in mothers of premature and medically fragile infants. In some studies, these mothers, especially with ongoing parenting support and interventions aimed at decreasing stress, have been described as being sensitive and contingently responsive despite their infants being less positively engaged in interactions. In addition, the quality of their interactions with premature infants is the same as that of mothers of full-term infants, especially within the second half of the first year (Korja et al. 2012; Montirosso et al. 2010). At the same time, mothers of premature infants, especially those with extremely low birth weight, have been described as more intrusive, controlling, and hyperstimulating. It is not clear whether this level of intrusiveness or unilateral engagement is an attempt to compensate for the infant's lack of response or engagement or is related to a higher level of maternal anxiety regarding their child's development (Bozzette 2006; Cox et al. 2000; Forcada-Guex et al. 2011). Mothers of premature infants have also been described as playing and smiling less; having less facial responsiveness but more vocal responses; having less matching and imitation of facial gestures; being less engaged in general, with fewer face-to-face interactions; and being less responsive to the infant's negative emotions, including sadness or anger (Korja et al. 2012; Malatesta et al. 1986; Schmücker et al. 2005). Some research has led to concern about co-regulatory processes in very preterm infants and their parents and has highlighted the need for early intervention to help these dyads (Sansavini et al. 2015).

ATTACHMENT

Attachment research in infants who are born prematurely or require a NICU stay has, for the most part, not shown an increased rate of insecure attachment (see Table 4–1) when compared with full-term infants. However, lower socioeconomic status and lower birth weight may be risk factors for insecure attachment (Korja et al. 2012; Wolke et al. 2014). More evidence is available to support a higher rate of disorganized attachment in these dyads (Cox et al. 2000; Pennestri et al. 2015; Wolke et al. 2014). It is possible that neurodevelopmental issues, such as increased prevalence of neurological sequelae, may be partly responsible for these findings. NICU admission in term infants has been found to cause a sixfold increase in the rate of disorganized attachment at age 36 months, independent of child neurodevelopmental factors, maternal sensitivity, or other parental factors (Pennestri et al. 2015). In effect, having and being separated from a medically ill infant can be traumatic experiences for parents that, if not resolved, may lead to patterns of avoidance and to frightened or frightening behavior that could result in disorganized attachment (Pennestri et al. 2015).

More recently, emphasis has been placed on the importance of emotional connection, resilience, and co-regulation rather than on outcomes such as attachment (Bergman et al. 2019). For this construct, the infant's first 1,000 minutes are deemed to be a critical period during which sensory inputs such as endocrine, olfactory, visual, tactile, and auditory facilitate emotional connection that is "analogous to the force between two magnets." Bergman et al. (2019) proposed that premature birth or early separation can break this force, causing avoidance behavior between the mother and infant.

Although treatment of maternal psychological distress and postpartum depression is widely assumed to reduce parenting stress and facilitate an improved parent–child relationship, data do not support this contention (Horwitz et al. 2015). Forman et al. (2007), in a study on psychotherapy to help mothers with postpartum depression interact with their infants, showed that at 18-month follow-up, mothers with depression who received interpersonal psychotherapy still rated their children lower on attachment security, higher on behavioral problems, and more negatively on temperament than did mothers without depression. By contrast, interventions utilizing video feedback in mothers with postpartum depression improved parent–infant interactions without changing ratings of maternal depression (Field 2010). These data suggest that treatment of maternal psychological distress is not sufficient for addressing parent–infant relational problems and that interventions must also focus on parent–infant interactions.

PARENT–INFANT PSYCHOTHERAPY

Currently, developmental care programs are the primary support for the mental health of NICU infants. However, mental health professionals have increasingly recognized and implemented dyadic and family interventions. Infant mental health interventions in the NICU target the relationship between infants and caregivers as one of the main external environmental contexts for infants, given the extensive evidence of its role in mitigating distress and its long-term effects on the child's psychological, mental, and physical health. Various philosophies of intervention use different ports of entry (see Table 4–1) to create change in the dyadic (parent–infant) or family system. Some approaches focus on understanding and changing the negative parental representational mind toward their infant or toward themselves as parents. As discussed earlier, these representations can be affected by many factors, such as the parents' history with their own caregivers; past traumas in their lives; current traumas, such as birth trauma, prematurity, or medical illness in their infant; conflicts with their partner or other close family members; and other psychosocial traumas. Others focus on helping parents see the infant for who the infant is, thus becoming more observant and increasing their reflective functioning (see Table 4–1) and, as a result, responding to the infant in a more contingent and sensitive way. Interventions might target observed interactions between parents and infants, such as the way parents hold, feed, soothe, play with, and look at their infant. This is a strength-based work aimed at helping parents becoming more confident, competent, and sensitively responsive.

Attention is also paid to the dynamics within the parental couple and family, including siblings and extended family involved in helping with childcare. Parents are supported by receiving developmental guidelines or practical and strategic help with other psychosocial and case management matters that enables them to be at the bedside. For example, financial difficulties, worries about job security, lack of somewhere to stay near the hospital, difficulty in commuting, and childcare concerns for other children in the family may affect parents' ability to be physically or emotionally present at their infant's bedside. Infant mental health interventions should be informed by the cultural context of each family. In the next section we first describe an adaptation of an evidence-based model of intervention in the NICU and then an approach that is not a psychotherapy intervention but aims at reestablishing the emotional connection and mutual co-regulation between NICU infants and their parents.

Child–Parent Psychotherapy

Child–parent psychotherapy (CPP) is a relationship-based dyadic intervention for infants and young children that aims to restore an optimal developmental trajectory for parents and children who have experienced a traumatic event or are experiencing challenges in their attachment relationship (Lakatos et al. 2019). CPP is an evidence-based treatment that enhances healing for infants and their caregivers through a relational and trauma-informed model of care. Although CPP is more of a longer-term treatment model, Lakatos et al. (2019) modified the intervention to match the length of stay for infants and families in the NICU. CPP may involve just 1 or 2 sessions or up to 10 sessions for families, based on their needs. In their pilot program, the authors used the six modalities of CPP: facilitating developmental progress, providing reflective developmental guidance, encouraging appropriate protective behavior, providing emotional support and empathic communication, interpreting the feelings and actions of parents and infants, and providing crisis interventions, case management, and concrete assistance. This is an ongoing pilot study, and the authors have not currently published any results for their intervention.

Family Nurture Intervention

FNI targets infants born between 26 and 34 weeks' postmenstrual age (PMA) and their parents, with a view that premature birth and the resulting separation are traumatic for infants and mothers and can disrupt the emotional connection and autonomic co-regulation between them. FNI focuses on autonomic emotional connection and emotional communication between parents and infants rather than on attachment and bonding. It was designed based on the polyvagal theory, in which the autonomic state provides a neurophysiological platform for optimal co-regulation between infants and caregivers. This can lead to regulation of the physiological state and social engagement through vagal effects on heart rate, facial gestures, and gaze, among others (Porges et al. 2019). FNI uses a series of techniques to promote closeness and emotional connection, some of which are not necessarily new or unique to FNI but are used to develop the emotional and physical connection and autonomic co-regulation in the parent–infant dyad. FNI is frequently carried out by trained nurture specialists and consists of components such as teaching mothers to talk to their infant for prolonged periods of time; express various emotions, including sadness; improve eye contact; use firm touch; swap a cotton cloth between herself and the baby to help with olfactory connection; and hold when appropriate (skin-to-skin and non-skin-to-skin). Mothers implement these measures with support and help from the nurture specialist to develop calmness for both herself and her baby. These are called *calming sessions*. Furthermore, FNI involves educating the family about the emotional needs of the premature infant and supporting the mother and infant to continue the calming cycles (Porges et al. 2019). FNI has been shown to increase maternal sensitivity levels at 36 weeks' PMA and high-frequency electroencephalogram results at 41 weeks' PMA, to decrease depression and anxiety at 4 months' corrected age, and to improve Bayley Scales of Infant Development–III scores at 18 months' corrected age. FNI has also been associated with fewer attention problems noted on the Child Behavior Checklist, a decreased risk for social emotional problems assessed using the Modified Checklist for Autism in Toddlers–Revised, accelerated brain maturity in frontal regions, and increased cardiac vagal nerve tone and autoregulation (Porges et al. 2019).

Treating Parental Psychological Distress

Early interventions to reduce distress of parents with premature infants consisted of supportive therapy and self-help techniques. Several studies assessed parent support by pairing new NICU mothers with a NICU "graduate" (Preyde and Ardal 2003; Roman et al. 1995) or examined self-help discussion groups led by a nurse and NICU graduate (Minde 2000). Other researchers have used journal writing or kangaroo care as a way to help parents come to terms with their NICU experience and to facilitate mother–newborn contact (Anderson et al. 2003). A relatively smaller number of studies evaluated intervention programs focused on reducing symptoms of parental anxiety (Cobiella et al. 1990; Kaaresen et al. 2008). However, early studies in this population neither included the well-documented treatment components known to be effective in treating PTSD nor focused on the trauma associated with having a medically fragile infant and loss of the parental role.

CRITICAL INCIDENT STRESS DEBRIEFING

Since the mid-1980s, single-session interventions have been developed for the prevention and treatment of both acute stress disorder and PTSD. This category of psychological interventions, often referred to as *critical incident stress debriefing*, was proposed as a form of crisis intervention rather than as a psychological treatment. Delivered shortly after the trauma exposure, often within 2–3 days, psychological debriefing involves encouraging participants to give a narrative account of the traumatic experience, including their related emotions and thoughts. Meta-analyses of studies of this approach have concluded that no evidence supports its efficacy, and some evidence suggests that it may, in fact, be harmful (Rose et al. 2003). As a result, this category of intervention is not recommended for routine use and has not been tested or validated in the NICU setting.

TRAUMA-FOCUSED COGNITIVE BEHAVIORAL THERAPY

Trauma-focused cognitive behavioral therapy (TF-CBT) is another category of interventions using a classic cognitive behavioral therapy (CBT) approach. It consists of several sessions delivered within 3–5 weeks of the traumatic exposure (Foa et al. 1995). Many RCTs have demonstrated the efficacy of comparable brief early CBT. TF-CBT has been shown to be effective in the treatment of acute stress disorder in civilian trauma survi-

Table 4–2.	Components of trauma-focused cognitive behavioral therapy

1. Psychoeducation about the typical trauma response

2. Cognitive restructuring to identify and challenge dysfunctional and erroneous cognitions about the trauma and replace these with functional and realistic cognitions

3. Self-distraction or thought stopping

4. Relaxation training, which may include controlled breathing, Progressive Muscle Relaxation, or hypnosis

5. Imaginal exposure (subject is instructed to recount a version of the traumatic event in the present tense, which is recorded and replayed to encourage subject to confront avoided aspects of the traumatic situation) or in vivo exposure to the stressful traumatic event

6. Structured writing therapy that encourages patients to reflect upon their coping strategies in response to the trauma and promotes social sharing and support, the lack of which is a major predictor of PTSD (van Emmerik et al. 2008)

Source.   Nemeroff et al. 2006.

vors and victims with mild traumatic brain injury and acute symptoms of PTSD in physically injured trauma victims (Schnurr et al. 2007; Sijbrandij et al. 2007). The core components of TF-CBT are shown in Table 4–2.

A recent meta-analysis of PTSD treatment in 70 studies concluded that TF-CBT was significantly better than waitlist/usual care or other techniques, including self-help booklets and non-trauma-focused supportive psychotherapy, in reducing the symptoms of PTSD (Bisson et al. 2013). There is also evidence that individual TF-CBT, eye movement desensitization and reprocessing (EMDR), stress management, and group TF-CBT are effective in treating PTSD. Other non-trauma-focused psychological treatments were not found to reduce PTSD symptoms as significantly; in particular, both TF-CBT and EMDR were superior at 1- and 4-month outcomes. In explaining the efficacy of the brief early TF-CBT programs in reducing symptoms of PTSD, anxiety, and depression, Foa and Kozak (1986) suggested that repeated imaginal exposure to the traumatic incident results in a reduction in fear based on the hypothesis that habituation to the emotional responses develops between sessions through imaginal reliving of the trauma. It is also believed that the irrational beliefs, commonly seen in PTSD, of being incompetent and helpless are corrected with cognitive restructuring and the acquisition of skills such as relaxation and anxiety reduction.

In considering the application of these techniques to the NICU situation, one important consideration is that this traumatic event is unlike many other single-incident traumas that lend themselves to the techniques of imaginal exposure, a core component of TF-CBT. In the NICU, the source of the trauma is deeply embedded with the parents' infant, and the traumatic stress may be a continuous and ongoing experience. As a result, intervention approaches in the NICU rely more heavily on so-called stress inoculation training techniques, which include relaxation training, thought stopping, cognitive restructuring, and roleplay (Nemeroff et al. 2006).

Two early treatments intended to both reduce and prevent the development of trauma-related symptoms in new mothers of premature infants have been evaluated (Table 4–3) (Bernard et al. 2011; Jotzo and Poets 2005). Bernard et al.'s (2011) brief CBT intervention consisted of three 45-minute sessions delivered during a 2-week period while the infant was still in the hospital. The intervention used a CBT model with the goal of reducing symptoms of depression, anxiety, trauma, and general distress. Specific CBT-based skills such as cognitive restructuring and relaxation techniques were taught, and the common thoughts and feelings of NICU parents, the characteristics of premature infants, and effective communication skills in the NICU setting were discussed. This intervention was evaluated in a pilot study with 56 mothers of premature infants. Although the intervention did not significantly reduce trauma symptoms, it did result in decreased depression symptoms. The authors hypothesized that their intervention either was too brief in nature or did not specifically target the mother's traumatic reactions.

Jotzo and Poets (2005) developed a trauma-focused intervention piloted with 25 mothers that started a few days after the birth of their infants. This intervention followed a primary prevention model consisting of an initial crisis intervention, meetings approximately two times per week, daily visits at critical times, such as surgery, and the opportunity to ask for additional appointments. Treatment components included

1. Reconstructing what happened immediately prior to and following the infant's birth
2. Introducing relaxation and calming techniques
3. Providing education about trauma and stress reactions
4. Providing support at times of emotional strife
5. Exploring coping mechanisms, such as personal resources, social support, and practical problem solving
6. Exploring the parents' perception of their infant and potential for avoidance behaviors
7. Eliciting the mother's detailed history regarding pregnancy and delivery in order to identify specific traumatic events
8. Discussing the parent–infant relationship and parental role
9. Exploring reactions to the NICU situation and encouraging parents to express criticisms

The authors found that their intervention resulted in significant reductions in all categories of trauma symptoms assessed using the Impact of

Table 4–3. Interventions specifically targeting parental PTSD

Authors	Population	Methods	Design	Outcomes	Results
Bernard et al. 2011	Single-site study of 56 mothers of NICU infants, <37 weeks and >1,000 g and expected to survive. A total of 305 mothers were eligible, but 196 not recruited due to hospital transfer. Another 7 mothers dropped out of the intervention group, leaving equal numbered groups.	Brief cognitive behavioral intervention. Three-session CBT-based intervention aimed to reduce general anxiety, depression, and PTSD in NICU parents. The intervention consisted of three 45- to 55-minute sessions of individual therapy focused on different skills (e.g., relaxation techniques, cognitive restructuring, and communicating effectively with NICU staff).	RCT. Control group received standard care, which included contact with physicians, nurses, social workers, and chaplaincy when requested.	DTS SASRQ BDI-II	Reduced level of depression symptoms ($P = 0.06$) Trend toward lower levels of trauma symptoms ($P = 0.23$) 86% of mothers found the intervention beneficial

Table 4–3. **Interventions specifically targeting parental PTSD** *(continued)*

Authors	Population	Methods	Design	Outcomes	Results
Jotzo and Poets 2005	Single-site study of mothers of NICU infants <37 weeks, with no congenital anomalies, and expected stay of ≥14 days. Of 217 mothers screened, 102 were eligible; 58 were included in the study and 50 in the analysis.	Trauma preventative psychological intervention. Trauma-focused treatment utilized early crisis intervention and extra support at critical times. Treatment included reconstructing what happened immediately before and after birth, introducing relaxation and calming techniques, normalizing stress and trauma reactions, and exploring coping strategies.	Sequential control group design. Control group mothers were able to ask for counseling by a minister in the hospital.	IES PLI-Q	Reduced IES symptoms: Overall trauma ($P=0.013$) Intrusion ($P=0.055$) Avoidance ($P=0.023$) Hyperarousal ($P=0.019$)

Table 4–3. Interventions specifically targeting parental PTSD *(continued)*

Authors	Population	Methods	Design	Outcomes	Results
Shaw et al. 2013, 2014	Single-site study of mothers of NICU infants 25–34 weeks, >600 g, with no congenital anomalies and expected to survive. Of 196 mothers screened, 157 were eligible; 105 were randomized to treatment and 98 were included in the analysis.	TF-CBT. Six-session intervention targeting PTSD, anxiety, and depression. Sessions lasted 45–50 minutes and were designed to teach relaxation, cognitive restructuring, trauma narrative, and changing negative perceptions of the infant and the parenting experience.	RCT. Control group received one 45-minute information session about the NICU environment and education about parenting premature infants.	DTD SASQR BDI-II BAI	4- to 5-week outcomes: Reduced level of trauma symptoms ($P=0.023$) Reduced level of depression symptoms ($P<0.001$) Trend toward lower levels of trauma symptoms ($P=0.23$) 6-month outcomes: Reduced level of trauma symptoms ($P<0.001$) Reduced level of depressive symptoms ($P=0.001$) Reduced level of anxiety
Horsch et al. 2016	Single-site study of 67 mothers of preterm infants, <32 weeks or <1,500 g, studied at 3 months' corrected age.	Expressive writing for 15 minutes a day for 3 consecutive days.	RCT. Control group received usual care.	PPQ EPDS SF-36	3- to 4-month outcomes: Reduced level of trauma symptoms ($P=0.013$) Trend toward lower level of depression symptoms ($P<0.605$)

Table 4–3. Interventions specifically targeting parental PTSD *(continued)*

Authors	Population	Methods	Design	Outcomes	Results
					6-month outcomes: Reduced level of trauma symptoms ($P=0.029$) Reduced level of depressive symptoms ($P=0.001$) Improved mental health on SF-36 ($P<0.001$)
Koochaki et al. 2019	Single-site study of 81 mothers of preterm infants (<2,500 g; <37 weeks). Of 90 mothers screened and randomized to treatment, 81 were included in the analysis.	Cognitive behavioral counseling. Group-based intervention with four mothers per group. All received education on infant care, health, infant behavior, and parent–infant interactions. Intervention group received education on emotions, stress relief, and how to use problem-solving skills, including self-talk.	RCT. Control group received education on infant care.	PTSD symptom scale	3-week outcomes showed decreased PTSD symptoms ($P=0.000$)

Table 4–3. Interventions specifically targeting parental PTSD *(continued)*

Authors	Population	Methods	Design	Outcomes	Results
Howland et al. 2017	Study of 19 mothers with infants in the NICU.	Relaxation guided imagery. Mothers listened to a 20-minute relaxation guided imagery recording at least once per day for 8 weeks.	Single sample study	PSS CES-D STAI-AD	Reduced levels of perceived distress (r=−0.38), anxiety (r=−0.43), and depression (r=−0.41)
Mendelson et al. 2016	Study of 27 mothers with infants in the NICU.	Mindfulness. Mothers viewed a 20-minute introductory video on mindfulness and listened to four mindfulness audio recordings.	Single sample study	PHQ-8 GAD-7 SASRQ	Reduction in SASRQ anxiety/arousal (P<0.001) but not on others including total scores. Reduction in PHQ-8 (P<0.01) Reduction in GAD-7 (P<0.1)

Note.   BAI=Beck Anxiety Inventory; BDI-II=Beck Depression Inventory, 2nd Edition; CBT=cognitive behavioral therapy; CES-D=Center for Epidemiologic Studies Depression Scale; DTS=Davidson Trauma Scale; GAD-7=Generalized Anxiety Disorder-7; IES=Impact of Event Scale; PDE-8=Peritraumatic Dissociative Experience Questionnaire; PHQ-8=Patient Health Questionnaire–8 ; SASRQ=Stanford Acute Stress Reaction Questionnaire; SF-36=Short Form Health Survey; STAI-AD=State-Trait Anxiety Inventory for Adults.

Event Scale (Jotzo and Poets 2005). However, it is not known whether the intervention impacted measures of parental coping, parental confidence, parent–infant interaction, or infant development.

In 2013, Shaw and colleagues published data from a successful RCT of a stepped collaborative-care intervention that incorporated the principles of TF-CBT, including psychoeducation, cognitive restructuring, Progressive Muscle Relaxation, and development of a trauma narrative to address parental trauma. It also included sessions designed to change mothers' negative perceptions of their infant and their parenting experience in order to decrease parental perceptions of child vulnerability (PPCV). Mothers in the intervention group reported greater reduction in trauma symptoms (Cohen's $d=0.41$, $P=0.023$) and depression (Cohen's $d=0.59$, $P<0.001$) versus mothers in the comparison group. Both conditions improved significantly in terms of anxiety, with no differences between groups. However, although sessions targeted infant redefinition and education about PPCV, they had no effect on mother–infant attachment or child functioning, and PPCV was lowered only in one group, the mothers who reported previous traumatic experiences at baseline (Shaw et al. 2013). At 6-month assessment, the differences between the intervention and comparison conditions were significant and sizable and became more pronounced when compared with 4- to 5-week outcomes: Davidson Trauma Scale (Cohen's $d=-0.74$, $P<0.001$); Beck Anxiety Inventory (Cohen's $d=-0.627$, $P=0.001$); Beck Depression Inventory II (Cohen's $d=-0.638$, $P=0.002$). Mothers showed increased benefits at 6-month follow-up, suggesting they continued to make use of the techniques acquired during the intervention phase (Shaw et al. 2014).

More recently, Koochaki et al. (2019) published findings from an Iranian RCT describing a group-based cognitive behavioral intervention to reduce PTSD symptoms in a sample of 90 NICU mothers. Both the intervention and control groups received eight counseling sessions twice weekly that included information about medical issues, nutrition, infant positioning, hygiene and infection, infant behavior, parent–infant interaction, and general care. The PTSD intervention group received interventions that were based on principles of CBT and included discussion of maternal feelings, education about stress and stress relief, the use of self-talk as a coping strategy, and problem-solving skills. Some of the more typical TF-CBT interventions, including the trauma narrative, were not included. Results showed significant benefits for the intervention group immediately following the intervention and at 3-week follow-up.

Overall, the results of these studies suggest that interventions that incorporate principles of TF-CBT provide an effective and cost-effective way to prevent and reduce symptoms of traumatic stress in mothers of premature infants in the NICU setting. In fact, a systematic review and meta-analysis of the effectiveness of trauma-focused psychological interventions for PTSD symptoms in women following childbirth—not necessarily including NICU experiences—concluded that these interventions were effective in reducing PTSD symptoms in both the short and medium term (Furuta et al. 2018). Brief, trauma-focused sessions resulted in significant decreases in symptoms of PTSD, depression, and anxiety that were sustained at 6-month follow-up (Shaw et al. 2013, 2014). Mothers who participated in the treatment rated these interventions very highly in terms of both usefulness and satisfaction.

Expressive Writing

Expressive writing has been used in several different populations exposed to traumatic events, including medical trauma, to help reduce the symptoms of psychological distress. Pennebaker and Beall (1986) proposed that expressing personal traumatic experiences in writing would help develop a more coherent narrative of the experience and thus foster temporal organization and a greater understanding of the events (Pennebaker and Francis 1996). The original instructions for the expressive writing were for patients to write for 15 minutes for 3 days in a row on their deepest thoughts and feelings about the traumatic event, but variations in this paradigm have been utilized in different studies (Table 4–4). Subsequent research has shown a range of positive outcomes, including both physical and psychological health, in both healthy and clinical populations (Frattaroli 2006).

Table 4–4.   Sample expressive writing prompts

What were the most emotional or troubling experiences?

What happened and in what order?

Who was there?

How did you feel, then and now?

Why do you believe it happened?

What have you learned?

Horsch et al. (2016) used expressive writing in an innovative study of 67 mothers with very premature infants who were by then 3 months old. Using the original instructions of Pennebaker and Beall (1986), participants were instructed to write about the experience of their child's birth and NICU hospitalization, making associations to their childhood and to past and current personal relationships as well as aspects of their past, current, and future hoped-for identities. Study findings showed significant decreases in maternal posttraumatic stress, as measured on the Perinatal PTSD Questionnaire (Quinnell and Hynan 1999), and symptoms of depression, measured using the Edinburgh Postnatal Depression

Scale (Cox et al. 1987) 1 and 5 months after the intervention. This work built on earlier reports of the efficacy of journal writing in mothers of premature infants (Barry and Singer 2001; Macnab et al. 1998).

Mindfulness

Mendelson et al. (2016) described a small pilot study of 27 NICU mothers who were offered a mindfulness intervention delivered using video and audio recordings. Mothers watched a 20-minute introductory video that explained the concepts of mindfulness and listened to audio recordings of mindfulness practices. Parents were assessed 2 weeks following the intervention and were found to have used the recordings at least one or two times and up to four times per week. The intervention was associated with a decrease in symptoms of depression, anxiety, and trauma, and all participants reported having a positive experience. Participants also reported improved sleep. Howland et al. (2017) also found that relaxation guided imagery was effective in reducing self-reported measures of distress, including perceived stress, state anxiety, and depressive symptoms, in a sample of 20 mothers of hospitalized preterm infants at 8-week follow-up.

Multicomponent Interventions

Thus far we have reviewed the evidence on primarily single-component interventions. However, much of the programmatic work done to support parental mental health during and after a NICU hospitalization has actually been part of multicomponent interventions with differing combinations and approaches. Table 4–5 reviews a number of multicomponent programs and their effects on parental or infant well-being. As mentioned, components of NICU and post-NICU programs that may be used to improve parental mental health include parent education; parent-specific psychological support; integration of the parent into infant care, including mitigation of pain and stress; provision of sensory experiences and participation in routine care; and treatment focusing on dynamics in the parent–infant relationship. Programs vary in the length and timing of their implementation, although the trend has been toward earlier intervention beginning during the NICU admission.

Conclusions and Future Directions

Optimal care for infants and the parent–infant dyad in the NICU should include a combination of developmental care interventions and treatments to address any parental psychological distress and parent–infant relational problems. Although developmental care is now routinely used

Table 4–5. Multicomponent programs and their impacts on infant and family well-being

Program	Education (parent or staff)	Parent (or staff) psychological support	Infant sensory experience	Parent–infant bonding intervention	Outcomes
Infant Health and Development Program (Martin et al. 2008; McCarton et al. 1997; McCormick et al. 2006)	Parent education from discharge to 3 years that gives regular anticipatory guidance on infant development	Home visits, parent group meetings			Improved IQ in infants at 36 months and lower behavior problem scores at 5 and 8 years Improved IQ scores and higher math achievement but no differences in behavior scores at 18 years Higher rates of maternal employment and less emotional distress
Early Developmental Mother–Child Intervention Program (Gianni et al. 2006)	Education about observing and interpreting preterm infant behavior to promote infant social-cognitive skills from discharge to 1 year	Intervention to help mothers verbalize feelings of grief, guilt, and anxiety			Improved scores in personal-social, eye-hand coordination, and reasoning subscales at 36 months of age in formerly preterm infants

Table 4–5. Multicomponent programs and their impacts on infant and family well-being *(continued)*

Program	Education (parent or staff)	Parent (or staff) psychological support	Infant sensory experience	Parent–infant bonding intervention	Outcomes
Mother–Infant Transaction Program (Kaaresen et al. 2008; Milgrom et al. 2010, 2013; Newnham et al. 2009; Nordhov et al. 2010; Olafsen et al. 2008; Rauh et al. 1990)	Education on reading infant cues, infant behavior, and appropriate sensitive responses and about massage and kangaroo care	Mothers given opportunities to express feelings of grief and guilt Mothers log changes and development in their infant to help redefine prognosis	Massage and kangaroo care		Improved parent responsiveness, more positive view of infant, and mothers less stressed by and more sensitive to infants Increased length of mother–infant interaction, fewer difficult regulatory behaviors, improved cognitive development at 3 and 9 years White matter brain development
COPE (Melnyk et al. 2006, 2009)	1. Information on appearance and behavior of preterm infants	Journaling about infant characteristics and milestones			Decreased parental depression and anxiety

Table 4–5.   Multicomponent programs and their impacts on infant and family well-being *(continued)*

Program	Education (parent or staff)	Parent (or staff) psychological support	Infant sensory experience	Parent–infant bonding intervention	Outcomes
COPE *(continued)*	2. Information on parental role in the NICU and the best ways to support infant development 3. Activities to help parents identify infant cues 4. Information on infant states, transition to home, and ways to enhance the parent–infant relationship 5. Anticipatory guidance on infant development				Improved confidence in parental role Increased positive parent–infant interactions Increased knowledge of infant behavior Decreased length of hospital stay and health care savings

Table 4–5. Multicomponent programs and their impacts on infant and family well-being *(continued)*

Program	Education (parent or staff)	Parent (or staff) psychological support	Infant sensory experience	Parent-infant bonding intervention	Outcomes
Promoting Mother's Ability to Communicate (Feely et al. 2008)	Taught to read infant cues and respond appropriately; use of video feedback	CBT for maternal anxiety and sensitivity training. Mothers taught to recognize feelings of anxiety and use deep breathing			Intervention feasible and acceptable to parents. Results failed to show efficacy in reducing parental anxiety and PTSD
Cues and Care, adapted from COPE (Zelkowitz et al. 2008, 2011)	Mothers taught to identify infant cues and respond sensitively	Mothers taught to recognize anxiety and distress and given strategies to relieve symptoms			No statistically significant differences in maternal outcomes (sensitivity, stress, anxiety, depression, PTSD)
Child–Parent Psychotherapy (Lakatos et al. 2019)	Developmental guidance and interpretation of infant cues	Provide emotional support with reflective listening, reframing the birth experience, help processing grief, crisis intervention, and case management	Encourage physical contact between parents and the infant, particularly skin-to-skin care	Encourage appropriate protective behavior, validating parental role, addressing stress and trauma that may negatively impact infant–parent attachment	Results as yet unpublished

Table 4–5. Multicomponent programs and their impacts on infant and family well-being *(continued)*

Program	Education (parent or staff)	Parent (or staff) psychological support	Infant sensory experience	Parent–infant bonding intervention	Outcomes
Close Collaboration with Parents (Ahlqvist-Bjorkroth et al. 2017, 2019)	Learning for parents and medical staff to interpret infant behavior Support with family-centered transition to home	Medical providers identify needs of the family; group reflective sessions between staff and trained psychologists; support for transition to home		Medical provider and parent work together to strengthen parents' capacity	Decreased symptoms of depression in mothers of preterm infants
Hospital to Home (Rice et al. 1977)	Education on delivering sensory experiences by parents to infants		Infant massage, vestibular stimulation, auditory stimulation, eye-to-eye contact		Greater weight gain, improved BSID developmental scores, greater maturational development by reflex measures when used by parents once home

Table 4–5. Multicomponent programs and their impacts on infant and family well-being *(continued)*

Program	Education (parent or staff)	Parent (or staff) psychological support	Infant sensory experience	Parent–infant bonding intervention	Outcomes
Auditory, Tactile, Visual, and Vestibular (Medoff-Cooper et al. 2015; White-Traut et al. 1993)			Auditory stimuli via a female human voice, light stroking, and eye-to-eye contact; rocking stimuli in specific sequence		Lower infant heart and respiratory rates, improved feeding interactions and oral feeding, improved behavioral states and reduced length of stay
Hospital-Home Transition: Optimizing Prematures' Environment (Vonderheid et al. 2016; White-Traut et al. 2013, 2014, 2015)	Maternal participatory guidance sessions		Auditory stimuli via a female human voice, light stroking, eye to eye contact, and rocking stimuli in a specific sequence		Improved mother–infant interaction and responsiveness during play, longer periods of alert state, improved infant weight gain, more orally directed behaviors, fewer acute care visits after discharge

Table 4–5. Multicomponent programs and their impacts on infant and family well-being *(continued)*

Program	Education (parent or staff)	Parent (or staff) psychological support	Infant sensory experience	Parent–infant bonding intervention	Outcomes
Family Nurture Intervention (Beebe et al. 2018; Hane et al. 2015; Porges et al. 2019; Welch et al. 2012, 2015, 2016)	Education on interactions with infant, including sensory experiences and how to calm infant, and on transition to home	Family support sessions involving support network if possible	Sensory inputs of smell, firm sustained touch, kangaroo care, vestibular input, taste, temperature	Calming interactions (calming cycle) between mother and infant using physical contact, speaking to infant, expressing emotions	Improved mother–infant face-to-face communication and touch and maternal caregiving behavior, reduction in maternal depression and anxiety at 4 months Improved neurodevelopmental outcomes in infants Improved attention, social-relatedness, cognitive and language scores at 18 months Improved autonomic regulation and more mature cardiac function Decreased maternal depression and anxiety

BSID=Bayley Scales of Infant Development; CBT=cognitive behavioral therapy; COPE=Creating Opportunities for Parent Empowerment.

in different formats in many NICUs, less attention has been given to recognizing symptoms of trauma connected to the NICU experience and to helping parents and infants establish optimal relationships. Some approaches, such as Creating Opportunities for Parent Empowerment (Melnyk et al. 2006), have robust effects on parenting confidence and parent–infant interactions and have also been found to help reduce parental symptoms of depression and anxiety. Others, such as Promoting Mothers' Ability to Communicate (Feely et al. 2008), that were specifically designed to address the symptoms of parental anxiety, were not found to have any significant impact on anxiety or PTSD distress.

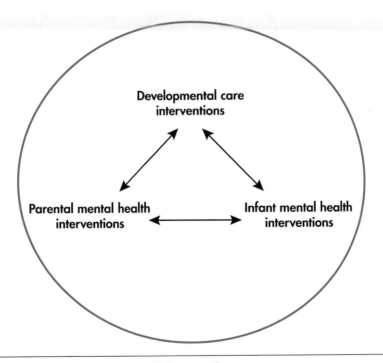

FIGURE 4–2. **NICU mental health interventions.**

By contrast, interventions with the goal of reducing parental trauma have by and large not included components to address the parent–infant interaction or other elements of developmental care, with the exception of Jotzo and Poets (2005), Shaw et al. (2013, 2014), and Koochaki et al. (2019), who created interventions specifically to address parental PTSD that included sessions on the parent–infant relationship, parental role, and concept of infant redefinition. However, none of these studies published specific results on infant outcomes, although Horwitz et al. (2015) reported no significant findings regarding PPCV. Although a unified intervention (Figure 4–2) addressing both parental psychological distress

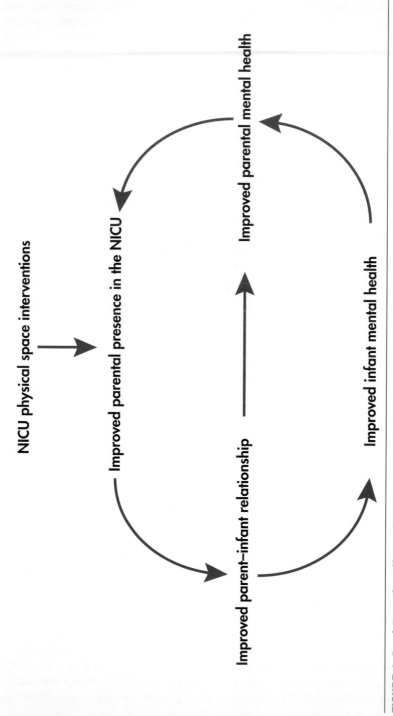

FIGURE 4–3.   Interactive effects of NICU psychological interactions.

and infant developmental issues in the NICU may be a future goal, the current state of our knowledge base suggests that developmental care and interventions to target both parental psychological distress and parent–infant relational difficulties must be implemented to maximize outcomes.

What has not yet been studied is the potential synergistic effect of these categories of interventions (Figure 4–3). For example, given that alterations in the expected parental role have consistently been found to be most strongly associated with symptoms of parental trauma, a developmental care intervention that helps reestablish a NICU-appropriate role for parents of premature infants would be expected not only to enhance infant outcomes but also potentially decrease parental trauma. It also has not been established how best to integrate and coordinate care in NICUs that offer both developmental care and interventions for parental psychological distress. Future studies should investigate this issue, given that the overlapping goals of each category are so similar. As indicated by Benzies et al. (2013), the thoughtful development of large, multisite RCTs that could test multiple components of interventions, including those that show promise in improving parental and child outcomes, may be useful. The principles outlined by Melnyk et al. (2002) provide a useful foundation for future study (Table 4–6).

Table 4–6. **Recommendations for informational and behavioral interventions for parents of low birth weight premature infants**

Health care providers should, early in the infant's care, provide parents with information regarding premature infant characteristics and how to become involved with their child's care.

Parenting interventions should begin early, with the goal of helping parents establish a pattern of positive parent–infant interactions.

Symptoms of parental anxiety and depression should be assessed and targeted before they impact the parent–infant relationship.

Parental beliefs should be assessed to identify those most likely to benefit from behavioral/informational programs.

Interventions should be feasible, timely, and cost effective if they are to be implemented as part of routine clinical care.

Source. Melnyk et al. 2002.

References

Afand N, Keshavarz M, Fatemi NS, Montazeri A: Effects of infant massage on state anxiety in mothers of preterm infants prior to hospital discharge. J Clin Nurs 26(13–14):1887–1892, 2017

Ahlqvist-Bjorkroth S, Boukydis Z, Axelin AM, et al: Close Collaboration With Parents intervention to improve parents' psychological well-being and child development: description of the intervention and study protocol. Behav Brain Res 325(pt B):303–320, 2017

Ahlqvist-Bjorkroth S, Axelin A, Korja R, et al: An educational intervention for NICU staff decreased maternal postpartum depression. Pediatr Res 85(7):982–986, 2019

Ahn HY, Lee J, Shin HJ: Kangaroo care on premature infant growth and maternal attachment and post-partum depression in South Korea, J Trop Pediatr 56(5):342–344, 2010

Aite L, Bevilacqua F, Zachary A, et al: Seeing their children in pain: symptoms of posttraumatic stress disorder in mothers of children with an anomaly requiring surgery at birth. Am J Perinatol 33:770–775, 2016

Als H: Toward a synactive theory of development: promise for the assessment and support of infant individuality. Infant Mental Health J 3(4):229–243, 1982

Als H: A synactive model of neonatal behavioral organization: framework for the assessment of neurobehavioral development in the premature infant and for support of infants and parents in the neonatal intensive care environment. Phys Occup Ther Pediatr 6(3/4):3–53, 1986

Anderson GC, Chiu SH, Dombrowski MA, et al: Mother–newborn contact in a randomized trial of kangaroo (skin-to-skin) care. J Obstet Gynecol Neonatal Nurs 32(5):604–611, 2003

Arnon S, Diamant C, Bauer S, et al: Maternal singing during kangaroo care led to autonomic stability in preterm infants and reduced maternal anxiety. Acta Paediatrica 103(10):1039–1044, 2014

Axelin A, Lehtonen L, Pellender T, et al: Mothers' different styles of involvement in preterm infant pain care. J Obstet Gynecol Neonatal Nurs 39:415–424, 2010

Badr LK, Abdallah B, Kahale L: A meta-analysis of preterm infant massage: an ancient practice with contemporary applications. MCN Am J Matern Child Nurs 40(6):344–358, 2015

Barlow J, Herath NI, Bartram Torrance C, et al: The Neonatal Behavioral Assessment Scale (NBAS) and Newborn Behavioral Observations (NBO) system for supporting caregivers and improving outcomes in caregivers and their infants. Cochrane Database Syst Rev (3):CD011754, 2018

Barry LM, Singer GH: Reducing maternal psychological distress after the NICU experience through journal writing. J Early Interv 24(4):287–297, 2001

Baudesson de Chanville A, Brevaut-Malaty V, Garbi A, et al: Analgesic effect of maternal human milk odor on premature neonates: a randomized controlled trial. J Hum Lact 33(2):300–308, 2017

Beebe B, Myers MM, Lee SH, et al: Family nurture intervention for preterm infants facilitates positive mother–infant face-to face engagement at 4 months. Dev Pychol 54(11):2016–2031, 2018

Beheshtipour N, Baharlu SM, Montaseri S, et al: The effect of the educational program on Iranian premature infants' parental stress in a neonatal intensive care unit: a double-blind randomized controlled trial. Int J Community Based Nurs Widwifery 2(4):240–50, 2014

Benzies KM, Magill-Evans JE, Hayden KA, Ballantyne M: Key components of early intervention programs for preterm infants and their parents: a systematic review and meta-analysis. BMC Pregnancy Childbirth 13(suppl 1):S10, 2013

Bergman NJ, Ludwig RJ, Westrup B, et al: Nurturescience versus neuroscience: a case for rethinking perinatal mother–infant behaviors and relationship. Birth Defects Res 111(15):1110–1127, 2019

Bergomi P, Chieppi M, Maini A, et al: Nonpharmacological techniques to reduce pain in preterm infants who receive heel-lance procedure: a randomized controlled trial. Res Theory Nurs Pract 28(4):335–348, 2014

Bernard RS, Williams SE, Storfer-Isser A, et al: Brief cognitive-behavioral intervention for maternal depression and trauma in the neonatal intensive care unit: a pilot study. J Trauma Stress 24(2):230–234, 2011

Bisson JI, Roberts NP, Andrew M, et al: Psychological therapies for chronic post-traumatic stress disorder (PTSD) in adults. Cochrane Database Syst Rev (12):CD003388, 2013

Böll S, Almeida de Minas AC, Raftogianni A, et al: Oxytocin and pain perception: from animal models to human research. Neuroscience 007(1).149 161, 2018

Borghini A, Pierrehumbert B, Miljkovitch R: Mother's attachment representations of their premature infant at 6 and 18 months after birth. Infant Ment Health J 27(5):494–508, 2006

Boundy E, Dastjerdi R, Spiegelman D, et al: Kangaroo mother care and neonatal outcomes: a meta-analysis. Pediatrics 137(1): e20152238, 2016

Bourgeois JP, Jastreboff PJ, Rakic P: Synaptogenesis in visual cortex of normal and preterm monkeys: evidence for intrinsic regulation of synaptic overproduction. Proc Natl Acad Sci USA, 86(11):4297–4301, 1989

Bozzette M: A review of research on premature infant–mother interaction. Newborn Infant Nurs Rev 7:49–55, 2006

Brazelton TB: Neonatal Behavioral Assessment Scale (Clinics in Developmental Medicine No. 50). Philadelphia, JP Lippincott, 1973

Browne JV, Talmi A: Family based intervention to enhance infant–parent relationships in the neonatal intensive care unit. J Pediatr Psychol 30(8):667–677, 2005

Burnett AC, Anderson PJ, Cheong J, et al: Prevalence of psychiatric diagnoses in preterm and full-term children, adolescents and young adults: a meta-analysis. Psychol Med 41 (12): 2463-74, 2019

Chamberlain C, Gee G, Harfield S, et al: Parenting after a history of childhood maltreatment: a scoping review and map of evidence in the perinatal period. PLoS One 14(3), 2019

Champagne F, Diorio J, Sharma S, et al: Naturally occurring variations in maternal behavior in the rate are associated with differences in estrogen-inducible central oxytocin receptors. Proc Natl Acad Sci USA 98(22):12736–12741, 2001

Charpak N, Ruiz-Pelaez JG, Charpak Y, et al: Kangaroo Mother Program: an alternative way of caring for low birth weight infants? One-year mortality in a two cohort study. Pediatrics 94:804–810, 1994

Chen YS, Tan YJ, Zhou LS, et al: Clinical effect of maternal voice stimulation in alleviating procedural pain in hospitalized neonates. Zhongguo Dang Dai Er Ke Za Zhi 21(1):58–63, 2019

Chidambaram AG, Manjula S, Adhisivam B, et al: Effect of kangaroo mother care in reducing pain due to heel prick among preterm neonates: a crossover trial. J Matern Fetal Neonatal Med 27(5):488–490, 2014

Chik YM, Ip WY, Choi KC: The effect of upper limb massage on infants' venipuncture pain. Pain Manag Nurs 18:50–57, 2017

Chiu SH, Anderson GC: Effect of early skin-to-skin contact on mother-preterm infant interaction through 18 months: randomized controlled trial. Int J Nurs Stud 46(9):1168–1180, 2009

Choi HJ, Kim SJ, Oh J, et al: The effects of massage therapy on physical growth and gastrointestinal function in premature infants: a pilot study. J Child Health Care 20(3):394–404, 2016

Chorna OD, Slaughter JC, Wang L, et al: A pacifier-activated music player with mother's voice improves oral feeding in preterm infants. Pediatrics 133(3):462–468, 2014

Cobiella CW, Mabe PA, Forehand RL: A comparison of two stress-reduction treatments for mothers of neonates hospitalized in a neonatal intensive care unit. Child Health Care 19:93–100, 1990

Cox JL, Holden JM, Sagovsky R: Detection of postnatal depression: development of the 10-item Edinburgh Postnatal Depression Scale. Br J Psychiatry 150:782–786, 1987

Cox SM, Hopkins J, Sydney H: Attachment in preterm infants and their mothers: neonatal risk status and maternal representations. Infant Mental Health J 21(6):464–480, 2000

Croy I, Mohr T, Weidner K, et al: Mother–child bonding is associated with the maternal perception of the child's body odor. Physiol Behav 198:151–157, 2019

D'Agata AL, Young EE, Cong X, et al: Infant Medical Trauma in the Neonatal Intensive Care Unit (IMTN): a proposed concept for science and practice. Adv Neonatal Care 16(4):E1–E2, 2016

Davidson J, Ruthazer R, Maron JL: Optimal timing to utilize olfactory stimulation with maternal breast milk to improve oral feeding skills in the premature newborn. Breastfeed Med 14(4):230–235, 2019

De Alencar AE, Arreas IC, de Albuquerque EC, Alves JG: Effect of kangaroo mother care on postpartum depression, J Trop Pediatr 55(1):36–38, 2009

De Bernardo G, Svelto M, Giordano M, et al: Supporting parents in taking care of their infants admitted to a neonatal intensive care unit: a prospective cohort pilot study. Ital J Pediatr 43(1):36, 2017

Diego MA, Field T, Hernandez-Reif M: Procedural pain heart rate responses in massaged preterm infants. Infant Behav Dev 32:226–229, 2009

Domanico R, Davis DK, Coleman F, et al: Documenting the NICU design dilemma: parent and staff perceptions of open ward versus single family room units. J Perinatol 30(5):343–351, 2010

Dudek J, Colasante T, Zuffiano A, et al: Changes in cortical sensitivity to infant facial cues from pregnancy to motherhood predict mother–infant bonding. Child Dev 91(1):e198–e217, 2018

Erkul M, Efe E: Efficacy of breastfeeding on babies' pain during vaccinations. Breastfeed Med 12:110–115, 2017

Ettenberger M, Cardenas CR, Parker M, Odell-Miller H: Family centered music therapy with preterm infants and their parents in the neonatal intensive care unit (NICU) in Colombia: a mixed-methods study. Nordic J Music Therapy 26(3):207–234, 2017

Feely N, Zelkowitz P, Charbonneau L, et al: Assessing the feasibility and acceptability of an intervention to reduce anxiety and enhance sensitivity among mothers of very low birth-weight infants. Adv Neonatal Care 8(5):276–284, 2008

Feldman R, Eidelman AI, Sirota L, Weller A: Comparison of skin-to-skin (kangaroo) and traditional care: parenting outcomes and preterm infant development. Pediatrics 110(1):16–26, 2002

Field T: Postpartum depression effects on early interactions, parenting, and safety practices: a review. Infant Behav Dev 33(1):1, 2010

Field T: Preterm newborn pain research review. Infant Behav Dev 49:141–150, 2017

Finelli J, Zeanah CH, Smyke A: Attachment disorders in early childhood, in Handbook of Infant Mental Health. Edited by Zeanah CH. New York, Guilford, 2019, pp 452–465

Foa EB, Kozak MJ: Emotional processing of fear: exposure to corrective information. Psychol Bull 99:20–35, 1986

Foa EB, Hearst-Ikeda D, Perry KJ: Evaluation of a brief cognitive-behavioral program for the prevention of chronic PTSD in recent assault victims. J Consult Clin Psychol 63:948–955, 1995

Fontana C, Menis C, Pesenti N, et al: Effects of early intervention on feeding behavior in preterm infants: a randomized controlled trial. Early Hum Dev 121:15–20, 2018

Forcada-Guex M, Borghini A, Pierrehumbert B, Ansermet F: Prematurity, maternal posttraumatic stress and consequences on the mother–infant relationship. Early Hum Dev 87(1):21–26, 2011

Forman DR, O'Hara MW, Stuart S, et al: Effective treatment for postpartum depression is not sufficient to improve the developing mother–child relationship. Dev Psychopathol 19(2):585–602, 2007

Franck LS, Oulton K, Ndereitu S, et al: Parent involvement in pain management for NICU infants: a randomized controlled trial. Pediatrics 128(3):510–518, 2011

Frattaroli J: Experimental disclosure and its moderators: a meta-analysis. Psychol Bull 132(6):823, 2006

Furuta M, Horsch A, Ng ES, et al: Effectiveness of trauma-focused psychological therapies for treating post-traumatic stress disorder symptoms in women following childbirth: a systematic review and meta-analysis. Front Psychiatry 9:591, 2018

Gehl MB, Alter CC, Rider N, et al: Improving the efficiency and effectiveness of parent education in the neonatal intensive care unit. Adv Neonatal Care 20(1):59–67, 2020

Gianni ML, Picciolini O, Ravasi M, et al: The effects of an early developmental mother–child intervention program on neurodevelopment outcome in very low birth weight infants: a pilot study. Early Hum Dev 82(10):691–695, 2006

Gilkerson J, Richards JA, Warren SF, et al: Language experience in the second year of life and language outcomes in late childhood. Pediatrics 142(4), 2018

Gilmore KJ, Meersand P: Normal Child and Adolescent Development: A Psychodynamic Primer. Washington, DC, American Psychiatric Publishing, 2014

González-Serrano F, Lasa A, Hernanz M, et al: Maternal attachment representations and the development of very low birth weight premature infants at two years of age. Infant Ment Health J 33(5):477–488, 2012

Grossmann KE, Bretherton I, Waters E, et al: Maternal sensitivity: observational studies honoring Mary Ainsworth's 100(th) year. Attach Hum Dev 15(5–6):443–447, 2013

Hall RA, Hoffenkamp HN, Tooten A, et al: Longitudinal associations between maternal disrupted representations, maternal interactive behavior and infant attachment: a comparison between full-term and preterm dyads. Child Psychiatry Hum Dev 46(2):320–331, 2015

Hall SL, Famuyide ME, Saxton SN, et al: Improving staff knowledge and attitudes toward providing psychosocial support to NICU parents through an online education course. Adv Neonatal Care 19(6):490–499, 2019

Hane AA, Myers MM, Hofer MA, et al: Family nurture intervention improves the quality of maternal caregiving in the neonatal intensive care unit: evidence from a randomized controlled trial. J Dev Behav Pediatr 36(3):188–196, 2015

Harrison TM: family centered pediatric nursing care: state of the science. J Pediatr Nurs 25:335–343, 2010

Hart B, Risley TR: American parenting of language-learning children: persisting differences in family child interactions observed in natural home environments. Dev Psychol 28(6):1096–1105, 1992

Hernandez-Reif M, Diego M, Field T: Preterm infants show reduced stress behaviors and activity after 5 days of massage therapy. Infant Behav Dev 30(4):557–561, 2007

Holditch-Davis D, White-Traut RC, Levy JA, et al: Maternal satisfaction with administering infant interventions in the NICU. J Obstet Gynecol Neonatal Nurs 42(6):641–654, 2013

Holditch-Davis D, White-Traut RC, Levy JA, et al: Maternally administered interventions for preterm infants in the NICU: effects on maternal psychological distress and mother–infant relationship. Infant Behav Dev 37(4):695–710, 2014

Holsti L, Grunau RE, Oberlander TF, et al: Specific newborn individualized developmental care and assessment program movements are associated with acute pain in preterm infants in the neonatal intensive care unit. Pediatrics 114(1):65–72, 2004

Horsch A, Tolsa JF, Gilbert L, et al: Improving maternal mental health following preterm birth using an expressive writing intervention: a randomized controlled trial. Child Psychiatry Hum Dev 47(5):780–791, 2016

Horwitz SM, Leibovitz A, Lilo E, et al: Does an intervention to reduce maternal anxiety, depression and trauma also improve mothers' perceptions of their preterm infants' vulnerability? Infant Ment Health J 36(1):42–52, 2015

Howland LC, Jallo N, Connelly CD, Pickler RH: Feasibility of a relaxant guided imagery intervention to reduce maternal stress in the NICU. J Obstet Gynecol Neonatal Nurs 46(4):532–543, 2017

Hunter ML, Blake S, Simmons C, et al: Implementing a parent education program in the special care nursery. J Pediatr Health Care 33(2):131–137, 2019

Huot RL, Thrivkraman KV, Meaney MJ, et al: Development of adult ethanol preference and anxiety as a consequence of neonatal maternal separation in Long Evans rats and reversal with antidepressant treatment. Psychopharmacology 158(4):366–373, 2001

Im H, Kim E: Effect of Yakson and Gentle Human Touch versus usual care on urine stress hormones and behaviors in preterm infants: a quasi-experimental study. Int J Nurs Stud 46:450–458, 2009

Johnston C, Fillon F, Campbell-Yeo M, et al: Kangaroo mother care diminishes pain from heel lance in very preterm neonates: a crossover trial. BMC Pediatr 8:13, 2008

Johnston C, Campbell-Yeo M, Fernandes A, et al: Skin-to-skin care for procedural pain in neonates. Cochrane Database Syst Rev (1):CD008435, 2014

Jones R, Jones L, Feary AM: The effects of single-family rooms on parenting behavior and maternal psychological factors. J Obstet Gynecol Neonatal Nurs 45(3):359–370, 2016

Jotzo M, Poets CF: Helping parents cope with the trauma of premature birth: an evaluation of a trauma-preventive psychological intervention. Pediatrics 115:915–919, 2005

Kaaresen PI, Ronning JA, Tunby J, et al: A randomized controlled trial of an early intervention program in low birth weight children: outcome at 2 years. Early Hum Dev 84(3):201–209, 2008

Koochaki M, Mahmoodi Z, Esmaelzadeh-Saeieh S, et al: Effects of cognitive-behavioral counseling on posttraumatic stress disorder in mothers with infants hospitalized at neonatal intensive care units: a randomized controlled trial. Iran J Psychiatry Behav Sci 12(4):e65159, 2019

Korja R, Savonlahti E, Haataja L, et al: Attachment representations in mothers of preterm infants. Infant Behav Dev 32(3):305–311, 2009

Korja R, Latva R, Lehtonen L: The effects of preterm birth on mother–infant interaction and attachment during the infant's first two years. Acta Obstet Gynecol Scand 91(2):164–173, 2012

Kotzer AM, Zacharakis SK, Raynolds M, Buenning F: Evaluation of the built environment: staff and family satisfaction pre- and post-occupancy of the children's hospital. HERD 4(4):60–78, 2011

Krueger C, Parker L, Chiu SH, Theriaque D: Maternal voice and short-term outcomes in preterm infants. Dev Psychobiol 52(2):205–212, 2010

Lahav A, Skoe E: An acoustic gap between the NICU and womb: a potential risk for compromised neuroplasticity of the auditory system in preterm infants. Front Neurosci 8(381):1–8, 2014

Lakatos PP, Matic T, Carson M, Williams ME: Child-parent psychotherapy with infants hospitalized in the neonatal intensive care unit. J Clin Psychol Med Settings 26(4):584–596, 2019

Lariviere J, Rennick JE: Parent picture-book reading to infants in the neonatal intensive care unit as an intervention supporting parent–infant interaction and later book reading. J Dev Behav Pediatr 32(2):146–152, 2011

Lee S, Kimble LP: Impaired sleep and well-being in mothers with low-birth-weight infants. J Obstet Gynecol Neonatal Nurs 38(6):676–685, 2009

Leerkes EM, Crockenberg SC, Burrous CE: Identifying components of maternal sensitivity to infant distress: the role of maternal emotional competencies. Parent Sci Pract 4:1–23, 2004

Lester BM, Hawes K, Abar B, et al: Single-family room care and neurobehavioral and medical outcomes in preterm infants. Pediatrics 134(4):754–760, 2014

Lester BM, Salisbury AL, Hawes K, et al: 18-Month follow-up of infants cared for in a single-family room neonatal intensive care unit. J Pediatr 177:84–89, 2016

Loewy J: NICU music therapy: song of kin as critical lullaby in research and practice. Ann NY Acad Sci 1337(1):178–185, 2015

Lund LK, Vik T, Lydersen S, et al: Mental health, quality of life and social relations in young adults born with low birth weight. Health Qual Life Outcomes 10: 146, 2012

Lundstrom JN, Mathe A, Schaal B, et al: Maternal status regulates cortical responses to the body odor of newborns. Front Psychol 4(597):1–6, 2013

Maayan-Metzger A, Kedem-Friedrich P, Bransburg Zabary S, et al: The impact of preterm infants' continuous exposure to breast milk odor on stress parameters: a pilot study. Breastfeed Med 13(3):211–214, 2018

Macho P: Individualized developmental care in the NICU: a concept analysis. Adv Neonatal Care 17(3):162–174, 2017

Macnab AJ, Beckett LY, Park CC, Sheckter L: Journal writing as a social support strategy for parents of premature infants: a pilot study. Patient Educ Couns 33(2):149–159, 1998

Mäkelä H, Axelin A, Feeley N, Niela-Vilén H: Clinging to closeness: the parental view on developing a close bond with their infants in a NICU. Midwifery 62:183–188, 2018

Malatesta CZ, Grigoryev P, Lamb C, et al: Emotion socialization and expressive development in preterm and full-term infants. Child Dev 57(2):316–330, 1986

Marshall-Baker A, Lickliter R, Cooper RP: Prolonged exposure to a visual pattern may promote behavioral organization in preterm infants. J Perinatol Neonat Nurs 12(2):50–62, 1998

Martin A, Brooks-Gunn J, Klebanov P, et al: Long-term maternal effects of early childhood intervention: findings from the Infant Health and Development Program (IHDP). J App Develop Psychol 29(2):101–117, 2008

McCarton CM, Brooks-Gunn J, Wallace IF, et al: Results at age 8 years of early intervention for low-birth-weight premature infants. The Infant Health and Development Program. JAMA 277(2):126–132, 1997

McCormick MC, Brooks-Gunn J, Buka SL, et al: Early intervention in low birth weight premature infants: results at 18 years of age for the Infant Health and Development Program. Pediatrics 117(3):771–780, 2006

Medoff-Cooper B, Rankin K, Li Z, et al: Multi-sensory intervention for preterm infants improves sucking organization. Adv Neonatal Care 15(2):142–149, 2015

Melnyk BM, Feinstein NF, Fairbanks E: Effectiveness of informational/behavioral interventions with parents of low birth weight (LBW) premature infants: an evidence base to guide clinical practice. Pediatr Nurs 28(5):511–516, 2002

Melnyk BM, Feinstein NF, Alpert-Gillis L, et al: Reducing premature infants' length of stay and improving parents' mental health outcomes with the Creating Opportunities for Parent Empowerment (COPE) neonatal intensive care unit program: a randomized, controlled trial. Pediatrics 118(5):e1414–e1427, 2006

Melnyk BM, Feinstein NF: Reducing hospital expenditures with the COPE (Creating Opportunities for Parent Empowerment) program for parents and premature infants: an analysis of direct healthcare neonatal intensive care unit costs and savings. Nurs Adm Q 33(1):32–37, 2009

Mendelson T, McAfee C, Dania AJ, et al: A mindfulness intervention to reduce maternal distress in neonatal intensive care: a mixed methods pilot study. Arch Women's Ment Health 21:791–799, 2016

Miles MS, Funk SG, Carlson J: Parental Stressor Scale: neonatal intensive care unit. Nurs Res 42(3):148–152, 1993

Milgrom J, Newnham C, Anderson PJ, et al: Early sensitivity training for parents of preterm infants: impact on the developing brain. Pediatr Res 67(3):330–335, 2010

Milgrom J, Newnham C, Martin PR, et al: Early communication in preterm infants following intervention in the NICU. Early Hum Dev 89(9):755–762, 2013

Minde K: Prematurity and serious medical conditions in infancy: implications for development, behavior, and intervention, in Handbook of Infant Mental Health. Edited by Zeanah CH. New York, Guilford, 2000, pp 176–194

Montirosso R, Borgatti R, Trojan S, et al: A comparison of dyadic interactions and coping with still-face in healthy pre-term and full-term infants. Br J Dev Psychol 28(Pt 2):347–368, 2010

Moradi S, Arshdi-Bostanabad M, Seyedrasooli A, et al: The effect of empowerment program on maternal discharge preparation and neonatal length of hospital stay: a randomized controlled trial. Iran J Nurs Midwifery Res 23(3):172, 2018

Neel ML, Yoder P, Matusz PJ, et al: Randomized controlled trial protocol to improve multisensory neural processing, language and motor outcomes in preterm infants. BMC Pediatr 19(1):81, 2019

Nemeroff CB, Bremner JD, Foa EB, et al: Posttraumatic stress disorder: a state-of-the-science review. J Psychiatr Res 40:1–21, 2006

Newnham C, Milgrom J, Skouteris H: Effectiveness of a modified mother–infant transaction program on outcomes for preterm infants from 3 to 24 months of age. Infant Behav Dev 32(1):17–26, 2009

Nordhov SM, Kaaresen PI, Ronning JA, et al: A randomized study of the impact of a sensitizing intervention on the child-rearing attitudes of parents of low birth weight preterm infants. Scand J Psychol 51(5):385–391, 2010

Nugent JK, Keefer CH, Minear S, et al: Understanding Newborn Behavior and Early Relationships: The Newborn Behavioral Observations (NBO) System Handbook. Baltimore, MD, Brookes, 2007

Nugent JK, Bartlett JD, Valim C: Effects of an infant-focused relationship-based hospital and home visiting intervention on reducing symptoms of postpartum maternal depression. Infants Young Child 27(4):292–304, 2014

O'Brien K, Robson K, Bracht M, et al: Effectiveness of family integrated care in neonatal intensive care units on infant and parent outcomes: a multicentre, multinational, cluster-randomised controlled trial. Lancet Child Adolesc Health 2(4):245–254, 2018

Ohlsson A, Jacobs SE: NIDCAP: a systemic review and meta-analyses of randomized controlled trials. Pediatrics 131:e881–e893, 2013

Olafsen K, Kaaresen P, Handegard B, et al: Maternal ratings of infant regulatory competence from 6 to 12 months: influence of perceived stress, birth weight, and intervention: a randomized controlled trial. Infant Behav Dev 31(3):408–421, 2008

Ortenstrand A, Westrup B, Broström EB, et al: The Stockholm Neonatal Family Centered Care Study: effects on length of stay and infant morbidity. Pediatrics 125(2):e278–e285, 2010

Pennebaker JW, Beall SK: Confronting a traumatic event: toward an understanding of inhibition and disease. J Abnorm Psychol 95(3):274–281, 1986

Pennebaker JW, Francis ME: Cognitive, emotional, and language processes in disclosure. Cogn Emot 10(6):601–626, 1996

Pennestri MH, Gaudreau H, Bouvette-Turcot AA, et al: Attachment disorganization among children in neonatal intensive care unit: preliminary results. Early Hum Dev 91(10):601–606, 2015

Picciolini O, Porro M, Meazza A, et al: Early exposure to maternal voice: effects on preterm infants' development. Early Hum Dev 90(6):287–292, 2014

Pineda RG, Stransky KE, Rogers C, et al: The single patient room in the NICU: maternal and family effects. J Perinatol 32(7):545–551, 2012

Pineda RG, Neil J, Dierker D, et al: Alterations in brain structure and neurodevelopment outcome in preterm infants hospitalized in different neonatal intensive care unit environments. J Pediatr 164(1):52–60, 2014

Pineda R, Guth R, Herring A, et al: Enhancing sensory experiences for very preterm infants in the NICU: an integrative review, J Perinatol 37(4):323–332, 2017

Porges SW, Davila MI, Lewis GF, et al: Autonomic regulation of preterm infants is enhanced by Family Nurture Intervention. Dev Psychobiol 61(6):942–952, 2019

Porter RJ, McAllister-Williams RH, Jones S, et al: Effects of dexamethasone on neuroendocrine and psychological responses to L-tryptophan infusion. Psychopharmacology 143(1):64–71, 1999

Preyde M, Ardal F: Effectiveness of a parent "buddy" program for mothers of very preterm infants in a neonatal intensive care unit. CMAJ 168(8):969–973, 2003

Procianoy RS, Mendes EW, Silveira RC: Massage therapy improves neurodevelopment outcome at two years corrected age for very low birth weight infants. Early Hum Dev 86(1):7–11, 2010

Provenzi L, Santoro E: The lived experience of fathers of preterm infants in the neonatal intensive care unit: a systematic review of qualitative studies. J Clin Nurs 24(13–14):1784–1794, 2015

Provenzi L, Fumagalli M, Scotto di Minico G, et al: Pain-related increase in serotonin transporter gene methylation associates with emotional regulation in 4.5-year-old preterm-born children. Acta Paediatr 00:1–9, 2019

Puthussery S, Chutlyami M, Tseng PC, et al: Effectiveness of early intervention programs for parents of preterm infants: a meta-review of systematic reviews. BMC Pediatr 18(1):223, 2018

Quinnell FA, Hynan MT: Convergent and discriminant validity of the perinatal PTSD questionnaire (PPQ): a preliminary study. J Trauma Stress 12(1):193–199, 1999

Raiskila S, Axelin A, Toome L, et al: Parents' presence and parent–infant closeness in 11 neonatal intensive care units in six European countries vary between and within the countries. Acta Paediatr 106(6):878–888, 2017

Rauh VA, Nurcombe B, Achenbach T, et al: The mother–infant transaction program: the content and implications of an intervention for the mothers of low-birthweight infants. Clin Perinatol 17(1):31–45, 1990

Reynolds LC, Duncan MM, Smith GC, et al: Parental presence and holding in the neonatal intensive care unit and associations with early neurobehavioral. J Perinatol 33:636–641, 2013

Rice R: Neurophysiological development in premature infants following stimulation. Dev Psychol 13(1):69–76, 1977

Roa E, Ettenberger M: Music therapy self-care group for parents of preterm infants in the neonatal intensive care unit: a clinical pilot intervention. Medicines (Basel) 5(4):134, 2018

Roberts KL, Paynter C, McEwan B: A comparison of kangaroo mother care and conventional cuddling care. Neonatal Netw 19(4):31–35, 2000

Roman LA, Lindsay JK, Boger RP, et al: Parent-to-parent support initiated in the neonatal intensive care unit. Res Nurs Health 18:385–394, 1995

Rose S, Bisson J, Wessely S: A systematic review of single-session psychological interventions ('debriefing') following trauma. Psychother Psychosom 72(4):176–184, 2003

Rowe ML: Child-directed speech: relation to socioeconomic status, knowledge of child development and child vocabulary skill. J Child Lang 35(1):185–205, 2008

Sanders MR, Hall SL: Trauma-informed care in the newborn intensive care unit: promoting safety, security and connectedness. J Perinatol 38(1):3–10, 2018

Sansavini A, Zavagli V, Guarini A, et al: Dyadic co-regulation, affective intensity and infant's development at 12 months: a comparison among extremely preterm and full-term dyads. Infant Behav Dev 40:29–40, 2015

Scala M, Seo S, Lee J, Park J, et al: Effect of reading to preterm infants on measures of cardiorespiratory stability in the neonatal intensive care unit. J Perinatology 38:1536–1541, 2018

Schechter DS, Myers MM, Brunelli SA, et al: Traumatized mothers can change their minds about their toddlers: understanding how a novel use of video-feedback supports positive change of maternal attributions. Infant Ment Health J 27(5):429–447, 2006

Schlez A, Litmanovitz I, Bauer S, et al: Combining kangaroo care and live harp music therapy in the neonatal intensive care unit setting. Isr Med Assoc J 13(6):354–358, 2011

Schnurr PP, Friedman MJ, Engel CC, et al: Cognitive behavioral therapy for posttraumatic stress disorder in women: a randomized controlled trial. JAMA 297:820–830, 2007

Shah PS, Herbozo C, Aliwalas LL, et al: Breastfeeding or breast milk for procedural pain in neonates. Cochrane Database Syst Rev 12:CD004950, 2012

Shah SR, Kadage S, Sinn J: Trial of music, sucrose, and combination therapy for pain relief during heel prick procedure. J Pediatr 190:153–158, 2017

Shaw RJ, St John N, Lilo EA, et al: Prevention of traumatic stress in mothers with preterm infants: a randomized controlled trial. Pediatrics 132(4):e886–e894, 2013

Shaw RJ, St John N, Lilo E, et al: Prevention of traumatic stress in mothers of preterms: 6-month outcomes. Pediatrics 134(2):e481–e488, 2014

Schmücker G, Brisch KH, Köhntop B, et al: The influence of prematurity, maternal anxiety, and infants' neurobiological risk on mother–infant interactions. Infant Ment Health J 26(5):423–441, 2005

Sijbrandij M, Olff M, Reitsma JB, et al: Treatment of acute posttraumatic stress disorder with brief cognitive behavioral therapy: a randomized controlled trial. Am J Psychiatry 164(1):82–90, 2007

Slade A: Parental reflective functioning: an introduction. Attach Hum Dev 7(3):269–281, 2005

Solomon J, George C: The measurement of attachment security and related constructs in infancy and early childhood, in Handbook of Attachment: Theory, Research, and Clinical Applications. Edited by Cassidy J, Shaver P. New York, Guilford, 2016, pp 366–396

Spinelli M, Frigerio A, Montali L, et al: 'I still have difficulties feeling like a mother': The transition to motherhood of preterm infants mothers. Psychol Health 31(2):184–204, 2016

Spittle AJ, Anderson PJ, Lee KJ, et al: Preventive care at home for very preterm infants improves infant and caregiver outcomes at 2 years. Pediatrics 126(1):e171–e178, 2010

Stern D: The Motherhood Constellation. A Unified View of Parent–Infant Psychotherapy. Karnac Books, 1998, pp 11–41

Stevens DC, Helseth CC, Thompson PA, et al: A comprehensive comparison of open-bay and single-family room neonatal intensive care units at Sanford Children's hospital. Herd 5(4):23–39, 2012

Tallandini MA, Scalembra C: Kangaroo mother care and mother–premature infant dyadic interaction. Infant Ment Health J 27(3):251–275, 2006

van Emmerik AA, Kamphuis JH, Emmelkamp PM: Treating acute stress disorder and posttraumatic stress disorder with cognitive behavioral therapy or structured writing therapy: a randomized controlled trial. Psychother Psychosom 77:93–100, 2008

Vasquez-Ruiz S, Maya-Barrios J, Torres-Narváez P, et al: A light/dark cycle in the NICU accelerates body weight and shortens time to discharge in preterm infants. Early Human Dev 90:535–540, 2014

Victoria NC, Murphy AZ: The long-term impact of early life pain on adult responses to anxiety and stress: historical perspectives and empirical evidence. Exp Neurol 275(pt 2):261–273, 2016

Vinall J, Grunau RE: Impact of repeated procedural pain-related stress in infants born very preterm. Pediatric Research 75(5): 584-87, 2014

Vohr B, McGowan E, McKinley L, et al: Differential effects of the single-family room neonatal intensive care unit on 18- to 24-month Bayley scores of preterm infants. J Pediatr 185:42–48, 2017

Volpe JJ: Dysmaturation of premature brain: importance, cellular mechanisms and potential interventions. Pediatr Neurol 95:42–66, 2019

Vonderheid SC, Rankin K, Norr K, et al: Health care use outcomes of an integrated Hospital-to-Home Mother–Preterm Infant intervention, J Obstet Gyn Neonatal Nurs 45(5):625–638, 2016

Walker SM: Biological and neurodevelopmental implications of neonatal pain. Clin Perinatol 40(3):471–491, 2013

Welch MG, Hofer MA, Brunelli SA, et al: Family nurture intervention (FNI): methods and treatment protocol of a randomized controlled trial in the NICU. BMC Pediatr 12:14, 2012

Welch MG, Firestein MR, Austin J, et al: Family Nurture Intervention in the neonatal intensive care unit improves social-relatedness, attention, and neurodevelopment of preterm infants at 18 months in a randomized controlled trial. J Child Psychol Psychiatry 56(11):1202–1211, 2015

Welch MG, Halperin MS, Austin J, et al: Depression and anxiety symptoms of mothers of preterm infants are decreased at 4 months corrected age with Family Nurture Intervention in the NICU. Arch Womens Ment Health 19(1):51–61, 2016

White-Traut RC, Nelson MN, Silvestri JM, et al: Patterns of physiologic and behavioral response of intermediate care preterm infants to intervention. Pediatr Nurs 19(6):625–629, 1993

White-Traut RC, Nelson MN, Silvestri JM, et al: Effect of auditory, tactile, visual and vestibular intervention on length of stay, alertness and feeding progression in preterm infants. Dev Med Child Neurol 44(2):91–97, 2002

White-Traut R, Norr KF, Fabiyi C, et al: Mother–infant interaction improves with a developmental intervention for mother-preterm infant dyads. Infant Behav Dev 36(4):694 706, 2013

White-Traut R, Rankin KM, Pham T, et al: Preterm infants' orally directed behaviors and behavioral state responses to the integrated H-HOPE intervention. Infant Behav Dev 37(4):583–96, 2014

White-Traut RC, Rankin KM, Yoder JC, et al: Influence of H-HOPE intervention for premature infants on growth, feeding progression and length of stay during initial hospitalization. J Perinatol 35(8):636–641, 2015

Wolke D, Eryigit-Madzwamuse S, Gutbrod T: Very preterm/very low birthweight infants' attachment: infant and maternal characteristics. Arch Dis Child Fetal Neonatal Educ 99(1):F70–F75, 2014

Woodward LJ, Bora S, Clark CA, et al. Very preterm birth: maternal experiences of the neonatal intensive care environment. J Perinatol 34(7):555–561, 2014

Wyly MV: Infant Assessment. New York, Routledge, 2018

Zeanah CH, Keener MA, Stewart L, et al: Prenatal perception of infant personality: a preliminary investigation. J Am Acad Child Psychiatry 24(2):204–210, 1985

Zelkowitz P, Feeley N, Shrier I, et al: The Cues and Care Trial: a randomized controlled trial of an intervention to reduce maternal anxiety and improve developmental outcomes in very low birthweight infants. BMC Pediatrics 8:38, 2008

Zelkowitz P, Feeley N, Shrier I, et al: The Cues and Care randomized controlled trial of a neonatal intensive care unit intervention: effects on maternal psychological distress and mother–infant interaction. J Dev Behav Pediatr 32(8):591–599, 2011

Zero to Three Infant Mental Health Task Force Steering Committee: Definition of Infant Mental Health. Washington, DC, National Center for Clinical Infant Programs, 2001

Zhang S, Su F, Chen W: The analgesic effects of maternal milk odor on newborns: a meta-analysis. Breastfeed Med 13(5):327–334, 2018

CHAPTER 5

Individual Trauma-Based Intervention for Mothers of Premature Infants

Emily A. Lilo, Ph.D., M.P.H.

Tonyanna C. Borkovi, M.B.B.S.

Angelica Moreyra, Psy.D.

Sarah M. Horwitz, Ph.D.

Richard J. Shaw, M.D.

In this chapter, we describe the development and implementation of a brief manualized individual treatment intervention based on principles of trauma-focused cognitive behavioral therapy (TF-CBT). The goal of the intervention is to prevent and reduce posttraumatic stress in mothers of preterm infants. Building on earlier work using a trauma-informed treatment model (Bernard et al. 2011) and incorporating principles of developmental care, we designed and evaluated the intervention with these goals in mind:

1. Prevention and treatment of symptoms of depression, anxiety, and posttraumatic stress in mothers of preterm infants
2. Enhancement of infant developmental outcomes and reducing the prevalence of overprotective parenting patterns

3. Implementation with mothers of premature infants in the busy and high-stress environment of a level-IV NICU
4. Delivery by bachelor's degree–level staff without extensive mental health training or experience

Feasibility

The issue of feasibility was of particular importance in the development of the treatment intervention. Feasibility depended to a great extent on timing. We recognized that the intervention should be delivered soon enough after birth to be effective but so soon as to preclude participation of parents who are already stretched thin. Parents of preterm infants are under exceptional levels of stress in the NICU, and we were concerned about whether mothers would be receptive or willing to participate in an intervention that was certain to place additional demands on their time. Based on past experience, we found that a family's first 2 weeks in the NICU can be especially overwhelming and that mothers likely will have already experienced profound stress and trauma in the NICU setting during those first 1–2 weeks following the birth of their infant. Therefore, we aimed to begin the intervention within 1–2 weeks after birth, early enough to start addressing mothers' emotional needs but allowing them enough time to settle into a routine in the NICU in which they would be able to tolerate a more intensive trauma-focused intervention.

When planning the frequency of treatment sessions, we continued to pay particular attention to the perceived time burden and convenience of our intervention, with the hope of minimizing additional stress placed on mothers and increasing the practicality of participation. Ultimately, we designed the intervention to consist of two sessions per week, each lasting 45–50 minutes, delivered over the course of 3 weeks. In our first series of sessions, most mothers did not consistently complete two sessions per week; thus, the intervention was typically completed in 4–6 weeks. Most of these mothers found that committing to two sessions a week was difficult due to competing demands, including appointments with specialists and the care team, needs of other children and family, work, and other emotional and physical strains on top of caring for their premature infant and for themselves.

The availability of resources, particularly access to psychological support services in the NICU, posed an additional challenge to feasibility. Although a handful of academic medical centers may have psychologists assigned to the NICU, this is typically the exception rather than the rule. In fact, for many NICUs, psychiatric consultation is often provided by psychiatry consultation services and limited to mothers with severe postpartum depression or psychotic disorders. Although social workers are able to provide psychological support to families, the sheer magnitude of their caseloads often leaves little time to provide targeted therapeutic interventions to address psychological needs. Given these challenges, we designed the treatment intervention to be highly structured so it could potentially be delivered by a variety of staff members, including bachelor's degree–level staff, peer mentors, social workers, or nurse educators, without extensive mental health training or experience. In the first randomized controlled trial (RCT) of our intervention, therapists included graduate-level psychology students in their first or second year of clinical training and one licensed social worker, all of whom had participated in our 8-hour in-person training, supplemented by at-home practice assignments and a NICU preparation tour.

Evidence-Informed Care

To optimize and evaluate its effectiveness in an RCT, we developed the intervention as a structured manualized treatment that could be delivered with high fidelity. In the design of our manual, we focused on adapting existing treatment models with content specific to the NICU environment. We looked to evidence-based interventional techniques that had been proven effective in addressing symptoms of anxiety, depression, and posttraumatic stress.

We anticipated that the intervention would be effective for a group of mothers with mild to moderate symptoms, but this would not preclude referral of highly symptomatic mothers for more intensive psychiatric treatment, including the potential use of psychiatric medications. Although our primary focus was on preventing and reducing symptoms of posttraumatic stress, we anticipated additional benefits with respect to symptoms of postpartum anxiety and depression.

TRAUMA-FOCUSED COGNITIVE BEHAVIORAL THERAPY

Evidence to support the use of TF-CBT is found in numerous studies of individuals who have undergone traumatic experiences, including military trauma, sexual abuse, physical trauma, and exposure disasters (Chard et al. 2013; Nemeroff et al. 2006; Resick and Schnicke 1992). In addition, prior work in the Stanford NICU had shown some effectiveness for a brief three-session intervention based on principles of CBT for parents of preterm infants (Bernard et al. 2011). Although this early study showed promising effects on parental depression, its limited success in addressing anxiety and posttraumatic stress suggested the need for a longer and more comprehensive intervention.

Our intervention also drew on findings from the PTSD model, specifically research showing that parental PTSD has been associated with decreased maternal ability to cope with stressors in the NICU, distorted maternal perceptions of their infant (Schechter et al. 2005), increased feelings of detachment and separation from their infant (Brisch et al. 2003), and negative influences on their parenting (Ross and McLean 2006). We integrated specific interventions based on TF-CBT (Nemeroff et al. 2006; Resick and Schnicke 1992), with the expectation that if mothers were able to reduce their trauma-related symptoms, they would have greater confidence in their coping ability, feel more bonded and attached to their infants, and improve their parenting ability.

Previous reviews of evidence-based trauma treatment, including TF-CBT and cognitive processing therapy, suggest that core components of effective treatment should include psychoeducation, cognitive restructuring, relaxation training, and exposure (Nemeroff et al. 2006; Resick and Schnicke 1992). Our intervention incorporated psychoeducation as a way to help mothers better understand their trauma and help normalize their response to the NICU experience. We provided education on the symptoms of PTSD and some of the feelings and thoughts commonly experienced by NICU parents. Cognitive restructuring was incorporated to help mothers identify and differentiate feelings from thoughts and recognize and challenge erroneous and maladaptive cognitions. Progressive Muscle Relaxation (PMR) and deep breathing were used to reduce symptoms of anxiety, and the mothers participated in a two-part trauma narrative exercise for exposure.

MATERNAL SENSITIVITY AND PARENT–INFANT INTERACTION

Several core features differentiate the traumatic nature of a NICU experience from more classic single-incident trauma. These include the way a mother perceives her pregnancy and birth experience, the status of her infant's health and well-being, the nature of the mother–infant relationship, and the mother's perception of her own current and future parenting role and capacity. With this in mind, we thought treatment should specifically incorporate and address these issues in addition to traditional principles of TF-CBT. The concept of *infant redefinition* is one that is seen in many developmental care interventions and is highly relevant in terms of helping a parent process and address symptoms of trauma. Our treatment manual addresses the notion of infant redefinition through strategies that address feelings of parental disempowerment or disengagement.

Sameroff's (1983, 1993) transactional model assumes that developmental outcomes are the result of the complex interaction between individual context and experiential context over time. To enhance a mother's ability to care for her infant, it is presumed she needs to integrate new information about the child's prematurity and health status into previously held beliefs about the imagined birth and parenting experience and may need to accept the loss of the "perfect" child (Hagan et al. 2004; Kersting et al. 2004; Miles 1989). Mothers need not only to learn about their preterm infants' appearance, behaviors, and how to care for them but also to grieve their own feelings of loss for the perfect child, perfect pregnancy, and perfect birth experience. They must work toward acceptance of their child and their early parenting experiences in order to be more emotionally available to their new infant. The mothers' own traumatic experiences may lead to emotional responses that prevent them from recognizing the developmental gains their infants are making and may lead them to adopt overprotective parenting styles. It becomes important in the NICU for mothers to be able to address their traumatic experiences and understand how their emotional and cognitive responses create barriers to recognizing their infant's current medical status and development.

The process of infant redefinition adapts material from the program *Creating Opportunities for Parent Empowerment* (Melnyk et al. 2001). The goal is enhancing optimal parenting and the mother–infant relationship by changing mothers' perceptions of their infant after birth and of their own parenting experience (Sameroff and Fiese 2000). Infant redefinition is based on the assumption that if parents no longer see their child as abnormal and difficult, they will be better able to engage in more normative caregiving interactions. Core components of current evidence-based treatments that address these issues are shown in Table 5–1.

OVERPROTECTIVE PARENTING AND VULNERABLE CHILD SYNDROME

A crucial component of the NICU experience is its potentially lasting impact on parenting style. Parents with symptoms of PTSD often adopt patterns of overprotective parenting that may have adverse effects on the feeding and sleep patterns and subsequently on the academic and emotional development of the child (Martin et al. 2008; McCormick et al. 1996; Pierrehumbert et al. 2003). To address this issue, our treatment manual includes psychoeducational material on vulnerable child syndrome (VCS), which may develop as an outcome of parental trauma (discussed further in Chapter 7).

Manual Development

We developed the individual treatment with the following goals:

1. Prevent and reduce parental posttraumatic stress, anxiety, and depression
2. Provide parents early education on recognizing infant cues, along with techniques to help challenge their negative perceptions regarding their infant's development and their personal parenting ability
3. Provide psychoeducation around optimal and developmentally appropriate parenting to limit patterns of overprotective parenting.

Table 5–1.   Intervention components to enhance maternal sensitivity and parent–infant interaction

---

Teaching the mother about infant characteristics and behavioral states.

Educating the mother about how to be sensitive to her infant's cues.

Encouraging the mother to observe changes in her infant and communicating ways the infant has become stronger and more competent.

Redefining the parenting experience by helping the mother to recognize the changes she has experienced in her parenting role.

Helping the mother anticipate future changes she can expect in her infant and parent–infant interactions.

Increasing the mother's feelings of comfort and confidence and promoting positive interaction by teaching her different activities to bond with, care for, and soothe her infant (including Containing Touch).

Introducing the concept of overprotective parenting and educating the mother on ways to minimize its occurrence.

Following a literature review, we designed six sessions to include the most relevant components of existing effective treatments (Table 5–2). The goals of each session were determined and documented. For sections of the manual that were primarily educational, such as teaching relaxation techniques, we scripted the language so that skills could be taught consitently. For sessions that were necessarily more individualized to each participant, such as identifying the most traumatic portion of the infant's hospitalization, topics were identified in outline format. The first draft of the manual was reviewed and approved by a scientific advisory board that included experts in PTSD in women, treatment development, parent–child attachment, neonatology, and implementation strategies.

Session 1: Introduction to the NICU

The goals of Session 1, which is primarily psychoeducational in nature, are as follows:

1. Develop and build rapport
2. Provide an opportunity for the mother to share her observations of her infant
3. Educate the mother about the appearance and behaviors of premature infants
4. Provide activities the mother can do with her infant in the NICU to encourage the infant's development
5. Teach the technique of deep breathing

This first session focuses on normalizing the experience of the parents and their reactions to the NICU environment.

Table 5–2.   Session content of the treatment manual

Session	Content of session
1: Introduction to the NICU and baby development	Develop rapport.
	Provide an opportunity for the mother to share her observations about her infant.
	Educate the mother about the appearance and behaviors of the premature infant.
	Discuss things the mother can do for her infant.
	Teach the mother deep breathing
2: Cognitive restructuring	Empathize with and normalize reactions of parents in the NICU setting.
	Help the mother identify emotions and the relationship between events, thoughts, and emotions.
	Teach the mother techniques: Examining the Evidence, What Would I Tell a Friend?, Positive Self-Statements.
	Assign an ABC-B Worksheet with Examining the Evidence exercise.
3: Stress, triggers, and self-care	Brief review of ABC-B Worksheet.
	Help the mother accurately label her thoughts and emotions in response to events.
	Reinforce the idea that changing thoughts can change the intensity or type of emotions experienced.
4: Loss and the trauma narrative	Educate the mother about symptoms of loss.
	Help the mother relax physically by teaching Progressive Muscle Relaxation.
	Help the mother create the trauma narrative.
5: Processing the trauma narrative	Have the mother read her trauma narrative with affective expression.
	Identify the mother's most challenging cognitions and emotions associated with her traumatic experience.
	Challenge self-blame and irrational thoughts.
6: Avoiding overprotective parenting and preparing for home	Redefine the infant: identify ways the infant has changed.
	Redefine the parenting experience: identify new things the mother can do with her infant.

Table 5–2.   Session content of the treatment manual *(continued)*

Session	Content of session
6: Avoiding overprotective parenting and preparing for home (*continued*)	Introduce the concept of overprotective parenting and how to limit its occurrence.
	Introduce infant states, engagement and disengagement, and associated caregiving.
	Help the mother anticipate further changes in her infant and in parent–infant interactions.

INTRODUCTION TO TREATMENT

The first session is best scheduled at the infant's bedside so that the infant's presence helps generate thoughts and feelings related specifically to the mother–infant dyad. The therapist can show curiosity and interest by commenting on the infant's appearance and any personal items that the parent may have placed in the incubator, with the goal of building rapport. Learning and remembering the infant's name in future sessions and inquiring about the infant's progress can also be helpful in this regard. In this session, set expectations about the frequency and anticipated length of the total treatment and convey that because each session builds upon the skills learned in the previous session, the treatment will be most helpful and effective if the mother completes all six sessions.

GETTING TO KNOW THE MOTHER AND HER PREGNANCY AND BIRTH EXPERIENCE

To set the mother at ease, the session starts with questions about her background, pregnancy, and delivery. Specific questions include

- Can you tell me what your pregnancy and the delivery were like?
- How are you feeling physically?
- Are you getting support from family and friends?
- Do you have any other children?

In many cases, this may be the first time the mother has been asked to relate her story of the birth experience, and her responses will give the therapist insight into the traumatic aspects of her NICU experience. The mother may become emotional, and the therapist should show interest and empathy with her story. Although the goal in this session is not to spend time processing the mother's experiences, the session provides important insights that will be revisited, for example, when learning cognitive restructuring exercises (Session 2) and writing trauma narratives (Sessions 4 and 5).

APPEARANCE AND BEHAVIORS OF THE INFANT

Next, the focus shifts to the infant, with questions about the infant's appearance and behavior. Specific questions include

- Now, let's talk about [baby's name]. Does your baby's name have any special significance?
- Do they look like anyone in your family?
- Does anything about your baby remind you of anyone?
- Does anything surprise you or stand out for you about your baby's appearance or behavior?

Questions about the infant's name and family likenesses may generate some interesting history that is unique to the mother's family and will help convey a sense of interest in the mother and build rapport. Such questions can begin to help the mother think of her infant as a member of her family rather than as a patient in a hospital. Typically, at this phase of a mother's NICU experience, most of the questions that have been asked about her infant by friends and family have focused on medical status, updates, and prognosis. By asking mothers these more personal questions, the therapist can not only gain a sense of the mother's attachment and bond with the infant but also encourage the mother to reflect on her own bond with her baby regardless of medical status and prognosis.

Questions about her infant's appearance and behavior provide an opportunity to educate the mother about common characteristics of preterm infants and how they differ from full-term infants with respect to their appearance and behavior. At this point in the session, the therapist reviews the "Common Characteristics of Premature Infants" handout (Table 5–3) and uses it to spark a conversation on what the mother may have noticed about her infant's appearance and behavior, while also normalizing these observations. The therapist should discuss any of the items on the handout that the mother checked and emphasize that the infant's lack of responsiveness, changes in breathing, and muscle weakness are normal and expected phenomena of preterm infants. The therapist should also reassure the mother that her infant will be growing and developing each day and will increasingly come to resemble the infant she had expected. This is also a time to acknowledge the anxieties the mother may have about aspects of the infant's development.

THINGS THE MOTHER CAN DO WITH HER INFANT

This section focuses on helping empower mothers to be active in their infant's care. Many mothers feel completely powerless in the NICU, un-

Table 5–3.   Common characteristics of premature infants

Appearance	They are small and thin.
	Their skin color may be blotchy.
	Their muscles are weak, and they may appear floppy.
	They have many tubes and wires attached to them.
Behavior	They sleep a lot.
	Their cries may be very weak or inaudible.
	Their movements may be jerky, and they may stick out their arms and legs in a brisk and rigid manner, as if startled.
Interactions	When awake, they may look groggy or "out of it."
	The monitor may alarm for different reasons.
	They may not always respond to talking or stroking because they are generally less active, alert, and responsive.

Source.   Adapted from Shaw and Horwitz 2013.

sure of how to look after their baby, and often displaced by the NICU staff who have much greater comfort and familiarity with the care of pre-term infants. The substantial gap between what the mother had antici-pated about her caretaking role and responsibilities and the reality of having an infant who is not breastfeeding or cannot be handled, a con-cept referred to as an *alteration in the expected parental role*, has been shown in multiple studies to be strongly associated with maternal depression and symptoms of posttraumatic stress (Holditch-Davis et al. 2003; Pier-rehumbert et al. 2003; Vanderbilt et al. 2009).

As a result of the medicalization of routine infant care, many of the activities that mothers may anticipate, such as breastfeeding, changing diapers, and holding their infants, are either not possible or much more complicated. In many cases, mothers of premature infants may not be producing milk at the time of delivery or struggle to pump as often as needed to increase milk production. What is more, the infant may not have the developmental readiness to latch on to the mother's breast or suckle. In addition, the numerous monitors and lines, as well as the need to keep the infant in the incubator, may act as barriers preventing the mother from holding and comforting her infant. However, the therapist can use the fol-lowing text in the session to help empower the mother to understand her own unique importance and provide her with techniques to take on the parental role:

> We have found that parents in this environment often feel distressed be-cause they are not sure what they can do with their baby, or what their role is supposed to be. Especially in the beginning, it might feel as though the NICU nurses are the experts, but it is important for you to remember that

> you also play a crucial role. _____ (baby's name) has been hearing your
> voice and feeling you since before they were born. It is your touch, smell,
> and voice that will help provide your baby with the most comfort. As you
> spend more time with _____ (baby's name), you will become the ex-
> pert on your baby.
>
> Next, we are going to be talking about things you can do for _____
> (baby's name) at this time.
>
> What types of interactions have you had with _____ (baby's name)
> so far?

The next handout, entitled "Things Parents Can Do With Their Baby
in the NICU" (Figure 5–1), provides suggestions about what mothers can
do to become involved in their baby's care when they are with their baby
in the NICU as well as in between visits. This includes engaging in Containing Touch and skin-to-skin care, learning their baby's cues, being a
soothing voice and touch, and eventually helping with breast, bottle, or
gastrostomy-tube feeding. Mothers are also given advice on how to communicate more effectively with the NICU staff so that they feel empowered to ask for what they need.

The therapist should thoroughly discuss each point, which activities
the mother has tried, and what successes and difficulties she and her infant have had. Point out that she can ask the nurse whether her infant is
ready to be touched, handled, or held and that their baby may be more
receptive to stimulation on some days than on others. The techniques that
should be reviewed with the mother include the following:

- **Containing Touch:** This is a technique with which mothers can
  touch and comfort their infant while the infant is in the incubator.
  When the infant is lying face down, the mother can place one hand
  on top of the infant's head and the other on the infant's bottom, using
  a gentle but firm touch rather than stroking, and guide her hands inward as though bringing her palms together. When the infant is lay-
  ing face up, the mother can place one hand on top of the infant's head
  and her other hand either under the infant's feet or over the infant's
  chest. The therapist should demonstrate this technique either with
  the mother's infant, if appropriate, or with a baby doll and encourage the mother to demonstrate the technique after the instruction.
- **Getting involved with caregiving tasks:** In an effort to reestablish
  the parental role, the therapist discusses bedside care activities in
  which the mother can participate. These include taking the baby's temperature, changing the diaper, swaddling, positioning, applying Aqua-
  for, and breast- or bottle feeding.
- **Reading the infant's cues and states:** An important part of developmental care is educating parents on how to read and interpret their
  infant's cues. Awareness of when to interact and stimulate the infant
  and when to soothe and decrease stimulation is an important skill

When you are with your baby you can:	In between visits you can:

Provide multisensory stimulation
 	
Visual
☐ Get up close to your baby and look at them
☐ Observe your baby's behavior and learn to read their cues
☐ Hold eye contact while feeding, holding, and massaging
 	
Voice
☐ Talk, hum, and sing to your baby as much as you can
 	
Touch
☐ Skin-to-skin holding (kangaroo care)
☐ Provide Containing Touch
☐ You can provide touch simply to show love
☐ Ask your nurse if you can help with caregiving tasks, including:
  - taking the temperature
  - changing the diaper
  - swaddling
  - positioning
  - applying Aquafor® (infant massage)
  - breast and bottle feeding
 	
Motion
☐ Wrap your baby up in a blanket and gently rock baby back and forth
☐ Hold your baby swaddled in your arms or lap
	Document
	☐ Write in your Baby Diary
	
	Connect
	☐ Leave something with your smell on it for your baby
	☐ Leave a picture of you for your baby
	☐ Carry a picture of your baby
	
	Visualize
	☐ Imagine how your milk is nourishing your baby
	
	Share
	☐ Share observations with the nurses and doctors on anything about your baby that concerns you
	
	Communicate
	☐ Ask questions about:
	  - your baby's medical status
	  - changes in your baby
	  - things you can do to care for your baby
	  - things you will soon be able to do with your baby

FIGURE 5–1.   Things parents can do with their baby in the NICU.
Source.   Adapted from Shaw and Horwitz 2013.

that is not often obvious to parents of newborns. Parents who attempt to engage their infant while the infant is not in a receptive state may experience the infant as being rejecting or may think of themselves as being an ineffective parent, with potential negative consequences on the parent–infant relationship. The following text from the manual illustrates how this concept can be explained to parents:

> All babies have six states (or levels of energy and awareness) that they progress through, from deep sleep to wide awake. Knowing how to recognize these states is important because _____ (baby's name) is ready for different types and levels of stimulation

and engagement at each state. If you try to get _____ (baby's name) to interact with you during times other than in the state which we call "Calm Alert," your baby may seem to either ignore you or become overstimulated; your baby may be too sleepy or too fussy, they may fall asleep, look drowsy and unfocused, or show stress cues. You should not take this personally, but instead realize that they were simply not at the right level of alertness or calmness to interact with you at that moment. When your baby is closer to full term, they will be able to interact with you more easily.

"Sleep and Awake States" (Figure 5–2) is a handout that describes the concept of infant states as ranging from deep sleep to light sleep, drowsy, calm alert, active alert, and fussing/crying. The therapist uses this handout to educate the mother about infant states of awareness and appropriate responses. The mother should also be encouraged to consult with her bedside nurse for help on how to master these techniques.

State	Description	What Parent Can Do
DEEP SLEEP	• Quietly sleeping with little movements • Breathing is usually regular • Baby is resting and growing the most	✓ At times, leave baby in bed with no extra stimulation ✓ Provide Containing Touch ✓ Hold Skin-to-Skin
LIGHT SLEEP	• Eyelids may flutter or open briefly • Breathing is often irregular • May move face and body	✓ At times, leaving baby with no extra stimulation will help them sleep ✓ Provide Containing Touch ✓ Hold Skin-to-Skin ✓ Reposition if appears uncomfortable

FIGURE 5–2.   Sleep and awake states.
Source.   Adapted from Shaw and Horwitz 2013.

- **Importance of holding baby skin-to-skin:** *Kangaroo care* is the technique of placing the infant upright on the parent's bare chest so that there is skin-to-skin contact between the infant and parent (Figure 5–3). This is a routine practice in most NICUs, and mothers are usually taught this technique by the bedside nurse. Videos are available online that demonstrate kangaroo care.[1] In this session, the therapist discusses the principles and benefits of skin-to-skin contact, which include increasing the infant's ability to regulate temperature, heart rate, and respiration (Anderson 2003; Ludington-Hoe et al. 2003). The therapist emphasizes how this helps solidify the parental role by explaining how the infant is soothed by the warmth of the mother's body, her smell, the sensations of rising and falling on her chest, and hearing her heartbeat and her voice. Kangaroo care also provides an opportunity for the mother to bond with her baby in an environment where there are otherwise many obstacles to intimate bonding. Additionally, it has been suggested that when the mother holds her infant skin to skin, she is exposed to the same microbes that her infant has been exposed to, and her body begins to produce antibodies that will then be present in her breast milk. This helps protect the infant until they can produce their own antibodies. The therapist should advise the mother to spend at least 30 minutes per day in skin-to-skin contact with her infant at times that the nurse believes to be suitable. If skin-to-skin care is not permitted for medical reasons, the parent can still be taught how to handle, position, and swaddle the infant, with guidance from the bedside nurse.

BENEFITS OF SKIN-TO-SKIN CONTACT

Infants in the NICU who engage in skin-to-skin contact have been shown to go home sooner.

Infants who are placed skin-to-skin with their mother or father become more relaxed and less agitated; their temperature, heart rate, and respiration rate stabilize. This positive change in your baby may be seen on the monitor.

Your baby will feel soothed by the warmth of your body, your smell, feeling the gentle rise and fall of your chest, and hearing your heartbeat and your quiet voice.

When an infant is placed in an isolette, they are exposed to bacteria different from their mother's. When the mother holds her infant skin-to-skin, the mother is then exposed to the bacteria too. She begins to produce antibodies, which can be found in her breast milk, which will help protect her baby.

Fathers can do it too!

FIGURE 5–3.   The importance of skin-to-skin contact.
Source.   Adapted from Shaw and Horwitz 2013.

---

[1]Nationwide Children's Hospital in Columbus, Ohio, for example, offers an instructional video on their website.

Teaching the mother how to do kangaroo care is also important early on because she can share this skill with her partner. Mothers, fathers, or any identified caregivers can use kangaroo care to feel more engaged in the care process and to strengthen bonding and attachment with their baby.

COMMUNICATING IN STRESSFUL SITUATIONS

Many parents are intimidated by the NICU environment. First-time parents in particular may lack the skills to advocate effectively for themselves or for their infant or do not know how best to interact with NICU staff to gain important information about their infant's medical condition. To address this, our intervention teaches parents different styles of communication and how to best communicate with the nursing and medical staff to have their concerns and questions addressed. The types of communication include passive, aggressive, and assertive/effective communication (Figure 5–4).

How to use appropriate, effective, and direct communication

Use "I" statements - Be direct, be brief

The best way to communicate directly is to use "I" statements. This means you say three pieces of information: how you feel, the situation that made you feel that way, and how the staff can help you.

Try to be **direct**, keep it **short**, and state exactly how you **feel** and how the staff can best **help**.

Remember, your friends and family are trying to help support you, but it is important for you to tell them what is helpful and what is not.

"I feel_____ when _____ happens. Can you _____?"

        (Emotion)   **(Event)**   **(Action/request)**

FIGURE 5–4. Communicating in the NICU.
Source. Adapted from Shaw and Horwitz 2013.

The therapist should discuss what state the infant is currently in and use the handout to illustrate possible statements. The therapist emphasizes and models how to use direct, short "I" statements when communicating with staff. Examples of language that parents can use include the following:

- "I'm worried about holding my baby; can you please help me hold them?"
- "I feel confused when you give me lots of information all at once. Can you explain it to me again?"

- "I feel frustrated when you take control of everything. Can you please include me in your decision-making process?"

INTRODUCING THE BABY DIARY

The Baby Diary is a core component of treatment and is used to help with the process of infant redefinition. The Baby Diary both helps mothers connect with their infants during the NICU hospitalization and provides a valuable record of the family's experiences for future reference. The Baby Diary helps mothers begin to think about their baby as a member of their family as opposed to a patient in the hospital. It is divided into different sections: "Visiting Log," "Milestones for Baby," "Milestones for Mother," "Baby Observations," and "Mother's Experiences."

The Visiting Log provides a guide for mothers on ways they can engage with routine care, advocate for their baby, and bond with their baby at bedside. Often, mothers or caregivers feel out of place at bedside in the NICU and may hesitate to ask to be involved in routine care. They may have concerns that they cannot properly care for their baby. The Visiting Log provides ideas for what mothers can do at bedside and prompts them to ask for additional ways in which they can be involved in their baby's care. The "Milestones for Baby" and "Milestones for Mother" sections of the diary allow mothers to document their baby's achievements as well as their own parenting achievements while in the NICU. Many parents make "baby books" for their infants to document many of that child's "firsts." In the NICU setting, parents may begin to lose sight of how their baby is achieving milestones and "firsts." However, whether documented or not, their baby is still reaching these milestones. This section of the diary gives parents opportunities to reflect on what their baby can and does do, even while in the hospital. It also allows mothers to recognize what they have been able to accomplish as a parent during their baby's time in the NICU.

The mother is encouraged to make entries in the Baby Diary, including the times that she visits, developmental milestones that she notices in her infant, and milestones in her own growth as a parent. The diary includes a section where she can write observations and reflections. Mother and therapist review the Baby Diary at several points during the treatment, and by looking back at observations of her baby and herself earlier in the treatment, the mother is able to notice important developmental changes. These observations can help the mother redefine her infant as engaging in a process of growth and development rather than as a fragile and vulnerable child. Similarly, this may help the mother redefine herself as competent and effective in her parenting role. The Baby Diary provides a keepsake for the mother to look through in the future with her child, friends, and family and reflect on how much her family has grown from their time in the NICU.

RELAXATION TRAINING

Techniques of deep breathing, PMR, meditation, and mindfulness have all been shown to be useful techniques as part of TF-CBT. In this session, the mother is introduced to the technique of deep breathing, with the goal of building a skill she can use later when processing some of her more painful and traumatic NICU experiences. The therapist frames this exercise as one of the first techniques they will practice to promote self-care and stress reduction, a topic they will cover in more detail in a later session. Encouraging self-care at this stage gives the mother an effective coping mechanism that she can use when things become overwhelming.

Using a script, the therapist first demonstrates techniques of ineffective breathing and then, by contrast, demonstrates slow, deep abdominal breathing. Because many mothers of premature infants have had cesarean sections, the technique should be modified as needed to avoid causing or increasing physical pain. Mothers can also be referred to numerous breathing videos and mobile applications available for downloading. The therapist can suggest possible times to practice breathing exercises, including during breastfeeding, pumping, or while engaging in kangaroo care, and should ask the mother to propose how many times she can commit to practicing breathing exercises.

WRAP UP

Before concluding the session, the therapist should review any questions or concerns and confirm the date and time for their next session. The therapist may want to plan how best to remind the mother about the upcoming session. The mother should also be reminded to start making entries in her Baby Diary, to practice deep breathing, and to start or continue engaging in her infant's care in consultation with the bedside nurse.

LESSONS LEARNED FROM SESSION 1

Session 1 serves several main purposes: building rapport between therapist and mother, establishing a framework for treatment, and most importantly, empowering the mother to feel comfortable and competent in the NICU environment. We recognize that some parents may be reluctant initially to engage in an intervention that might imply the need for mental health support. Even after engaging, NICU mothers may be hesitant to open up to the therapist due to feelings of avoidance commonly seen in individuals who have gone through a traumatic experience. Many mothers avoid efforts to address their thoughts and feelings due to fears that the resulting emotions will be too overwhelming.

In this first session, the therapist should focus on the relationship between the mother and her infant in order to keep her engaged in treatment. One way to do this is to provide information and guidance about how she can become more involved in her infant's care. Generally, we have found that once a mother feels comfortable with her therapist, she will often openly share aspects of her experience. However, some mothers may need more time to feel fully engaged. The therapist can help in these situations by ensuring that the mother is getting something that she finds useful out of the experience.

Session 2: Cognitive Restructuring

Session 2 focuses on helping to normalize the mother's feelings and teaching her techniques to cope with negative thoughts and feelings. Many mothers experience a profound sense of loss following a premature birth and may have unresolved feelings of anger, guilt, frustration, and sadness. Some mothers may feel that they are not entitled to have these emotions because it detracts from their focus on their new baby. The goals of the second session are

1. To continue to build rapport
2. To build in a routine of using the Baby Diary
3. To normalize the emotions and reactions in the NICU setting, particularly feelings of guilt and responsibility
4. To help mothers identify the relationship between events, thoughts, and emotions and to challenge negative or unhelpful thoughts using classical CBT techniques

CHECK-IN

The therapist begins the session by checking in to see if the mother has been practicing the deep breathing techniques from the first session. The therapist should also review any entries the mother has made in the Baby Diary. If the mother has not made any entries, the therapist spends some time helping her enter examples of any caregiving behaviors she may have tried as well as anything new she may have noticed about her baby or her relationship with her baby. It is also helpful to address the barriers that prevented the mother from completing the Baby Diary in an effort to understand if the mother is resistant to the intervention. This may occur if she experiences uncomfortable emotions when completing her diary or avoids focusing on her relationship with her baby. The purpose of the Baby Diary is to help the mother think about her infant as an important member of her family rather than as a patient in the hospital. This begins to lay a foundation for the parent–child relationship and develops the mother's attachment with her child. Encouraging the mother to get into the habit of making entries regularly is important as part of the process of infant redefinition.

COGNITIVE RESTRUCTURING

The therapist begins to address some thoughts and feelings the mother has had throughout her NICU experience by reviewing some common thoughts and feelings of NICU parents (Figure 5–5). The therapist asks the mother if she can relate to any specific concerns and feelings on the list and to bring up any that are not on the list. It is important to pay close attention to the mother's most salient thoughts and feelings and to validate her experiences. Ask the mother to provide examples of a time that she felt these emotions and to link them to her experiences in the NICU. This introduces the concept that her traumatic experiences have a profound effect on her thoughts and feelings.

In the next section, the therapist introduces the concept of cognitive restructuring by explaining the connection between thoughts, feelings, and events.

> One of the things we have learned from the research is that every time something happens, people will try to interpret the event and its significance. We do this automatically, without thinking, and often are not aware of what we are telling ourselves or that we have attached meaning to the event. However, even though an event may appear small or insignificant, the way we interpret the event can have a large effect on the way we feel.

To help explain this concept, the therapist walks the mother through an ABC-B Worksheet, providing an example of how a mother would feel if a good friend did not acknowledge her when walking past her in the street (Figure 5–6). The example demonstrates that some aspects of a situation cannot be changed (a friend ignoring her), but the way in which we interpret the situation can help to change our own feelings about it and inform how we might choose to respond.

> This example illustrates how our interpretation of each situation influences the way we feel and behave. It also illustrates how there is almost always more than one way to interpret a situation. In this example, if you thought that your friend was ignoring you, you would feel angry or hurt. However, if you thought she was worrying about something important, or was ill, you might even feel sympathetic or concerned. This then could also affect how you might interpret and respond to the situation. In short, when something happens, we have an automatic thought about it, the thought leads to a feeling, and this feeling leads to a behavior. This process happens in a split second. When you have negative thoughts like this, it may create a cycle of negative thoughts and feelings.

The mother is asked to identify an example from her own experiences in the NICU and to use the ABC-B Worksheet to work through it. The therapist should help the mother use Figure 5–5 to select an emotion or

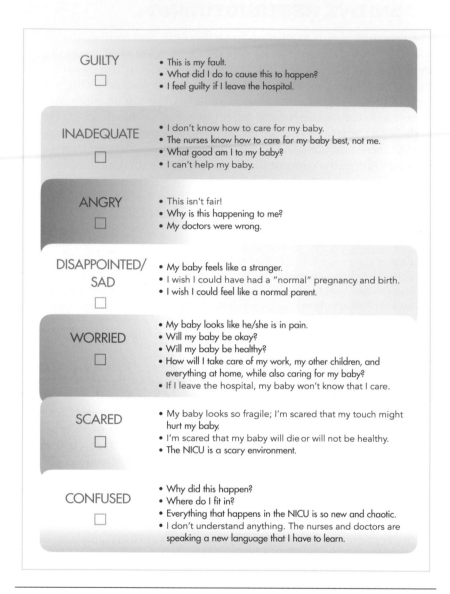

FIGURE 5–5.   Common thoughts and feelings of NICU parents.
Source.   Adapted from Shaw and Horwitz 2013.

thought that has stayed with her since it happened. The goal of this part of the session is to help the mother work through the ABC-B Worksheet, identifying the thoughts and feelings associated with her experience, and then come up with alternative thoughts. Mothers sometimes struggle to think of alternative ways of looking at the concepts of blame and guilt

ABC-B Worksheet

Activating event, Belief, Consequence - Behavior

1. AUTOMATIC REACTION

Activating event	Belief (thought)	Consequence (feeling)	Behavior
While crossing the street, I saw someone I know, but they did not say, "Hello."	• She must not like me. • I must have offended her at some point. • She's too stuck up to acknowledge me. • I'm a loser; other people saw me waving at her and getting no response.	• Embarrassed • Ashamed • Anxious • Sad • Angry	• Avoid her in the future • Confront her • Don't wave at people in the future

2. ALTERNATIVE EXPLANATIONS:

3. RESTRUCTURED / ALTERNATIVE REACTION

Same Activating event	NEW Belief (thought)	NEW Consequence (feeling)	NEW Behavior
While crossing the street, I saw someone I know, but they did not say, "Hello."			

How do you feel now? _____

FIGURE 5–6. ABC-B Worksheet.

Source. Adapted from Shaw and Horwitz 2013.

and may rely on the therapist to help develop a more positive interpretation. Emphasize that the goal of cognitive restructuring is not to alter the situation, feeling, or outcome but to offer alternative possible ways of interpreting the event. This practice can help the mother learn how to consider alternative explanations and thereby encourage different emotions and reactions in herself.

After coming up with alternative thoughts, the therapist should ask the mother how she would feel in light of these alternative explanations for what might have happened. The therapist should try to guide her toward verbalizing feelings that are more positive, for example, "more confident, less scared, and less guilty." The goal is not to eliminate unwanted or unhelpful feelings but to make those feelings more manageable by changing their intensity. In each session, mothers are asked to rate the intensity of their emotions on a scale of 0–10 (10 being the highest). After completing this exercise, the therapist asks the mother to rate the intensity of her emotions after considering alternative explanations.

Finally, the therapist should help the mother think about what new behaviors would result from these new thoughts and feelings. For example, if the mother correctly interprets her infant's decreased engagement as a reflection of the infant's resting state and not of disinterest, she will feel both competent and more connected with her infant. This is a good time to remind the mother about the states of infant readiness covered in Session 1 and, using this example, to show the mother that she has the power to change her interpretation of her infant's behavior.

EXAMINING THE EVIDENCE

In this section, the therapist introduces two additional techniques geared toward changing overwhelming and unwanted thoughts. The first is called "Examining the Evidence." The therapist uses an example with the mother based on the common situation of having an infant under the bilirubin lights (Figure 5–7).

> Sometimes when you are upset, it is hard to evaluate the evidence for your own thoughts. However, using a technique we call "Examining the Evidence," rather than simply taking your thoughts at face value, you can learn how to evaluate the evidence behind your negative thoughts. With this technique, you ask yourself what the facts really are and what those facts support. It is important that you evaluate only the facts that would stand up in a court of law. After you have looked at all the evidence, it is then possible to come up with a more rational and helpful way of evaluating your situation.

After working through this example, the therapist should choose a thought based on something the mother has expressed or explore possible thoughts she may be experiencing but has not yet voiced, and then choose the one most suitable. The therapist then helps the mother create lists of evidence that supports her thought or belief and evidence that does not. The manual provides a list of common negative thoughts as well as evidence against them (Figure 5–7). Once the mother has finished working through the handout and it is clear that the evidence against the negative thought outweighs the evidence supporting it, the therapist should ask the mother if seeing this has had any impact on her thought. The therapist should prompt the mother to realize that she can have a different perspective about her unhelpful thinking, which in turn can lead to a change in her feelings.

EXAMINING THE EVIDENCE

Example:

Belief (thought): _The bilirubin lights are a sign that my baby has taken a turn for the worse._

Evidence for	Evidence against
My infant needs special treatment for jaundice.	Jaundice is common, even in full-term babies.
	All the doctors and nurses report that this is treatable and will not have any lasting negative effects.

Your turn:

Belief (thought): _____

Evidence for	Evidence against
This is all my fault.	I did everything I could to ensure a healthy pregnancy.
I will never be able to take my baby home.	My baby is gaining weight and growing.
I do not feel I am getting to be a mother.	My baby is comforted by my voice and touch.

FIGURE 5–7. Examining the Evidence handout.
Source. Adapted from Shaw and Horwitz 2013.

WHAT WOULD I TELL A FRIEND?

Using the "What Would I Tell a Friend?" technique, the therapist reviews people's tendency to be much harsher judges of themselves than of others. Showing the mother how critical she may be of herself can help her begin to develop a greater feeling of empathy toward herself. By reflecting upon how she might respond to a friend in a similar situation, the mother learns how to exercise more cognitive flexibility and develop new ways of interpreting her situation.

Using the example we have just discussed, tell me what you would tell a friend if they were in the same situation as you are now. What would you say to help them feel better?

Most mothers quickly comment on how much kinder and sympathetic they would be toward their friend and how they would come up with useful alternative interpretations of the situation not dissimilar to those identified in the "Examining the Evidence" section. The therapist should strongly encourage the mother to keep practicing these techniques, explaining that it takes practice to achieve mastery.

POSITIVE SELF-STATEMENTS

The last portion of this session, "Positive Self-Statements," focuses on a technique that does not use thought replacement but is designed to help mothers feel empowered and encouraged.

If you are still having trouble coming up with a more rational, positive thought to replace a negative thought that keeps popping into your head, another technique to use is making a positive statement about yourself and your strengths to help you feel better about the situation. You could say to yourself, no matter what the negative thought is, "This is hard right now, but I can handle this."

The therapist should review possible rational positive self-statements with the mother (Figure 5–8). The therapist can ask if any of these particularly resonate with her, and they can work together to come up with additional examples she may find useful. Ask the mother to choose one self-talk statement that stands out for her and to practice saying it to herself over the course of the next week as an assignment.

WRAP UP

Before concluding the session, the therapist should check in to see if the mother has any questions or is still concerned about any of the things they have discussed. Ensure the mother feels comfortable practicing the cognitive restructuring exercises. She should also be encouraged to continue working on the Baby Diary and using the deep breathing techniques.

LESSONS LEARNED FROM SESSION 2

Session 2 is an important session in which mothers are taught the foundations of cognitive restructuring. These techniques will be used later in the intervention, when the mother starts to process her traumatic experience by writing a trauma narrative. For many mothers, this may be one of the first times they have discussed their NICU experience, and they

Positive Self-Statements

1. This is hard right now, but I can handle this.

2. I'm doing everything I can to help my baby.

3. I'm going to be a great mom.

4. The nurses are always here to help teach me how to care for my baby.

5. I can deal with anything thrown into my life.

6. This challenge will help me grow.

7. My baby is soothed by my touch and voice.

8. It feels good / will feel good when I hold my baby.

9. I can picture my baby big and strong.

10. I will love my baby no matter what.

11. I can imagine having my baby home, with all this in the past.

12. _____

FIGURE 5–8. Positive Self-Statements handout.
Source. Adapted from Shaw and Horwitz 2013.

may be hesitant to acknowledge feelings of anger or sadness. Many report not feeling comfortable sharing their thoughts and feelings out of fear of being judged or misunderstood. Many are preoccupied with feelings of guilt and blame that are rarely discussed in the NICU setting. The idealized view of new motherhood is of a period of all-consuming joy and happiness, but one in which the focus is on their baby. Even in the NICU, the primary focus is on the outcome of the infant. Many mothers do not feel they have the right to focus on their own emotional experience. This session sends them an important message and provides an opportunity to address these concerns while teaching them new skills for identifying, processing, and managing overwhelming and unhelpful thoughts and emotions.

Session 3: Stress, Triggers, and Self-Care

One of the core components of trauma-focused treatment is providing education about the concept of PTSD. Normalizing the presence of trauma symptoms, which may include nightmares or symptoms of anxiety, can be a great relief for mothers with an infant in the NICU. Session 3 explains the concept of traumatic stress, how triggers precipitate strong emotions, and the connection between stress and its physical and emotional effects. The session concludes with information on self-care to help manage those effects. The session's goals include

1. Reviewing the Baby Diary
2. Reviewing cognitive restructuring techniques learned in Session 2
3. Providing education about the symptoms of PTSD
4. Providing psychoeducation about triggers for PTSD symptoms and helping the mother identify her own triggers
5. Providing techniques to manage triggers
6. Explaining the physical effects of stress
7. Discussing ways to improve self-care

CHECK-IN

The therapist begins the session by checking in to see if the mother has been using the previous session's skills and if she has tried completing any additional cognitive restructuring worksheets on her own. Mother and therapist also review the Baby Diary. If she has not completed the Visiting Log or other sections in the diary, the therapist should take the time to help her do this. If she has completed an ABC-B Worksheet as assigned in Session 2, the therapist should review this with her. If not, the therapist should complete a worksheet with her, choosing a relevant example, to ensure the mother feels comfortable with the technique.

SYMPTOMS OF TRAUMATIC STRESS

This section starts with some educational material about the concept of trauma and how it is relevant to the mother's NICU experience:

> Many parents who have a baby in the NICU have very high levels of anxiety and may find themselves having uncomfortable thoughts or feel-

ings. One reason for this is that memories of the premature birth, as well as the experience of seeing your baby in pain or in a fragile or vulnerable state, can be extremely traumatic and can lead to emotional distress. For these reasons, many professionals are beginning to think of the experience of having a premature baby as a traumatic event, similar to the trauma of having a serious accident or of being assaulted or mistreated or similar to someone who has been traumatized in a war. However, one important difference for parents who have a baby in the NICU is that the trauma is an ongoing experience, often with multiple traumatic experiences related to their baby's medical complications.

It can also be common for parents to feel anxious when they leave their baby, even if it is just for a few minutes. On the other hand, some parents find it extremely difficult just being in the hospital and facing the various traumatic experiences that can happen there and as a result may find excuses to avoid coming in to see their baby.

Does it make sense to you to think of the experience of _____'s premature birth and their hospitalization in the NICU as a traumatic event?

The therapist asks the mother to reflect on her time in the NICU and to try to identify any specific traumatic experiences. After reflecting with her on what some of these experiences might be, the therapist describes the four categories of PTSD symptoms and provides the mother with a handout (Figure 5–9) where she can check off any symptoms she is currently experiencing or has experienced in the past.

If the mother endorses PTSD symptoms, the therapist should empathize with her and validate her experience. The therapist also explains how the mother can use the techniques learned in the first two sessions, particularly deep breathing and cognitive restructuring, to help manage her distressing thoughts or feelings. If the mother does not endorse any PTSD symptoms, reassure her that this can also be normal, letting her know that not everyone develops these symptoms and that they sometimes manifest at different times for different people. The therapist should provide psychoeducation about the role of avoidance as a symptom of PTSD, including avoiding potentially relevant symptoms of anxiety, distress, or guilt.

TRIGGERS

In this section, the therapist explains the concept of triggers, their relevance, and how they operate, using the example of a car accident:

Let me give you an example that's unrelated to the NICU but to which most people could relate. If someone has a traumatic experience, such as being in a head-on car collision, they may later go into a heightened state of fear or anxiety—perhaps even break out in a sweat or notice that their heart is racing—if something happens to remind them of the car accident. For example, driving on the same street where the accident hap-

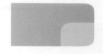

Symptoms of Traumatic Stress
(check all that apply)

Reexperiencing

☐ **Nightmares**
Disturbing dreams about your baby's birth or medical treatment in the hospital

☐ **Flashbacks**
The traumatic experience is replayed in your mind, like a recording of what happened, which may include visual images, sounds, smells, physical feelings, strong emotions. Flashbacks are likely to occur when something happens that reminds you of the trauma, or they can occur spontaneously, like when you are falling asleep or trying to relax.

☐ **Intrusive thoughts**
Thoughts that pop into your head uncontrollably and for no particular reason, and are difficult to block out, which can cause you to feel stressed

☐ **Emotional distress from trauma reminders**
Experiencing strong negative emotions when reminded of the traumatic event

☐ **Physical reactivity from trauma reminders**
Experiencing physical symptoms (such as pounding heart, rapid breathing, sweating) upon being reminded of the traumatic event

> A sense of reliving or reexperiencing the trauma is common for parents and can take many forms, including nightmares or flashbacks.
>
> Professionals believe these occur because the mind is trying to make sense of frightening memories or gain some control over them.

> Reexperiencing the trauma of hearing bad news about your baby's medical condition, or of witnessing your baby having painful procedures, may result in several common symptoms.
>
> If you are having upsetting dreams or intrusive thoughts and feelings, you are not alone; these are common for parents in your situation.

Negative thoughts and feelings

☐ **Negative feelings**
Emotions like sadness, guilt, anger

☐ **Negative thoughts**
Thinking negatively about the world, others, or yourself

☐ **Self-blame**
Blaming yourself for what happened

☐ **Difficulty experiencing positive emotions**
  ☐ Finding it hard to experience joy
  ☐ Struggling to connect emotionally with your baby

☐ **Decreased interest in activities**
Not doing things you used to enjoy

☐ **Difficulty recalling parts of the event**
Having difficulty remembering details from the event, such as the birth or your baby's admission to the NICU

Arousal and reactivity

☐ **Startle response**
Being easily startled by unexpected noises, such as the sound of the baby monitors, your phone ringing, or loud sounds from the street

☐ **Hypervigilance**
Always being on guard, alert, looking for threat

☐ **Risky or destructive behavior**
Doing things that are dangerous, like driving very **fast or drinking excessively**

☐ **Irritability**
Feeling easily annoyed or irritated

☐ **Difficulty concentrating**
Having difficulty concentrating on tasks

☐ **Difficulty sleeping**
Having difficulty falling or staying asleep

Another type of common reaction to traumatic stress is becoming very easily startled by unexpected noises, such as the sound of the baby monitors or loud sounds from the street.

A natural reaction to the intrusive memories and strong emotional reactions is the urge to push these thoughts and feelings away.

This natural tendency leads to a group of traumatic stress symptoms that mothers commonly experience, such as avoiding situations that remind them of the traumatic experience, including their baby's medical experiences.

Avoidance

☐ **External**
Avoiding things that remind you of the traumatic experience:
  ☐ Avoid visiting or calling the hospital
  ☐ Avoid doctors and nursery staff
  ☐ Avoid asking questions about your baby
  ☐ Avoid touching or caring for your baby

☐ **Internal**
Avoiding thoughts and feelings that remind you of the experience:
  ☐ Avoid thinking about your baby
  ☐ Avoid thinking about your experience

FIGURE 5–9. Symptoms of Traumatic Stress handout.
Source. Adapted from Shaw and Horwitz 2013.

pened or driving with oncoming traffic may trigger traumatic memories. In this case, the street where the accident took place and oncoming traffic would each be examples of triggers. Even watching someone drive a car on the television or seeing a picture of the street where the accident occurred might trigger the person to have the same feelings and reactions they had during the original accident. If we can identify the underlying thought, which in this case might be, "Other drivers will hit me" or "I am in danger," we can change the feelings and behaviors to cope with that trigger so that the person does not develop a phobia about driving on that specific street or generalize the fear to the point where they cannot drive at all.

The therapist reviews with the mother the list of common triggers for parents of premature infants and invites her to identify those are relevant for her (Figure 5–10).

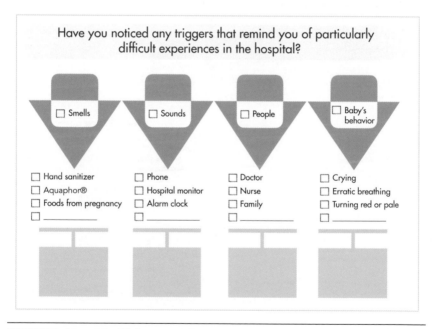

FIGURE 5–10.   Identifying your triggers.

Source.   Adapted from Shaw and Horwitz 2013.

If the mother has difficulty identifying triggers, the therapist should refer her back to some of the experiences described during Session 2 or provide her with some common examples (e.g., the monitor goes off; the neonatologist comes through the NICU doors). Other common triggers include the smell of hand sanitizer or receiving a phone call with the area code of the hospital. The therapist should make a note of the trigger(s) identified by the mother to use in the next section.

IMAGINING THE EXPERIENCE

After identifying the mother's triggers, the therapist leads her through an activity called "imagining the experience." In this exercise, the therapist discusses a stressful trigger that could lead to a hypothetically stressful experience but asks the mother to counter her automatic response of fear or anxiety using one of the strategies from her list of coping techniques.

> Let's use the trigger you picked earlier and see if we can work through it to make it more manageable by doing an exercise called "imagining the experience." Imagining the experience, as the name implies, involves choosing an experience or something that is a trigger for you and using our imagination to pretend that the experience is really happening. As I ask you to imagine one of your stressful triggers, we will rate your level of stress on a scale from 0 to 10, with 0 being the lowest level and 10 being the highest level, using the Feelings Thermometer Scale [Figure 5–11]. We will do a second rating of your level of stress at the end of the exercise to see if it has changed.
>
> As we go through this imagination exercise, we will be exploring your thoughts and feelings. An important part of this exercise will also be to help you figure out some new ways to cope with this imaginary situation. Let's take a look at your toolbox [Figure 5–12]. You can see that you already have some useful coping tools to help you with the triggers when they come up in real life.

The therapist establishes which trigger the mother wants to discuss and confirms that the mother is ready to engage in the exercise. Examples may include 1) the baby monitor alarm goes off while nurse is attending to another patient; 2) the infant appears to have difficulty breathing while she is holding them; 3) she gets an early morning phone call from the hospital; or 4) she gets to the hospital and finds that her baby is not in same location as the day before. Some mothers may be hesitant to engage in this exercise, so the therapist must remind the mother that she can stop at any time and that she has several tools to manage her emotions, such as deep breathing, if things get too stressful.

After confirming that the mother is ready to move forward, the therapist should ask her which coping tool from the toolbox she wants to use for the exercise. The therapist must then create a hypothetical scenario based on the trigger identified, starting out by inviting the mother to close her eyes to get into the moment and imagine the scenario. The therapist should start by asking the mother to imagine a point in the scenario before it becomes stressful and then proceed to the triggering event. The therapist asks her to close her eyes and start to imagine the scenario.

- Can you tell me what is coming into your mind as you imagine ____?
- Please tell me what you are feeling right now.
- Describe it in as much detail as you can.

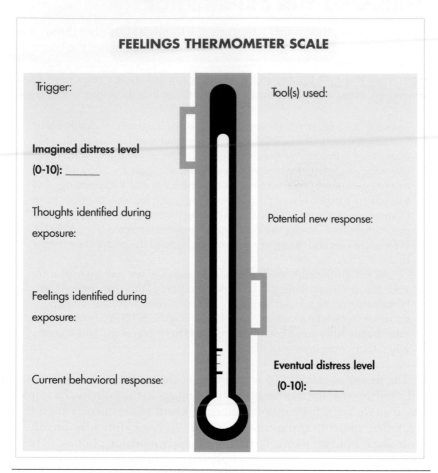

FIGURE 5–11.   Feelings Thermometer Scale handout.
Source.   Adapted from Shaw and Horwitz 2013.

If the mother is having difficulty describing her experience, the therapist should prompt her for more details about her thoughts and feelings.

- At this point, what is your level of distress on the 0–10 scale?
- What thoughts are going through your mind right now?
- What are you feeling right now?
- Without using your coping tools, how are you tempted to respond?
- What do you feel like doing?

The therapist should identify potentially unhelpful or unhealthy responses. If the mother's behavior reactions seem adaptive, the therapist should praise her and then increase the intensity of the current trigger

MOM'S TOOLBOX

☐ ABC-B exercise to find alternative thoughts

☐ Examining the Evidence

☐ What Would I Tell a Friend?

☐ Deep breathing and progressive muscle relaxation

☐ Positive Self-Statements (may refer back to favorites selected in session)

☐ Writing in journal or retelling story

FIGURE 5–12.   Mom's Toolbox handout.
Source.   Adapted from Shaw and Horwitz 2013.

by suggesting more distressing possibilities. The therapist then prompts the mother to try different coping strategies from her toolbox to control her anxiety:

> Now that we have imagined this unpleasant experience, let's use _____ (coping tool) from your toolbox rather than _____ (the unhealthy response). Can you think of some ways you could use this tool to change your thoughts or feelings or the way you are tempted to respond?

The therapist models how to use the coping tool, for example, doing an ABC-B Worksheet or a few rounds of deep breathing, and then asks the mother to put herself back in that moment with her eyes closed while the therapist asks the following questions:

• Can you picture yourself doing anything differently now?
• Can you describe to me what you are imagining right now?
• What are you thinking?
• What are you feeling?

If needed, the therapist should ask the mother what she could specifically say or do differently that would help her feel better or in more control. Some of the positive self-statements learned in Session 2 may be helpful, for example, "I am a good mother" or "I can handle this." To conclude, the therapist should ask the mother to rank her distress level again on a scale of 0–10 on the Feelings Thermometer (see Figure 5–11) to compare her scores. The therapist should also praise the mother for doing such a good job with a stressful activity and ask how she is feeling after completing this exercise.

PHYSICAL EFFECTS OF STRESS

After completing the "imagining the experience" exercise, the therapist describes the "Stress Triangle" to discuss the physical effects of stress and explains the importance of managing and reducing stress (Figure 5–13).

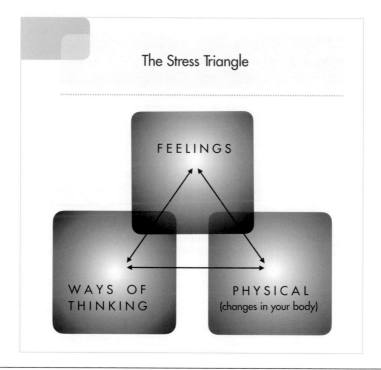

FIGURE 5–13.   The Stress Triangle handout.
Source.   Adapted from Shaw and Horwitz 2013.

We have talked today about common stress reactions in response to the NICU and your concern for your baby. Stress can affect us physically, by causing headaches, muscle aches, fatigue, or anxiety. This in turn can influence our thoughts and feelings in a negative way. Your feelings, your way of thinking, and changes in your body are all related. Let me give you an example of this. If you are feeling nervous or tense, it is likely that the muscles in your neck, shoulders, or jaw will tense up and possibly result in a headache. This might make it hard for you to sleep at night. Lack of sleep can result in your feeling even more stressed and less able to cope with the demands of having your baby in the NICU.

One way to reduce our stress is to change our negative thoughts using the techniques that we have discussed in our last two sessions. Another approach to stress is to find a way to relax physically, such as using the technique of deep breathing that we practiced in the first session.

The therapist concludes this section by reviewing the tips to reduce stress, boost self-care, and increase social support (Figure 5–14).

OVERCOMING BARRIERS TO SELF-CARE

Mothers often feel guilty about what has happened to their infant and blame themselves or think that others blame them for their infant's premature birth. These feelings may lead the mother to think she needs to overcompensate by constantly being at her infant's bedside. However, in reality, mothers and infants do better if mothers are less stressed and well rested. Mothers should be encouraged to take time for themselves without feeling that they are being selfish and should be told that self-care is a powerful way to enhance the well-being of their infant.

In this section, the therapist identifies barriers, including emotional, logistical, or financial concerns, that might impede the mother from engaging in self-care behaviors. The therapist helps her identify potential self-care behaviors as well as barriers to self-care (Figure 5–15). It is helpful to have the mother reflect on the self-care activities in which she engaged prior to her infant's admission to the NICU and to explore ways in which she can continue practicing self-care while in the NICU.

After determining what activities the mother is or wishes she were doing, the therapist uses the "Action Plan for Self-Care" worksheet to help her come up with a self-care plan. The therapist should pick one feasible activity, identify the barriers and solutions, and set goals. This may involve using skills from the toolbox to overcome specific barriers. Finally, the therapist helps the mother identify positive thoughts or self-statements that help her feel empowered to engage in a feasible plan of self-care.

WRAP UP

Before ending the session, the therapist should check in with the mother to see how she is feeling and if she has any questions or additional needs. The therapist encourages the mother to share what she is learning in these sessions with her family, encourages her to work on the Baby Diary, and reviews the tools she can use to manage negative thoughts or feelings. The therapist should also notify the mother that in the next session they will be working together to create a trauma narrative.

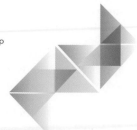

Rest and sleep

- Go to bed only when tired, and try to relax before bedtime.
- Get out of bed when you're unable to sleep. If you are not asleep within half an hour, do something relaxing until you feel sleepy again.
- Use the bed/bedroom for sleep only (no reading, watching TV, etc.).
- Try your best to go to bed at the same time every night and wake up at the same time every morning.
- Find more information at www.sleepfoundation.org.

If you are having trouble sleeping, here are some tips for improving your sleep:

- It is okay to take a break from breastfeeding to get a good night's sleep when you really need it; your rest benefits your baby too.
- Avoid caffeine, nicotine, and alcohol later in the day.
- Exercise, but not within 3 hours of bedtime.
- Establish a consistent sleep-wake schedule.

Talk to your friends and family

- Let them help you. ASK for support.
- Don't be shy to tell them what *is* helpful and what *isn't*.
- Ask them if they want to come visit your baby with you.
- Be open and honest with your partner. Talk about how you are feeling.

If you have other children

- Answer their questions honestly and simply.
- Make sure they know that they did not do anything to cause the baby to be born early.
- Talk with them about their feelings.
- Show them special and unique characteristics of their sibling with pictures.
- Make pictures, audio, or video recordings with them to bring to the baby.
- Set aside time just for them.

FIGURE 5–14.   Tips to reduce stress and increase support.

Source.   Adapted from Shaw and Horwitz 2013.

LESSONS LEARNED FROM SESSION 3

Some mothers are surprised or even a bit resistant to the idea that they may have had a traumatic experience and may hesitate to label what they have experienced as traumatic stress or PTSD. However, by the end of this session, mothers are more likely to acknowledge the traumatic nature of their experience, viewing PTSD not as mental illness but as a

---

Action Plan for Self-Care

Target activity:

Current barriers and challenges to doing the activity:

Ideas for how to work around the barriers and challenges:

I will use the following positive self-statements to encourage myself to take time for me:

My goal will be to do _____ for myself

_____ time(s) a day at the following time(s): _____.

FIGURE 5–15. **Action Plan for Self-Care handout.**
Source. Adapted from Shaw and Horwitz 2013.

normal reaction to an extraordinary and stressful situation. If the mother resists this concept, the therapist should not force the issue but find a way to support the mother's resilience. However, mothers often feel relieved and are comfortable accepting the notion that their NICU experience has been traumatic. The topic of traumatic stress is revisited in Sessions 4 and 5, so it is possible she will be able to more fully appreciate the traumatic aspects of her experience in the sessions to come.

Encourage the mother to engage in self-care by writing out a specific plan for self-care activities that she thinks are reasonably attained. Even mothers who are focused on time constraints or logistical issues can be convinced to try breathing exercises while pumping or breastfeeding or taking short walks outside the NICU. Emphasize the importance of caring for herself in order to properly continue providing care for her baby and highlight the importance of establishing regular eating and sleeping patterns, taking breaks from bedside, seeking support, and engaging in activities they may have enjoyed prior to their time in the NICU.

Session 4: Loss and Trauma Narrative

One of the core components of TF-CBT is the development of the trauma narrative. In this session, the mother writes a narrative of her experiences during her pregnancy, at the time of delivery, and during her infant's NICU hospitalization. This narrative will be read aloud and processed with the therapist in Session 5. Mothers consistently rate Session 4 and Session 5 as the most difficult because they are asked to recall traumatic memories. However, mothers also consistently report this to be the most beneficial part of the intervention. Session 4 builds on the concept of the NICU experience as traumatic, diving more deeply into the topics of trauma and loss. The goals of this session include

1. Reviewing the Baby Diary
2. Educating the mother about symptoms of loss
3. Developing the mother's trauma narrative
4. Providing instruction on the use of PMR

CHECK-IN

The therapist begins the session by reviewing the Baby Diary and asking if the mother has tried using any of her tools to manage any stressful situations that have arisen since the last session. The therapist then discusses the agenda for Session 4, explaining that they will first talk about loss and trauma, followed by a narrative exercise in which the mother will have a chance to tell her story. Be sure to acknowledge that although the idea of writing the trauma narrative might sound daunting, the therapist will be available to help and provide support.

LOSS

Premature birth is not only traumatic but also an experience of loss for the mother. She may feel cheated out of the experience of a normal pregnancy and birth and may have feelings of grief about the loss of the expected healthy child and early parenting experiences. The mother may also have concerns about her infant's long-term health and well-being. The therapist explains how traumatic events can lead to feelings of anger, depression, anxiety, and detachment, as well as the process of denial (Figure 5–16). The therapist reviews these pathways and explains that it is part of the normal process of grief and loss to move back and forth between these feelings or to have all of them simultaneously.

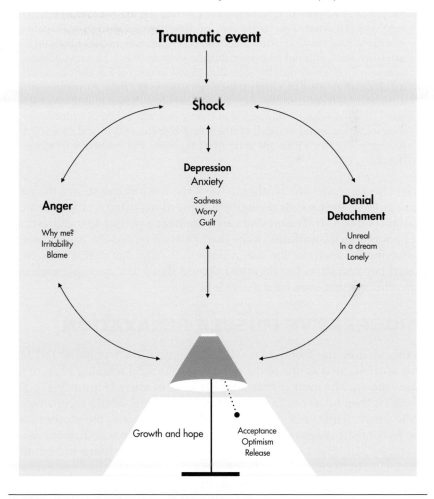

Responses to Trauma   There is a range of **three** general types of emotions that people tend to feel in response to a very upsetting experience. Most people go through some or all of these before they get to a state of acceptance or resolution. You may feel each of these different feelings at different times, and this is completely normal.

Traumatic event

Shock

Depression
Anxiety

Sadness
Worry
Guilt

Anger

Why me?
Irritability
Blame

Denial
Detachment

Unreal
In a dream
Lonely

Growth and hope | Acceptance
Optimism
Release

FIGURE 5–16.   **Responses to Trauma handout.**

Source.   Adapted from Shaw and Horwitz 2013. Design © Tonyanna C. Borkovi.

DEVELOPMENT OF THE TRAUMA NARRATIVE

After they discuss loss, the therapist explains to the mother that they will go through a series of questions about her pregnancy, birth, and NICU experience that will provide her with an opportunity to tell her story. The therapist explains that one of the evidence-based ways of coping with trauma is through writing or telling one's story, as well as through sharing the story with another person.

> I'm going to ask you to describe the events leading up to your baby's premature birth and the experiences that you have since had with your baby. I have a series of questions that I would like to ask you that will help us get started. This might feel a little different, since it will seem less like a conversation. After I ask you each question, I will be listening carefully, but I will not be responding to your answers. However, I am here to help if it becomes too stressful. Please answer the questions in as much detail as you can. Our research on women who have gone through a stressful or traumatic experience like yours has shown that telling the story of what actually happened is a very powerful way of processing their experience and one that mothers find helpful. In our next meeting, we are going to go through your story together and discuss it in more detail.

After checking with the mother to see if she has any questions, the therapist guides her through the narrative questions listed in the treatment manual (Table 5–4). The mother can write her responses to the questions on paper or on a computer, or the therapist can record the narrative and transcribe the material for use in Session 5. After the mother has completed her narrative, the therapist should thank her and acknowledge how difficult this exercise may have been.

PROGRESSIVE MUSCLE RELAXATION

In this section, the therapist teaches the mother the technique of PMR. This is often rated as one of the most enjoyable and relaxing parts of the intervention. The mother first rates her level of stress (Figure 5–17). The therapist then takes her through a session of PMR. Many recordings of PMR are available online. Following the PMR session, the mother rates her level of stress again. They then discuss a feasible schedule for her to practice PMR; good times to practice include while lying in bed after waking up in the morning or before going to sleep at night. The therapist explains how important it is for the mother to practice these new skills when she is not feeling stressed so she can master them and use them at times of future stress.

Table 5–4.   Trauma narrative questions from individual therapy manual

---

1. Could you tell me a little about your pregnancy?
2. When did you first find out that there was a possibility you might have a premature birth?
3. How did you feel when you first found out you were going to deliver early?
4. What do remember about your birth experience?
5. What do you remember about the first time you saw your baby? What were your first thoughts about your baby?
6. Please tell me about the first time you visited your baby in the NICU.
7. Please tell me about your experiences since your baby has been here in the hospital.
8. Do you remember any particularly difficult or stressful medical events or procedures?
9. Do you remember any particularly difficult or stressful conversations or interactions with any of the nurses or doctors?
10. Do you remember any particularly difficult or stressful experiences that happened to other parents or babies in the NICU?
11. Have you noticed any things in the NICU that cause you to feel particularly anxious or that you consider to be triggers for you?
12. Have you noticed any situations outside of the hospital that have caused you to experience a trigger?
13. Do you have any thoughts or beliefs about why your baby was born prematurely and why they needed to be in the NICU?
14. What impact has this experience had on you?
15. What impact has this experience had on your family and/or partner?
16. What worries do you have about how all this is going to affect your future? You can include concerns that may or may not seem rational to you.
17. How has this experience affected your view of yourself?
18. How has this experience affected your relationship with your partner?
19. How has this experience affected your view of other people in your life?
20. How has this affected your view of the world in general?
21. Is there anything else that I did not ask you about that you want to tell me about?

Source.   Adapted from Shaw and Horwitz 2013.

By regularly practicing Progressive Muscle Relaxation, you will really learn how to recognize when you feel tension in your body and then be able to let that tension go. It is good to write down the specific moments when you are going to practice so that it can be part of your schedule. Would you be willing to come up with a schedule for practicing your Progressive Muscle Relaxation?

Progressive Muscle Relaxation (PMR)

1. Find a comfortable, quiet place without any distractions.

2. Guide yourself through PMR or open a relaxation recording or application to guide you.

3. Notice any discomfort or tenderness you have in your body. Do not do anything that hurts, just skip whichever muscle is tender or sore. This is intended to be relaxing, so do not do anything that causes pain.

4. Observe your mind as it wanders, directing your thoughts back to focusing on tensing and relaxing your muscles.

5. Try to be mindfully engaged and relaxed without falling asleep.

Current stress rating (0–10): _____

Stress rating after muscle relaxation (0–10): _____

My goal will be to practice my **PMR** exercises _____ times a day/week

at the following time(s): _____

You can always practice these skills more often.
The more you practice, the more relaxed you will feel.

Good times to practice relaxation skills:

- When you wake up in the morning
- Before you go to bed at night
- Before a stressful event (such as visiting the NICU or a meeting with a doctor)
- After you leave the NICU
- After experiencing a nightmare or flashback
- When you are feeling anxious
- You can practice deep breathing—but **not** PMR—while holding or providing Containing Touch for your baby

FIGURE 5–17.   Progressive Muscle Relaxation handout.

Source.   Adapted from Shaw and Horwitz 2013.

WRAP UP

The therapist should check in once again with the mother to ensure that she is feeling stable after recounting or writing down her narrative. The therapist also reminds the mother that she has a variety of other tools in her toolbox, such as deep breathing exercises and the cognitive restructuring worksheets (e.g., ABC-B, What Would I Tell a Friend?, Examining the Evidence), should she feel increased stress or anxiety after completing the narrative activity. The therapist should thank the mother for her willingness to open up and share this very personal experience.

LESSONS LEARNED FROM SESSION 4

In this session, the therapist should give the mother the emotional space she needs to work through her story and resist the temptation to step in to reassure her or to help decrease her level of emotional distress during her narrative. The goal is for the mother to have as rich and intense an experience as possible to gain the maximum benefits from the intervention. Although the therapist should be supportive and empathetic, they should be careful not to derail or distract the mother from the emotionally difficult parts of her story. The therapist should also emphasize the importance of providing as much sensory detail as possible from all five senses. Encouraging the mother to either share or write her trauma narrative in the first person will assist her in accessing the emotions and thoughts she experienced during the time of the trauma.

If the mother appears detached or unemotional in the telling of her story, or if the narrative seems flat or lacking emotion, she may be experiencing emotional numbing or dissociation as part of her PTSD symptoms. The therapist should not pressure her to express more emotion during Session 4 but rather note this possibility and address it in Session 5 when the mother retells her story. Because the stories told by NICU mothers are often traumatic, the therapist should pay attention to their own reactions as well.

Finally, if the therapist is recording and transcribing the narrative, sufficient time should be allowed between Sessions 4 and 5 to carefully review it and note major themes or triggers (Table 5–5). However, Session 5 should be scheduled within 3–4 days if possible because developing the trauma narrative may trigger uncomfortable emotions the mother and she may require additional support.

Session 5: Reading and Processing the Trauma Narrative

The purpose of Session 5 is for the mother to process her emotions and identify potential triggers by reading her trauma narrative aloud in the presence of the therapist. Therapists who do not have a background in trauma treatment may require specific training and supervision with a mental health clinician to master the skills needed to conduct this session. The treatment manual has extensive in-session instructions and

Table 5–5.   Trauma narrative cue sheet from individual therapy manual

Major emotions noted in the narrative (e.g., anger, sadness, worry)

Significant omissions from the narrative (e.g., feeling excluded from the care of the infant, hearing bad news about the infant's prognosis, learning that her baby needs to have surgery or a procedure, witnessing unexpected traumatic medical events or procedures, unpleasant interactions with the staff, witnessing traumatic events occurring to other NICU babies)

Topics preceding or following lengthy pauses in the narrative

Themes noted in the narrative to be discussed in Session 5 (e.g., self-blame, guilt, things she wishes she had done differently, anger at doctor, concerns about her life being ruined)

Triggers identified

Source.   Adapted from Shaw and Horwitz 2013.

guidance about how to support the mother as she reads her trauma narrative. The goals of this session include

1. Having the mother read her trauma narrative aloud, with emotional expression
2. Identifying the mother's "stuck points" regarding her traumatic experiences
3. Discussing potential triggers and providing guidance to the mother on how to manage these
4. Challenging self-blame and irrational thoughts

CHECK-IN

The therapist begins the session by checking in to see if the mother has made any new entries in the Baby Diary and Visiting Log. If she has not been keeping up with these tasks, encourage her to do so, particularly because the intervention is nearing its conclusion. The Baby Diary entries are used in Session 6 to review the progress the mother and her infant have made.

READING THE TRAUMA NARRATIVE

The therapist explains that the mother will be asked to read her trauma narrative aloud, which will help her to process her experience:

> In our last meeting, we went through your experience of being here in the NICU, including your pregnancy and birth experience. You also told me how you felt the entire experience has affected you personally and how it has affected your family. I have had a chance to go through your story, and I have a transcript for us to use in today's session. What I'd

like us to do today is to ask you to read it aloud. The reason we're doing this is that research has shown that if a mother has had a particularly difficult or traumatic experience in the NICU, one way to deal with it is to first write about what happened and then process it by reading it aloud. Even though it may be difficult for you, my expectation is that it will help you better understand your feelings about what has happened during your baby's time in the NICU. Many mothers have a feeling of emotional release after reading their story. After you have read your narrative, I will ask you some questions.

The therapist instructs the mother not to focus too much on how she reads but on what she has to say and how the story makes her feel as she reads it.

Could you read this aloud for me now? As you are reading, try to put yourself back in the moment when these things were happening. Imagine that it's happening right now. Try to remember what it really felt like when it all happened. It's fine if you find yourself becoming emotional as you go over your story. In fact, please try to express your feelings as you read.

Detailed instructions are provided for the therapist for how to handle the narrative reading. The therapist should allow the mother to read the narrative in its entirety without interruption. Although the therapist can make supportive, encouraging comments, they should not help the mother process her experience until the entire narrative has been read. The therapist should listen carefully not only to what the mother reads but also to what she leaves out. If the therapist suspects that an important aspect of the story has been avoided, the mother should be asked for more detail about that portion of the experience once she has finished reading the entire narrative. Common traumatic experiences include complicated labor and delivery, loss of a twin, feeling excluded from the care of the infant, hearing bad news about the infant's prognosis, learning that the baby needs to have surgery or a procedure, witnessing unexpected traumatic medical events or procedures, having unpleasant interactions with the NICU staff, and witnessing traumatic events occurring to other babies in the NICU.

If the mother expresses a great deal of emotion while reading her narrative, the therapist should remain silent. Efforts to comfort her, such as offering her a tissue and other gestures, may interfere with the process. Therapists new to trauma therapy are often concerned that mothers will experience an overwhelming amount of affect. The therapist must allow the mother to fully experience the range of her emotions while sharing her narrative in order for the exercise to be effective and should model to the mother that she can experience overwhelming emotions without decompensating.

In some cases, the mother may read her narrative without any emotion. If this happens, the therapist should pause her early in her account and respond in the following way:

> Clearly, you are describing what must have been a very difficult and emotional experience. But it is interesting to me that you are not talking about your story in a very emotional way. Do you think this is true? Do you have any ideas about why you are not expressing your feelings? Do you think you might be consciously holding back your feelings?
>
> Many mothers are worried about losing control or feeling being overwhelmed by their emotions. However, research on mothers of premature infants has shown that it is helpful to let out the emotions. Let me give you an analogy. We can think about your emotions as though they were a bottle of soda that has been shaken. When the cap comes off, there is a rush, but it is temporary and eventually the soda flattens. If you were to quickly put the cap back on, the soda would retain its fizz. The soda, under pressure, has energy to it but cannot keep producing that energy when the cap is left off. We can look at your emotions in the same way. You feel the strength of the emotions when you open the lid, for example, when you start to think or write about your experiences. But if you keep the lid on, the emotions stay bottled up inside of you and you end up not being able to work through the experience. Think about some times when you have felt sad or angry. What happened after you allowed yourself to feel and express your emotions?

After addressing this issue, the therapist should ask the mother to continue with her account. If she now starts to experience more emotional distress, the therapist should sit quietly and not interfere with or minimize the emotions. In some cases, the mother may not be avoiding her emotions at all but experiencing them just as they were experienced at the time—that is, she may be in a state of dissociation. This should be noted and discussed in the next session. Should this occur during the session, grounding techniques can be used, such as encouraging the mother to open her eyes if they are closed, asking her to name objects she sees in the room, or asking her to touch the chair she is sitting in and describe what she feels. These grounding techniques will help her become more present focused and recognize that she is no longer living through the distressing situation and is in the safety of the room with the therapist.

PROCESSING THE NARRATIVE

After the mother finishes reading, the therapist should check in to see if she is ready to go on. The therapist then asks a series of questions meant to identify particularly stressful aspects of the experience, identify specific triggers, help the mother process the traumatic experiences, and remind her about the tools she can use to cope with her emotions.

- Could you tell me a little about the thoughts and feelings you had while you were reading your story?
- Did anything surprise you while you were reading your story?
- What was the most difficult or disturbing part of the story?
- Looking at the entire experience, what would you say was the most stressful part of the story?
- Were there any aspects of your experience that you found more difficult to remember or describe?
- Is there anything that you feel is important that was left out?

The therapist should share major themes and elements they noticed when reviewing the narrative and ask the mother to reflect on each. The therapist prompts her to discuss any relevant triggers and reminds her that she has the tools in her toolbox should she need them. If she still seems to be struggling, the therapist may consider doing an ABC-B Worksheet, Examining the Evidence exercise, or a session of PMR. However, these should not be used to avoid experiencing the emotions but rather to help the mother cope with them if they become too intense.

RESPONSIBILITY AND BLAME

In this section, the therapist focuses on the concepts of responsibility and blame, with the goal of addressing the common misconceptions mothers have about their role and responsibility in their child's premature birth and NICU experiences. The therapist clarifies that although the mother may feel responsible for the premature birth, in most cases she is not actually to blame. The therapist uses a cognitive restructuring exercise called 20/20 Hindsight (Figure 5–18) to help the mother acknowledge the human instinct to look at things with hindsight and identify elements that could have been done differently; this helps her realize that she probably did everything she possibly could have done to protect her baby. The handout prompts the mother to think about regrets she has about the experience and then to work through the Examining the Evidence and What Would I Tell a Friend? exercises to think about anything she could or would have done differently, which may help her realize that she is not to blame.

ACCOMPLISHMENTS, POSITIVES, AND PRIDE

The concept of posttraumatic growth describes how individuals who have had traumatic experiences may undergo a transformation that creates positive developments in their personality and worldview. In this section, the therapist helps the mother identify strengths and psychological growth she may have experienced. The goal is to help her see herself

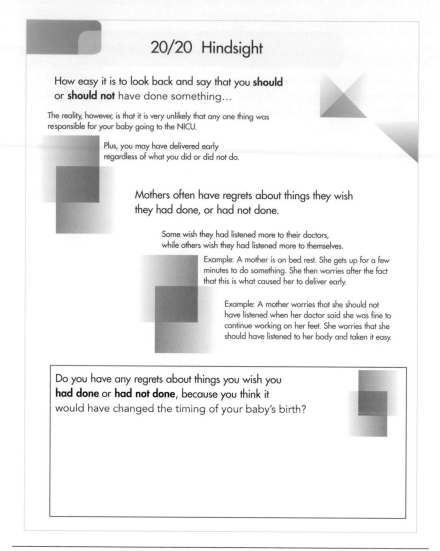

20/20 Hindsight

How easy it is to look back and say that you **should** or **should not** have done something...

The reality, however, is that it is very unlikely that any one thing was responsible for your baby going to the NICU.

Plus, you may have delivered early regardless of what you did or did not do.

Mothers often have regrets about things they wish they had done, or had not done.

Some wish they had listened more to their doctors, while others wish they had listened more to themselves.

Example: A mother is on bed rest. She gets up for a few minutes to do something. She then worries after the fact that this is what caused her to deliver early.

Example: A mother worries that she should not have listened when her doctor said she was fine to continue working on her feet. She worries that she should have listened to her body and taken it easy.

Do you have any regrets about things you wish you **had done** or **had not done**, because you think it would have changed the timing of your baby's birth?

FIGURE 5–18.　20/20 Hindsight handout.

Source.　Adapted from Shaw and Horwitz 2013.

as a survivor rather than a trauma victim. The therapist starts by helping the mother list specific accomplishments and things she may feel proud of during her time in the NICU (Figure 5–19).

　　The therapist comments on specific positive things the mother has been able to do, using her own words and phrases as much as possible and referencing prior conversations. Examples may include, "You got the best prenatal care you could; you did nearly everything your doctor

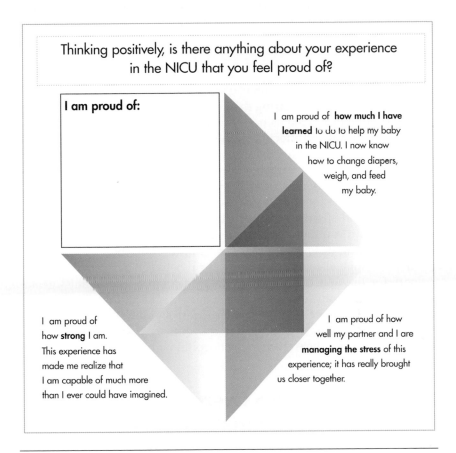

FIGURE 5–19.   **Accomplishments, positives, and pride.**
Source.   Adapted from Shaw and Horwitz 2013.

told you to do, even though you had to take care of numerous other responsibilities; and now, here in the NICU, you have been consistently trying to figure out how best to help your infant survive. On top of that, you have shown up for every one of our sessions together."

WRAP UP

To conclude, the therapist checks in with the mother to see how she is feeling and reminds her of the various tools in her toolbox to help her if she feels distressed. The therapist should also encourage her to rewrite her trauma narrative, repeatedly if possible, emphasizing that research has shown that this helps parents overcome symptoms of trauma. The therapist should ask the mother to bring her Baby Diary to the next session and inform her that the session will take place at her baby's bedside or, if the baby has been discharged, at her home.

LESSONS LEARNED FROM SESSION 5

Following this emotionally intense session, many mothers report feelings of great relief after sharing their experience with the therapist. This session is often described as both the most anxiogenic session and one of the most helpful and effective. If the mother still seems overwhelmed, the therapist may want to check in with her during the next few days. Mothers usually report that they found it helpful to share their narratives with their partners or other family members, so the therapist may want to encourage them to do so. Mothers state that sharing the narrative helped open up a dialogue with their partner and facilitated a deeper level of communication. Both parents may experience an outpouring of emotions during this process that can be quite cathartic.

The therapist also has tasks to perform between Sessions 5 and 6 to prepare for the final session, including calculating the infant's gestational age. If the baby is likely to be discharged and Session 6 will be conducted at the mother's home, the therapist should allow ample time because interruptions or unanticipated events may occur. It is also possible to have the mother return to the hospital with her infant for the final session.

Session 6: Avoiding Overprotective Parenting and Preparing for Home

Session 6 focuses on helping the mother prepare for her infant's discharge and begins a discussion about overprotective parenting, described earlier in the context of VCS (see Chapter 7). This session should take place at the infant's bedside if possible. The goals of this session include

1. Debriefing with the mother about the trauma narrative
2. Encouraging the process of infant redefinition by helping the mother realize how much has changed with respect to her infant's growth and development
3. Helping the mother realize how much has changed with respect to her parenting role and capacity
4. Educating the mother about how to recognize and avoid patterns of overprotective parenting
5. Educating the mother about ways to optimize her interactions with her infant
6. Wrapping up the treatment intervention

CHECK-IN

The therapist first checks in with the mother regarding her reactions to recounting and processing her trauma narrative in Session 5. The hope is that the experience was therapeutic and did not increase her feelings of guilt or distress, or if it did, that she found ways to manage those feelings and saw them eventually subside. The therapist also reinforces the importance of the different coping techniques the mother has learned to help with increased emotional distress. If she still seems distressed by the narrative, the therapist can conduct a deep breathing or PMR session or lead her through a cognitive restructuring exercise. It may be helpful to compare her current level of distress with that she experienced while telling her trauma narrative. The therapist should emphasize that although creating a trauma narrative brings up challenging thoughts and distressing emotions, the mother was able to successfully complete the narrative and used her coping strategies to remain engaged in her infant's care. The therapist can also discuss how even difficult and traumatic emotions dissipate over time and become more manageable.

SUCCESSFUL VERSUS OVERPROTECTIVE PARENTING

In this section, the therapist discusses the concept of overprotective parenting and its relevance to parents of premature infants. Parents typically have increased anxiety as a result of their traumatic experiences, which can lead them to be both overprotective and overly permissive as well as less likely to set appropriate limits. Although this tendency is both very common and understandable, it may result in future difficulties for the infant.

> Let's talk first about the tendency of parents to be overly anxious. The anxiety that mothers have is often rooted in the fact that their baby has had many difficult medical experiences and may in fact have been medically fragile. However, this belief that your baby is medically fragile may continue, even after your baby has made a full recovery and is no longer considered by doctors to be at any greater medical risk than a healthy full-term infant.
>
> The belief that their baby is medically fragile and the resulting anxiety can lead parents to be constantly on guard, always expecting the worst. Parents may end up being so overly cautious that they may not encourage their baby to take steps forward in the course of their normal development. This pattern of overly anxious parenting may cause their child to become excessively anxious or dependent, and it may ultimately limit their potential.

The therapist should pause to see if this makes sense to the mother and, if not, provide further explanation. The therapist asks if the mother could see herself falling into a pattern of overprotective parenting and then explains how feelings of guilt interfere with effective parenting:

> The second component of overprotective parenting is the tendency to be overly lenient. By this, we mean that parents have difficulty setting limits or saying "No" and may just give in to all of their child's demands. This tendency to be overly lenient is commonly motivated by feelings of guilt. Parents of premature babies often feel so guilty about the premature birth of their child and their child's early experiences in the NICU that it leads them to have difficulty saying "No" or being able to set age-appropriate boundaries as their children grow older.
>
> Examples of overly lenient parenting include difficulty finding the right balance between being available to respond to all of your baby's desires and encouraging your baby and child to adapt to accommodate your needs (e.g., for sleep or certain schedules). The tendency for mothers to be overly lenient and focused on the child's needs has been shown to be associated with a number of different behavioral problems in children when they get older. These include the child not accepting limits from other adults, such as teachers, or not having good sharing skills with playmates.
>
> Research shows that children need to learn how to accept appropriate limits and that their parents are their first and best teachers. By setting limits early, you help your child develop the self-control they will need as they get older.

The therapist explains that these behaviors lead to poor dynamics between parents and their children and often can lead to unhealthy emotional development (Figure 5–20) and illustrates ways in which overly anxious or overly lenient parenting can play out in a child's life. The therapist asks the mother to check off thoughts or feelings she can imagine herself having and then discusses the risks of such behaviors and ways to avoid these situations.

For some mothers, this discussion may seem premature or not relevant, and the issue of overprotective parenting may need to be reviewed at a later time (see Chapter 7). In this case, it is important to emphasize that knowledge about this topic may be useful in the future to prevent unhealthy outcomes for the child. This "plants the seed" for mothers to be mindful that their NICU experiences may make them more likely to develop overprotective parenting styles, and they should keep this in the back of their mind as their child develops.

> This may all seem a long way off, and not particularly relevant to you with your baby still here in the hospital; however, we have found that is much easier for parents to be aware of the pitfalls of overprotective parenting ahead of time and make a conscious effort to establish a successful parenting style from the beginning. Most parents who end up in a pattern of overprotective parenting realize it is not good for their grow-

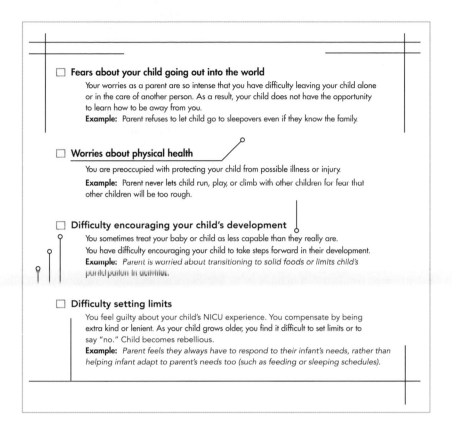

☐ **Fears about your child going out into the world**

Your worries as a parent are so intense that you have difficulty leaving your child alone or in the care of another person. As a result, your child does not have the opportunity to learn how to be away from you.

Example: Parent refuses to let child go to sleepovers even if they know the family.

☐ **Worries about physical health**

You are preoccupied with protecting your child from possible illness or injury.

Example: Parent never lets child run, play, or climb with other children for fear that other children will be too rough.

☐ **Difficulty encouraging your child's development**

You sometimes treat your baby or child as less capable than they really are.

You have difficulty encouraging your child to take steps forward in their development.

Example: Parent is worried about transitioning to solid foods or limits child's participation in activities.

☐ **Difficulty setting limits**

You feel guilty about your child's NICU experience. You compensate by being extra kind or lenient. As your child grows older, you find it difficult to set limits or to say "no." Child becomes rebellious.

Example: Parent feels they always have to respond to their infant's needs, rather than helping infant adapt to parent's needs too (such as feeding or sleeping schedules).

FIGURE 5–20. Long-term effects of overprotective parenting.

Source. Adapted from Shaw and Horwitz 2013.

ing child but do not know how to change their parenting style. Your awareness of this issue will really help you support your child in becoming a happy, competent, and independent person who realizes their full potential as they grow and develop.

TRIGGERS AND OVERPROTECTIVE PARENTING

To connect the concept of overprotective parenting with symptoms of posttraumatic stress, the therapist refers back to the topic of triggers and how they may prompt such responses (Table 5–6).

Let's take this a step further by really personalizing your awareness of parenting behaviors that could lead to a pattern of overprotective parenting. We are going to take another look at the triggers we have been

Table 5–6.   Triggers and overprotective parenting

Common child issues	Mother's response
Baby or child looks sad when mother tries to leave or put them to sleep	Mother feels guilty and decides not to follow through
Baby looks uncomfortable when doing "tummy time"	Mom gets scared and does not let baby practice "tummy time" anymore
Family makes plans to leave baby with a sitter	Mother either panics and will not go or spends the whole night obsessing about the baby being home
Baby coughs when swallowing a piece of sweet potato on first attempt	Mother gets scared and purees all of baby's food indefinitely
Baby catches a cold after mom takes baby with her to grocery store	Mother worries and rarely lets baby out of house
Baby develops rash	Mother panics and immediately rushes baby to doctor's office
Baby bumps head on coffee table while crawling on floor	Mother worries baby is seriously injured and rushes baby to emergency department

Source.   Adapted from Shaw and Horwitz 2013.

working with to see if your resulting behaviors might put you and _____ (baby's name) at risk for this pattern of parenting.

Using the handout, they discuss whether any of her specific triggers could be risk factors for overprotective parenting behaviors.

- What are you thinking, and how do those thoughts make you feel?
- How would you handle this situation?
- How would you handle the potential anxiety/panic/stress?

The therapist should praise the mother's desire to be nurturing and for her baby to be healthy, particularly if she is responding in an appropriate way. However, if her reaction to the situation is not appropriate (e.g., not putting her child down to sleep), the therapist should guide her through the exercise using a technique from her toolkit, such as an ABC-B Worksheet, and then have her reimagine her response, highlighting the changes in her parenting approach.

- Can you imagine yourself doing any of these things?
- Do you think if you could pause and go through the [tool chosen from the toolbox] we used during the triggers exercise that your response would be different?

- What might your new response be?
- How would you compare the impact your initial panicked response had on you with the impact of the new response (in which you pause and reflect)?

The therapist stresses that overprotective parenting can be avoided and how beneficial this would be. Encourage the mother to share this parenting information with her partner or any family members likely to have frequent contact with the child.

> Even though overprotective parenting is common with children who were born prematurely, it is also highly preventable. The first step is just being more aware of the natural tendency to be overly anxious or overly lenient and then trying to catch ourselves when we notice it happening. If we are able to do this, it is more likely we will be able to pause, reflect, and then respond in a thoughtful way. It may be a lifelong process, but it is one that will ultimately help promote your child's development and well-being.

DEVELOPING A SUCCESSFUL PARENTING STYLE

In this section, the therapist discusses developing a successful parenting style and identifies ways to promote a pattern of healthy parenting (Figure 5–21). The therapist explains that the mother may want to seek out more information on developmentally appropriate approaches to limit-setting and parenting strategies.

> I would now like you to read this next handout for ways to work toward a successful parenting style to raise a happy, competent child. By pushing yourself early on to go outside your comfort zone, either to let your children do things that make you a little anxious or to put aside the guilt and set appropriate limits for your child, you will be helping them in the long run. You are already doing many of the things on this list, which is fantastic.

The therapist asks the mother if she can imagine practicing any of the items on the list and praises and encourages her efforts to master these behaviors.

INFANT OBSERVATION

In this section, therapist and mother turn their attention to the infant. The sequence of the next few activities depends on the baby's state of readiness. If the infant is awake and alert, the therapist leads the mother through face-to-face interactions first and the infant observations sec-

Developing a Successful Parenting Style

There were, and may still be, times when it is scary how small and fragile your baby appears. However, your baby is growing, and will continue to grow, becoming bigger, stronger, and more resilient.

Unfortunately, for some parents, if the worried feelings take over, they may get stuck in seeing their baby as more immature and fragile than they really are. This can cause some parents to be over-protective and over-anxious, even when it is no longer necessary or helpful to the baby. Parents also sometimes feel so guilty for the early experiences of their baby that they are overly lenient to compensate.

Parents who fall into this pattern:

- won't leave their baby
- won't let their baby do things that they are developmentally ready to do (such as "tummy time," eating solid foods, or walking by themselves)
- treat their baby as sick or fragile (for example, frequently check baby for signs of illness)
- have difficulty setting appropriate limits or discipline as their baby gets older

Can you imagine falling into this pattern?

These ways of parenting often cause children to be difficult to control and overly dependent. Here are some ways to avoid the Overprotective Parenting pattern:

- Right now, try not to let feelings of worry or anxiety keep you from holding and interacting with your baby.
- Practice doing new things with your baby even if you are nervous.
- Pay attention to your baby's new strengths and abilities.
- Notice ways you may view your baby as more fragile and/or less competent than they are in fact becoming.
- Encourage your child to do as much as they can as they grow.
- Let your child experience the world, make mistakes, go out and get dirty, and know that you are supporting them.
- Get the support you need.
- If you find that after you bring your baby home, you experience distress that is troublesome, consider seeing a therapist; many parents find this is helpful after leaving the hospital. Your social worker or physician can give you a referral.
- When your baby gets older, it is crucial that you are able to set limits. Children gain self-control and security when parents set appropriate limits in loving and clear ways.

What is something that you could do with your baby now that may stretch your comfort and **encourage your child's competency?**

_ _

You can also list these in your Baby Diary under "My Caregiving Goals."

FIGURE 5–21.　Developing a Successful Parenting Style handout.

Source.　Adapted from Shaw and Horwitz 2013.

ond, or vice versa. If the infant is asleep, the therapist begins with the "preparing for home" discussion.

　　The infant observation exercise helps the mother realize how much she has learned about her baby as well as how much her baby has grown and progressed since birth. The therapist and mother start by observing the baby and then review the Baby Diary and Visiting Log. The therapist should spend a few minutes observing the baby and sharing what he or she sees, making specific comments comparing what the therapist sees now with what he or she saw at the beginning of the intervention, including differences in the infant's current behavior and appearance and the mother's comfort in interacting with and responding to her child. If the infant is not doing many new things (e.g., is still sleeping most of the time or is still sick and unable to be held), the therapist may ask the mother if anything about her baby or her experience feels different now from how they felt immediately after the baby's birth. Taking the time to reflect on the ways in which she and the baby have grown throughout their experience in the NICU is an important part of the therapeutic process; it allows the mother to recognize how much has changed over time in the NICU regardless of how close the baby is to discharge or what medical and developmental obstacles might remain.

The therapist and mother should review the "Important Milestones for Baby" and "Important Milestones for Mother" sections of the Baby Diary. If the mother has not completed much of the Baby Diary, the therapist should encourage her to do so now. They should go through the diary together, and the therapist should praise accomplishments noted by the mother, commenting enthusiastically on all of the milestones and accomplishments that have been reached. The mother should be encouraged to reflect on milestones yet to come and continue to recognize and celebrate such milestones for her baby and for herself as a parent.

FACE-TO-FACE INTERACTIONS

The therapist now leads the mother through two participant observer exercises to show her how much she has learned about reading her infant's cues and their needs. When the baby is awake and alert, the therapist starts by observing the infant and then explaining to the mother the concept of being a participant observer:

> Let's see how [baby's name] is doing right now. What state is your baby in right now? How comfortable do they seem?
>
> Now I would like you to hold and talk to [baby's name] in a specific sequence, which I will guide you through. When the interaction is done, I will be asking you some questions about how your baby experienced the interaction, and then how you experienced the interaction. You will want to go slowly and carefully so that you can be mindful of those observations.
>
> This exercise requires you to be a participant observer. The concept of being a participant observer is that you have to engage in the task at hand while at the same time trying to maintain an outside perspective on the situation, like a bird's eye view. While no one can do this all of the time, it is a helpful goal for mindful parenting.

At this point, the therapist should make sure the infant is in an alert state. If the infant is asleep, changing their diaper may help them wake up, or this exercise may have to wait until a later time.

> I would like you to sit down and get comfortable. Also, if you think [baby's name] should be swaddled, let's pause for a moment while you go ahead and swaddle them.
>
> Have you ever held [baby's name] up in front of you for a face-to-face interaction? That is what we are going to do. I would like you to start by holding [baby's name] upright. [The therapist can demonstrate by putting their hands out to demonstrate the correct positioning].
>
> Now I would like you to slowly raise [baby's name] so that they are about 1 foot away from your face.
>
> Can you softly talk to your baby?
>
> Once you have [baby's name] in a calm alert state, or as close as you think they are going to get in the next minutes, let me know and we will proceed. [Let mother talk to the baby for up to 60 seconds].
>
> Since their eyes are open right now, why don't we find out if they are ready to track your face? Can you lean your body slowly to one side while you talk to your baby, taking about 3–5 seconds to move from the center to the right?
>
> Now slowly back to the midline, about 3–5 seconds.
>
> Now slowly to the other side.
>
> Repeat for approximately 1 minute.

The therapist should remind the mother to slow down or speed up if necessary. If the infant does not engage, the therapist should ask if the infant normally does engage or if it would be better to repeat the exercise at a later time. The therapist should provide any other positive feedback possible if the mother does not comment on these issues while working through the handouts. It is also important to emphasize that the mother was able to interact with her baby like an expert and to help her see how much she has learned since her infant was born.

This face-to-face interaction is crucial in building the foundation for a secure attachment and bond between mother and child. It is important to recognize whether the mother is fixated on the medical aspects of the baby, for example, focused on the wires, leads, and the baby's vital signs. If so, the therapist should have her pause and begin to describe her infant's face, facial expressions, skin color, and body posture. This may help ground her in the moment and frame the face-to-face time as an interaction with her child rather than with a hospital patient.

PREPARING FOR HOME

The therapist and the mother now focus on preparing for the baby to go home. Discharge, while anticipated and desired, often triggers feelings of anxiety in new parents. It is important to help the mother appreciate that she is more competent and capable than she might feel. The language in this section may need to be adjusted depending on whether the infant has already been discharged or is still in the NICU and whether this is the mother's first child. Use this time to reflect on how the mother is an expert on her child not only in how much she knows about the baby's medical complexities but also in how well she has learned her baby's likes, dislikes, and cues.

The therapist guides the mother through a list of important things to consider with respect to her infant. The goal is to leave the mother feeling as though she knows her baby well and has the skills and tools to be an excellent caregiver. Fears and concerns brought up by the mother can be addressed using skills such as the Examining the Evidence or What Would I Tell a Friend? exercises.

In preparation for the child going home, the therapist provides information about important developmental milestones and about the typical growth and development of premature infants and how they differ from that of full-term infants. Together, mother and therapist calculate the infant's adjusted age to help estimate when the baby is expected to attain relevant milestones. The therapist should give positive support to the things the mother is most excited about and use these as a jumping-off point to discuss activities the parents can do to help with their child's development.

WRAP UP

The therapist ends the treatment intervention on a positive and empowering note, making sure the mother recognizes all the work she has put in throughout her time in treatment by recapping the process of identifying emotions and thoughts during her time in the NICU, the skills she learned to restructure her thoughts and the techniques to calm her mind and body, how she created and shared the trauma narrative, and, finally, how much her baby has progressed while in the NICU. The therapist encourages the mother to continue using the skills she has learned and practiced throughout her time in treatment as well as to continue to read and share her trauma narrative, should she want to. The mother should reflect on how she has been able to experience distressing emotions and move through those emotions without breaking down. The therapist should allow an opportunity to address any last questions or concerns the mother may have prior to concluding the session.

> We are coming to the end of our time together, so let's take a minute to leaf through your binder handouts and activities that we have done over the last few weeks. This way you will know all the resources that you have to refer to on your own.
> I have really appreciated having these meetings with you and getting to know you and your baby. You have done a lot of good work to

help process and cope with this experience. I encourage you to continue to talk with loved ones about how you are doing. If you find, over the next weeks or months, that you are feeling more distress than you would like as a result of this experience, you could always consider speaking with a professional. Your hospital social worker, your obstetrician, or your primary care doctor should be able to help with a referral to a therapist who will be able to give you more support. Many parents find that this is helpful after their baby has been in the hospital.

LESSONS LEARNED FROM SESSION 6

Because this is the last session, it is important that mothers feel they are set up for success. The goal of the session is to help them work through their fears and feel empowered and competent in caring for their child. The therapist will have built a strong rapport with the mother, who may admit to fears and anxieties not previously discussed. The therapist must hear and acknowledge those concerns. The mother also may wait until the last few minutes of the session to bring up these concerns, so the therapist should be ready to budget in some extra time if necessary and remind the mother about the tools she now has at her disposal. The session should end on a positive note, and the therapist should thank the mother for investing so much time and energy into the sessions to help her infant.

Additional Observations and Lessons Learned

ALTERATION IN THE EXPECTED PARENTAL ROLE

Research has repeatedly shown that one of the factors most strongly associated with psychological distress is the *alteration in the expected parental role* (Lilo et al. 2016). Mothers are abruptly thrown into the highly medicalized environment of the NICU, which is the opposite of what they had been expecting. They must become familiar with the concepts of neonatal jaundice, bilirubin lights, gastrostomy tubes, and continuous positive airway pressure, among others (see Chapter 1). In addition, they are confronted with an infant who often bears little resemblance to the traditional portrayal of a healthy newborn baby.

The NICU itself is an intimidating and uncomfortable environment. Parents frequently feel marginalized and excluded from their infant's care. Most routine caretaking tasks are provided by NICU nurses, leaving mothers feeling peripheral and redundant apart from their ability to pump and provide breast milk. Concerns about infection due to the infant's immature immune system and constraints on the mother's ability to have physical contact with her infant further contribute to feelings of estrangement and disrupt the normal process of maternal bonding.

ROLE OF THE NICU TEAM

NICU staff, many of whom have been there many years, frequently and inadvertently become desensitized to the traumatic nature of their work and may not appreciate how stressful it is for new parents to have an infant in the hospital (Colville et al. 2017; Mealer et al. 2009). Research has drawn attention to the issues of trauma and burnout in providers in intensive care units and how this may contribute to a lack of empathy for NICU parents. Although the staff are competent and kind, they often fail to appreciate the magnitude of the emotional experience on the parents of their patients. Research suggests that mothers can perceive comments made by NICU staff to be hurtful and judgmental (Lilo et al. 2016). Comprehensive programs of psychological consultation in the NICU should incorporate staff support and educational components to address these issues.

SENSITIVITY TO LOGISTICAL ISSUES

The importance of flexibility on the part of the intervention team has already been discussed. However, it is also important to keep in mind the logistical issues that come up in the context of having a premature infant in the NICU. Many families live a considerable distance from specialty NICU care, and geographical relocation of the family creates a significant burden, particularly for low-income families. Families who have long NICU stays, sometimes upward of 3 months, may have additional concerns related to finances. Parents may have to make difficult decisions about whether to return to work, which naturally further interferes with the bonding process. Fathers are routinely excluded from the care of the premature infant, depriving both partners of the opportunity to develop an emotional connection.

FLEXIBILITY

Part of the reason this intervention was so successful and well received was due to the flexibility we were able to provide to mothers. Although the sessions are useful and provide vital tools and treatments to help them cope, they can only do these things if the therapist can meet them where they are, both emotionally and physically. Although parents in the NICU can clearly benefit from mental health intervention, it is unrealistic to expect them to do this independently at a time of such significant stress. The flexibility of scheduling sessions at convenient times, often in the evenings, was instrumental in facilitating the efficacy of the intervention. During implementation of the RCT, many sessions were conducted on weekends and sometimes in the mother's home.

NORMALIZATION OF THE MOTHER'S EXPERIENCE

The normalization of the mother's experience and encouragement and support given to her by the therapist were also essential components of the project's success. It is critically important to de-pathologize the experience as much as possible, so it feels less like psychological treatment and more like support, and to emphasize that the mother's reactions to the traumatic experience of the NICU are normal and expected. Therapists continually reiterated not only that mothers' reactions were appropriate to the situation but also that it would be more unusual if they did not have significant symptoms of anxiety and guilt. For mothers who resist psychological support, destigmatize the mental health aspects of the intervention and reframe it as a way to build coping skills to better support their infants. Mothers should be praised for engaging in treatment and taking time to focus on their own health and well-being. Their ability to acknowledge and express their feelings was viewed as a strength in the context of a life-altering event. Mothers often comment on the strength of their relationship with the therapist and the feeling of support throughout the intervention. It was also important to emphasize that the mothers were not alone in their distress about having an infant in the NICU and that all parents are affected to some degree by their NICU experience.

MATERNAL SATISFACTION

Mothers who participated in the original RCT almost without exception commented on its usefulness and relevance (Shaw et al. 2014). They appreciated the opportunity to focus on themselves and on their feelings and concerns and to have their reactions validated. They also valued the coping strategies they were taught, and most found the therapists likable, knowledgeable, and supportive. None of the participants thought the use of a manualized or guided intervention felt forced or staged or inadequate to address their needs, and all participants thought the intervention should become part of the normal standard of care for the NICU, including for their partners.

DEVELOPING A PEER SUPPORT NETWORK

Given that isolation is one of the most common concerns of NICU parents, connecting parents with other parents or families in the NICU is another avenue to consider in terms of providing additional support and resources. Parents of infants in large NICU units seldom connect with each other, and with the trend in NICU design toward single-bed units, the potential for isolation may yet increase. The benefits of peer support between NICU parents is highlighted in the description of a group therapy intervention in Chapter 6.

Online Supplements

Readers interested in implementing our intervention in their NICUs can access the treatment manual and handouts described in this chapter, as well as other resources, via our companion page on the American Psychiatric Association Publishing website (www.appi.org/Shaw). For questions or additional information, readers are also welcome to contact the editor of this book, Richard J. Shaw (rjshaw@stanford.edu).

References

Anderson GC: Mother–newborn contact in a randomized trial of kangaroo (skin-to-skin) care. J Obstet Gynecol Neonatal Nurs 32(5):604–611, 2003

Bernard RS, Williams SE, Storfer-Isser A, et al: Brief cognitive-behavioral intervention for maternal depression and trauma in the neonatal intensive care unit: a pilot study. J Trauma Stress 24(2):230–234, 2011

Brisch KH, Bechinger D, Betzler S, Heinemann H: Early preventive attachment-oriented psychotherapeutic intervention program with parents of a very low birthweight premature infant: results of attachment and neurological development. Attach Hum Dev 5(2):120–35, 2003

Chard KM, Resick PA, Monson CM, Kattar KA: Cognitive Processing Therapy Veteran/Military Version Therapist's Group Manual. Washington, DC, U.S. Department of Veterans' Affairs, 2013. Available at: https://www.div12 .org/wp-content/uploads/2014/11/Group-CPT-Manual.pdf. Accessed July 9, 2020.

Colville GA, Smith JG, Brierley J, et al: Coping with staff burnout and work-related posttraumatic stress in intensive care. Pediatr Crit Care Med 18(7):e267–e277, 2017

Hagan R, Evans SF, Pope S: Preventing postnatal depression in mothers of very preterm infants: a randomised controlled trial. J Obstet Gynecol Neonatal Nurs 111(7):641–647, 2004

Holditch-Davis D, Bartlett T, Blickman A, Miles M: Posttraumatic stress symptoms in mothers of premature infants. J Obstet Gynecol Neonatal Nurs 32(2):161–171, 2003

Kersting A, Dorsch M, Wesselmann U, et al: Maternal posttraumatic stress response after the birth of a very low-birth-weight infant. J Psychosom Res 57(5):473–476, 2004

Lilo EA, Shaw RJ, Corcoran J, Storfer-Isser A: Does she think she's supported? Maternal perceptions of their experiences in the neonatal intensive care unit. Patient Exp J 3(1):15–24, 2016

Ludington-Hoe SM, Anderson GC, Swinth JY, et al: Randomized controlled trial of kangaroo care: cardiorespiratory and thermal effects on healthy preterm infants. Neonatal Netw 23(3):39–48, 2003

Martin A, Brooks-Gunn J, Klebanov P, et al: Long-term maternal effects of early childhood intervention: findings from the Infant Health and Development Program (IHDP). J Appl Dev Psychol 29(2):101–117, 2008

McCormick C, Workman-Daniels K, Brooks-Gunn J: The behavioral and emotional well-being of school-age children with different birth weights. Pediatrics 97(1):18–25, 1996

Mealer M, Burnham EL, Goode CJ, et al: The prevalence and impact of post traumatic stress disorder and burnout syndrome in nurses. Depress Anxiety 26(12):1118–1126, 2009

Melnyk BM, Alpert-Gillis L, Feinstein NF, et al: Improving cognitive development of low-birth-weight premature infants with the COPE Program: a pilot study of the benefit of early NICU intervention with mothers. Res Nurs Health 24:373–389, 2001

Miles M: Parents of critically ill premature infants: sources of stress. Crit Care Nurs Q 12:69–74, 1989

Nemeroff CB, Bremner JD, Foa EB, et al: Posttraumatic stress disorder: a state-of-the-science review. J Psychiatr Res 40(1):1–21, 2006

Pierrehumbert B, Nicole A, Muller-Nix C, et al: Parental post-traumatic reactions after premature birth: implications for sleeping and eating problems in the infant. Arch Dis Child Fetal Neonatal Ed 88(5):F400–F404, 2003

Resick PA, Schnicke MK: Cognitive processing therapy for sexual assault victims. J Consult Clin Psychol 60(5):748–756, 1992

Ross LE, McLean LM: Anxiety disorders during pregnancy and the postpartum period: a systematic review. J Clin Psychiatry 67(8):1285–1298, 2006

Sameroff A: Developmental systems: contexts and evolution, in Handbook of Child Psychology, 1st Edition. Edited by Kessen W. New York, Wiley, 1983, pp 238–294

Sameroff A: Models of development and developmental risk, in Handbook of Infant Mental Health. Edited by Zeanah C. New York, Guilford, 1993, pp 3–13

Sameroff A, Fiese BH: Transactional regulation: the developmental ecology of early intervention, in Handbook of Early Childhood Intervention. Edited by Shonkoff JP, Meisels SJ. Cambridge, UK, Cambridge University Press, 2000, pp 135–159

Schechter DS, Coots T, Zeanah CH, et al: Maternal mental representations of the child in an inner-city clinical sample: violence-related posttraumatic stress and reflective functioning. Attach Hum Dev 7(3):313–333, 2005

Shaw RJ, Horwitz SM: PROMOMS for Preemies: Prevention of Postpartum Traumatic Stress in Mothers With Preterm Infants (Treatment Manual Handouts). Unpublished manual, 2013

Shaw RJ, St John N, Lilo EA, et al: Prevention of traumatic stress in mothers of preterms: 6-month outcomes. Pediatrics 134(2):e481–e488, 2014

Vanderbilt D, Bushley T, Young R, Frank DA: Acute posttraumatic stress symptoms among urban mothers with newborns in the neonatal intensive care unit: a preliminary study. J Dev Behav Pediatr 30:50–56, 2009

CHAPTER 6

Group-Based Trauma Intervention for Mothers of Premature Infants

Angelica Moroyra, Psy.D.

Stephanie Seeman, Psy.D.

Emily Wharton, M.S.

Tonyanna C. Borkovi, M.B.B.S.

Richard J. Shaw, M.D.

As reviewed in previous chapters, parenting in the NICU may be a stressful, overwhelming, and isolating experience. Many parents of preterm infants endorse a sense of otherness related to the process of becoming a parent in the NICU. Society often dictates expectations of parenting roles and creates a familiar narrative that most parents count on when preparing for the birth of their child. Whether for the first or subsequent times, becoming a parent might mean having a baby shower, discovering the baby's sex, selecting a name prior to delivery, nesting (e.g., setting up a nursery), and taking home a healthy baby following delivery. With the introduction of social media, having a new baby also might include announcements of the pregnancy and the baby's arrival as well as frequent photo updates of milestones achieved. These are the parenting milestones many expectant parents fantasize about reaching. What becomes of the fantasy once reality deviates from the societal expectations of what it means to have a baby?

In our clinical experience, parents with preterm infants hospitalized in the NICU often endorse feeling left out of what it means to become a parent. Most people have not seen a photograph of a baby born preterm or the medical equipment required to sustain a preterm infant, and most may not have expected to spend the first few months with their newborn in a hospital. Consequently, arriving in the NICU can be quite shocking, and few feel prepared. Although NICU admissions are not uncommon, the experience itself remains alienating. A feeling of isolation echoes throughout the NICU and further widens the gap between the expected parental role and the reality of parenting in a hospital.

Because many families cycle through the NICU, there is little continuity and families can feel isolated. Most families come into the unit, wash up at the handwashing station, attend morning medical rounds, and spend the rest of their time at bedside with their infants. Parents may pass each other in the hospital hallways, exchange occasional waves or smiles if in a pod or open bay, and may even exchange pleasantries or medical updates while meeting in the shared family lounge.

Our team noticed that even when providing individualized treatment as described in Chapter 5, we were not tapping into a resource already present in the unit: other parents. Although all NICU experiences are unique to each family, many can relate to a cluster of NICU experiences, such as the trauma of a preterm delivery, exposure to their baby's medical procedures, and the impact of a prolonged hospital stay on their lives. In this chapter, we describe the process of adapting the individual trauma-focused cognitive behavioral therapy (TF-CBT) manual for use in a group intervention model. The goals of this project included 1) reducing feelings of isolation by providing an opportunity for mothers in the NICU to connect with other mothers, and 2) providing mothers with techniques and skills to understand and process their traumatic experiences, culminating with the opportunity to create and share a trauma narrative with social support present.

To develop the rapport and cohesion needed for mothers to write and share their trauma narrative in a group setting, a closed design was implemented: new participants could not join once a group began. Mothers joining a group had to meet the following criteria: having an infant born at or prior to 34 weeks' gestational age, having an infant who is likely to survive, and not being considered at high psychiatric risk (i.e., no psychotic symptoms or suicidal or infanticidal ideation). Adapting the individual intervention to a group intervention introduced several questions:

1. Can a group intervention provide the same or greater reduction in symptoms of anxiety, depression, and trauma compared with individual therapy?

2. Will enhancing social support for mothers in turn enhance coping styles and strategies in the NICU?
3. Can we support the process of developing trauma narratives in a group setting?

To address these questions, our team compiled literature reviews related to the benefits of group therapy, group models using components of trauma narrative therapy, and the relationship between social support and coping strategies. We also examined the risks and benefits of reading and processing a trauma narrative in a group setting. This chapter examines our proposed responses to these three questions and elaborates on the aims, strengths, and challenges of adapting an individual trauma-based intervention to a group-based model.

Benefits of Group Therapy

Several benefits of the group therapy format have been observed, such as cost effectiveness, increased social support, and greater accountability for participants attending sessions and completing homework (Castillo et al. 2016; Mott et al. 2013; Ready et al. 2008, 2012). Social support has in turn been linked to enhanced active coping styles, which act as protective factors in relation to symptoms of anxiety and depression (Roohafza et al. 2014).

The literature shows that patients rate TF-CBT groups highly in terms of satisfaction and perceived benefit (Mott et al. 2013; Sloan et al. 2013). Moreover, group therapy may provide patients with opportunities for mutual support, interpersonal feedback, and a sense of altruism (Yalom and Leszcz 2005). Several studies have demonstrated that group therapy provides increased social support through positive influence from peers and even results in greater accountability for attendance at group sessions (Mott et al. 2013; Ready et al. 2008, 2012). In a study of 20 veterans who engaged in exposure-based group therapy, more than 75% of the subjects said they had considered dropping out of the group, but in fact only 5% actually did (Mott et al. 2013); commitment to other group members was cited as the most common reason for continuing to attend sessions. Participants also rated the most helpful part of the therapy as the feedback and support they received from other group members.

Group therapy may provide the additional benefits of reducing feelings of isolation and alienation common in PTSD, establishing a sense of interpersonal safety through formation of trusting relationships, and providing an environment where individuals can see that others are experiencing similar issues (Yalom and Leszcz 2005). Studies of veterans in PTSD therapy groups found that participants benefit from validation and normalization by interacting with individuals who have had similar traumatic experiences (Ready et al. 2012; Smith et al. 2015). The Department of Veterans Affairs/Department of Defense's (2017) most recent and comprehensive clinical practice guidelines for PTSD have since recommended manualized group therapy over no treatment (Schwartze et al. 2019).

Although TF-CBT can be delivered in both group and individual formats (Barrera et al. 2013), most of the research on PTSD treatments has focused on examining the efficacy and effectiveness of TF-CBT in an individual format, with less focus on TF-CBT groups (Barrera et al. 2013). In our case, group therapy for parents of preterm infants may be a more efficient model than individual therapy because it has the potential to reach a larger number of people and may ultimately be more cost effective (Sloan et al. 2017).

Trauma-Focused Cognitive Behavioral Therapy Groups for PTSD

Trauma-focused groups and non-trauma-focused groups differ. Trauma-focused groups integrate memories of trauma into the therapeutic process in an attempt to alter the meaning of the trauma for each individual. Non-trauma-focused groups place more emphasis on the role of trauma as a contributor to present problematic behaviors, with less focus on the traumatic experience itself (Shea et al. 2009). Barrera et al. (2013) and Schwartze et al. (2019) published meta-analytic reviews of exposure-based group cognitive behavioral therapy (CBT) and group treatments for PTSD without an exposure component, respectively. They found substantial support for the exposure-based CBT, with medium to large effect sizes, and weaker evidence for approaches without exposure (Schwartze et al. 2019). Table 6–1 identifies eight studies that evaluated TF-CBT groups. Behavioral interventions included exposure to trauma memory, and cognitive work included attempts to modify the meaning attributed to the traumatic event (Shea et al. 2009).

Outcomes of Group-Based Trauma-Focused Cognitive Behavioral Therapy

TF-CBT groups have been shown to significantly reduce PTSD symptoms from pre- to posttreatment (Akbarian et al. 2015; Beck et al. 2009; Bradley and Follingstad 2003; Castillo et al. 2016; Falsetti et al. 2008; Hinton et al. 2011; Hollifield et al. 2007; Schnurr et al. 2003). Although several studies did not observe between-group differences following intent-to-treat analyses (Beck et al. 2009; Hollifield et al. 2007; Schnurr et al. 2003), dose-response and completers analyses revealed significant findings. An analysis of Vietnam veterans who had received an adequate

Table 6–1. Details of randomized controlled trials examining trauma-focused CBT groups

Authors	Treatment description	Sample	Trauma type	Control
Akbarian et al. (2015)	60- to 90-minute, 10-session CBT group that included psychoeducation, cognitive restructuring, imagined flooding, mindfulness training, PMR, and breathing retraining	N=40; mixed sexes; PTSD diagnosis	Mixed	MCC
Beck et al. (2009)	2-hour, 14-session CBT group; combination of cognitive restructuring and exposure-based treatment	N=44; mixed sexes; PTSD diagnosis	MVA	MCC
Bradley and Follingstad (2003)	2.5-hour, 18-session CBT group; combination of DBT and narrative exposure	N=49; females only; no PTSD diagnosis	Childhood sexual abuse	Waitlist
Castillo et al. (2016)	90-minute, 17-session CBT group; five imaginal exposure, five cognitive, and four behavioral skills lessons	N=86; females only; PTSD diagnosis	Mixed	Waitlist
Falsetti et al. (2008)	12-week exposure-based treatment focused on comorbid PTSD and panic attacks	N=62; females only; PTSD diagnosis	Mixed	Waitlist
Hinton et al. (2011)	Culturally adapted CBT for Latina women with PTSD	N=24; females only; PTSD diagnosis	Mixed	AMR
Hollifield et al. (2007)*	12-session CBT group; combination of cognitive restructuring, behavioral activation, and in vivo exposure	N=84; mixed sexes; PTSD diagnosis	Mixed	Acupuncture
Schnurr et al. (2003)	2-hour, 30-session CBT plus 5 booster sessions	N=360; males only; PTSD diagnosis	Combat	PCG

Note. AMR=applied muscle relaxation; CBT=cognitive behavioral therapy; DBT=dialectical behavioral therapy; MCC=minimal contact condition; MVA=motor vehicle accident; PCG=present-centered supportive group; PMR=Progressive Muscle Relaxation.
*Included more than two conditions. People diagnosed with PTSD were randomized to either an 1) empirically developed acupuncture treatment, 2) a group CBT, or 3) a wait-list control.

dose of treatment revealed that a TF-CBT group was more effective than a present-centered group[1] for reducing avoidance and numbing, as well as possibly reducing overall PTSD symptoms (Schnurr et al. 2003). Similarly, Beck et al. (2009) found that among those who completed treatment, 88.3% of those in the TF-CBT group did not meet criteria for PTSD at the end of treatment, compared with 31.3% of those in the control group.

Another study found that cognitive and exposure modules produced a greater reduction in PTSD symptoms than did a skills-based module that emphasized assertiveness training and relaxation techniques (Castillo et al. 2016). Individuals in TF-CBT groups also observed significant improvements in depression (Akbarian et al. 2015; Bradley and Follingstad 2003; Hollifield et al. 2007), anxiety (Akbarian et al. 2015; Hinton et al. 2011; Hollifield et al. 2007), panic (Falsetti et al. 2008), quality of life (Castillo et al. 2016), and emotion regulation skills (Hinton et al. 2011) over time.

Regarding methods of exposure, a meta-analytic review of exposure in group CBT found no significant differences in effect sizes between treatments that included in-group exposures and those that did not (Barrera et al. 2013). Additionally, treatments that involve imaginal exposure in written form appear to be just as effective as those that involve verbalized imaginal exposure within the group sessions (Sloan et al. 2016). However, Sloan et al. (2017) argued that building trust and cohesion among group members should take place prior to beginning the trauma-focused components of treatment. As a result, conducting imaginal exposure that is shared aloud may require a greater number of total treatment sessions (Beck et al. 2009).

A comparison of attrition rates suggests that TF-CBT can also be delivered effectively in a group format and seems to be tolerable to group members (Sloan et al. 2017). In fact, several studies combined group and individual treatment formats to ascertain whether a combination approach would increase tolerability of exposures and minimize dropout rates (Beidel et al. 2011; Chard 2005; Smith et al. 2015). These studies saw no difference in dropout rates between combined formats and strictly group formats, signifying that any considerable group component is not likely to worsen rates of attrition.

In sum, given the significant reductions in PTSD symptoms at posttreatment across the studies in Table 6–1, TF-CBT groups should be con-

---

[1]Present-centered group therapy is parallel to Yalom and Leszcz's (2005) model of group therapy. Characterized by a "here-and-now" focus, it emphasizes group cohesion and support and the process of interpersonal learning. It incorporates "nonspecific" and supportive types of interventions but does not include exposure, cognitive restructuring, or other elements of trauma-focused group therapy.

sidered an acceptable treatment for PTSD, especially in clinical settings where resources are limited. However, only one randomized controlled trial has compared individual- and group-based trauma-focused therapy. Using a cognitive-only version of cognitive processing therapy (CPT), which is typically a trauma and exposure-based intervention, the trial omitted the exposure component and focused solely on challenging trauma-related cognitions (Resick et al. 2017). These findings leave questions as to whether group-format TF-CBT would be expected to provide greater clinical benefits than individual-format TF-CBT for parents of preterm infants.

Trauma Narrative

One core component of TF-CBT is the writing and reading of the parent's trauma narrative (Cohen and Mannarino 2008). Patients are encouraged to write down the thoughts, feelings, and bodily sensations they experienced during a traumatic event along with the details of the situation. Trauma narratives are a standard component of most trauma-focused treatments.

Theories are numerous about the mechanism through which writing and reading a trauma narrative can reduce trauma symptoms. One of the most commonly cited is that retelling one's trauma story in a safe environment facilitates recovery through the process of habituation (Kaminer 2006). For many trauma survivors, the trauma memory itself has become a feared stimulus. They may avoid reminders of the traumatic memory, which reinforces their view of the memory as dangerous. Thus, by writing and rereading their trauma narratives, they become habituated to the associated anxiety and learn that revisiting the event is not dangerous. This process is believed to help overcome the avoidance of traumatic memories as the associated fear lessens (Cohen and Mannarino 2008).

Emotional processing theory (Foa and Kozak 1986) conceptualizes PTSD as a failure to sufficiently process a trauma memory as a result of excessively avoiding thoughts and situations that remind the individual of the trauma. These avoidance behaviors maintain individuals' negative and inaccurate beliefs about themselves and the world and prevent emotional processing from occurring. First, the trauma memory structure is believed to activate the perception that the world is entirely dangerous. Second, the way people remember how they behaved during and after a traumatic event, along with the inhibiting presence of PTSD symptoms, may lead to beliefs about their inability to cope as well as to feelings of incompetence (Foa 2011). In the case of traumatic experiences in the NICU, a mother may develop thoughts about the world ("my baby will never be safe in this world") or about herself ("I couldn't protect my baby, so I'm an incompetent mother").

In this model, creating and reading a trauma narrative aloud fosters emotional processing by confronting the trauma-related stimuli. Emotional processing theory hypothesizes that in vivo exposure to trauma reminders, imaginal exposure (repeated revisiting through recounting the traumatic memory aloud), and processing (discussing the revisiting experience) may disconfirm a trauma survivor's global negative beliefs (Foa and Kozak 1986).

Narrative exposure therapy proposes that by activating the fear structure involved in the trauma memory in a safe context, individuals can integrate new information that is incompatible with their fear (Schauer et al. 2011). This integration of new, contradictory information can reduce fear associated with the memory over time. Narrative exposure therapy also focuses on the role of the trauma narrative in organizing the memory of the event. Trauma survivors often have fragmented memories of the traumatic event and can feel confused about the timeline or may even actively avoid talking about the event and thus not have the opportunity to process their emotions or reconstruct their autobiographical memory (Schauer et al. 2011). Theories on expressive writing propose that writing about a traumatic event helps the individual provide structure, organization, and cohesion to the traumatic memory that was originally lacking (Pennebaker 1997; Smyth et al. 2001). It is hypothesized that trauma survivors with poor social support might be at increased risk of PTSD (Ozer et al. 2003) because they may not be encouraged or have the opportunity to discuss the event (Schauer et al. 2011). Furthermore, the linguistic process of labeling emotions has been found to control amygdalar activity and the fear response (Hariri et al. 2000). Thus, the therapist can help patients verbalize, label, and clarify their emotional experience of the trauma memory as a means of regulating their ongoing emotions related to the trauma (Schauer et al. 2011).

RISKS OF TRAUMA NARRATIVE IN GROUP THERAPY

A meta-analysis by Barrera et al. (2013) identified three primary concerns clinicians often have about the exposing of traumatic details in group settings. First is the fear that hearing the details of one member's trauma will vicariously traumatize other group members (Taylor et al. 1999). This concern is particularly relevant when similarities exist between the individuals' traumatic experiences (Beck and Coffey 2005) and is based on the theory of secondary traumatization, which posits that listening to someone recall a traumatic memory in therapy may cause clinicians to develop PTSD-like symptoms (Elwood et al. 2011). No empirical data currently support the occurrence of secondary traumatization in group therapy contexts (Barrera et al. 2013).

Barrera et al. (2013) also found group CBT with a trauma exposure component to be highly effective (effect size 1.13) in reducing PTSD symptoms. Given that this analysis focused on differences between pre and post effect sizes, it is possible that patients did experience an initial symptom exacerbation from hearing the trauma accounts of other group members but subsequently improved. This would be consistent with other studies of exposure-based group CBT that found a minority of patients experienced temporary symptom exacerbation that quickly returned to baseline (Ruzek et al. 2001).

A second concern that clinicians often have about group members sharing details of their traumas with one another is that they will compare others' traumas with their own. Clinicians fear patients may determine their own distress is unwarranted because another group member had it "worse" (Barrera et al. 2013). Alternatively, patients may conclude that their own trauma was worse and feel less hope for recovery. This is particularly relevant for mothers of premature infants because the current physical health of the infants may vary between families.

The third concern clinicians have is that group formats may not allow sufficient time for each patient to verbalize and process the details of their trauma. In other words, clinicians worry that the time constraint of processing multiple group members' traumatic material may result in an inadequate dose of exposure (Barrera et al. 2013). Group exposure therapies typically engage patients in two in-session imaginal exposures (Beck and Coffey 2005; Schnurr et al. 2003), which is fewer than the five to eight exposure sessions in prolonged exposure (Foa et al. 2007). Individual CPT, by comparison, only has two sessions explicitly devoted to the trauma account (Resick and Schnicke 1992).

BENEFITS OF TRAUMA NARRATIVE IN GROUP THERAPY

Despite these concerns, there are many potential benefits to using trauma exposure in the group therapy setting. One of the primary advantages group therapy offers is the experience of universality—helping group members feel they are not alone in their struggle (Yalom 1995). This may be especially important for trauma survivors, who often report feeling isolated (Nietlisbach and Maercker 2009). In the group therapy context, the sharing of a traumatic experience may engender a sense of commonality among participants. One study gathered 20 veterans' perspectives on the effectiveness and tolerability of 12 sessions of group-based exposure therapy for PTSD. The participants shared that hearing other group members' in-session imaginal exposures had a normalizing effect and indicated that receiving feedback from fellow veterans on their own imaginal exposures was the most helpful aspect (Mott et al. 2013).

Trauma-focused groups offer the opportunity for patients with similar experiences to come together, which may reduce the stigma and sense of isolation common in the experience of PTSD (Barrera et al. 2013). The supportive nature of a group environment may also help group members rebuild a sense of safety and trust that may have been lost as a result of the traumatic experience (Foa et al. 2008).

As much as groups introduce the possibility of one person's trauma story heightening another's, they also carry great potential for positive modeling, in which one member's positive experiences in therapy can powerfully inspire another's. The group setting may foster an increased willingness for participants to engage in trauma exposure exercises. Clinicians in one study observed that when one group member had a successful experience with exposure, that member served as a role model for others to follow (Beck and Coffey 2005). Similarly, another study found that the first group members to participate in exposures modeled how the exercises would be effective and tolerable (Mott et al. 2013). In summary, group interventions that targeted anxiety, depression, and PTSD symptoms have been widely efficacious, including those that have used trauma narratives as a focus of treatment.

Goals for Group Intervention for Mothers of Preterm Infants

The intention of the group intervention described in this chapter is to prevent or reduce symptoms of anxiety, depression, and posttraumatic stress in parents with preterm infants hospitalized in the NICU. The adaptation of the intervention to a group context retains the clinical underpinnings of the individual intervention, including the use of TF-CBT and CPT to address traumatic stress reactions. When creating a structured forum for mothers to connect and share their thoughts, feelings, stressors, and traumatic memories, many facets have been designed to facilitate a close group experience for participants. The logistics of meeting twice weekly (1.5 hours per session) for 3 consecutive weeks also enhances the likelihood that mothers can complete all six sessions prior to their infant's discharge from the NICU. By completing the intervention in only 3 weeks, the group model allows mothers several opportunities to connect and establish a sense of rapport within the group prior to discharge. The resulting sense of community allows for greater perceptions of social support throughout a historically isolating time for mothers in the NICU. Specific goals of the group-based intervention include

1. Targeting prevention or reduction of anxiety, depression, and trauma symptoms for mothers of preterm infants in the NICU

2. Creating a community of mothers with infants born preterm, subsequently increasing perceived social support
3. Providing an intervention to multiple mothers at any given time while in the NICU and increasing the likelihood mothers will be able to complete group intervention prior to discharge

Adaptations to the Individual Therapy Treatment Manual

In this section we describe the principal adaptations made from the individual therapy treatment manual.

SESSION 1: INTRODUCTION TO THE NICU

In the group adaptation, Session 1 focuses on setting the stage for mothers to participate in the group by way of discussing and setting the therapeutic framework for the intervention. Goals of the first session include instructing mothers on what to expect from each session as well as providing opportunities for them to connect with group members as they discover similarities in their experiences and begin to learn about each mother's infant and journey in the NICU. We begin the group intervention by first introducing mothers to each other:

> Take a look around you and say hello to the person next to you. You are all here because you had the privilege of having a baby but also the trauma of your baby arriving too early. Each of you is unique in your own experiences. All of your stories are different. But you are united by the fact that you are going through one of the most stressful and difficult experiences in your entire life.

This introduction signals to the mothers that each is uniquely suited to be a part of the group. It also launches the group with a sense of the mothers' connectedness to one another. From the beginning of the session, mothers are encouraged to create relationships with other members that may extend beyond the group. The facilitator helps establish group rules and guidelines tailored specifically to their individual group. This allows participants to establish boundaries within the group to promote an environment in which they feel safe and comfortable sharing vulnerable thoughts, feelings, and experiences. Figure 6–1 shows the group guidelines discussed at the beginning of Session 1.

By encouraging mothers to take ownership of the group by creating their own group guidelines and by building in opportunities to involve each mother in group activities (e.g., having them take turns reading handouts, introduce themselves, and share information about their infant and their infant's course in the NICU), the facilitator reinforces that

Group Rules and Guidelines

Confidentiality	Group discussions are confidential. What is said in group stays in group. Confidentiality is the norm for all mental health groups. Having a confidentiality agreement helps members feel comfortable coming to group and sharing.
Community	Socialization outside of the group is welcomed. The hope of this group is to create a sense of community and support among parents, in and outside of the group sessions. Social support can be a helpful tool when treating depression, anxiety, and posttraumatic stress.
Commitment	Attend all groups on time. Members are expected to make groups a priority and attend all sessions, arrive on time, and remain for the entire session unless there is an emergency. Members who are unable to attend a session are expected to call beforehand. Because this is a short-term treatment, attendance of all group sessions is important.
Consideration	Do not talk about group members who are not present. To create a safe and trusting environment, we ask that group members refrain from speaking about others when they are no longer in the group or are unable to attend.
Continuity	Complete Baby Diary entries and bring them to group. We may discuss Baby Diary entries during group sessions. The Baby Diary is an important part of group and is related to strengthening your relationship with your baby. Please try your best to complete diary entries prior to group sessions and be ready to discuss entries if you are comfortable doing so.
Consultation	Please do not share any of the skills learned or handouts provided with other mothers in the NICU. Skills learned in this group should be monitored and guided by a trained professional.

FIGURE 6–1.   Group Rules and Guidelines handout.
Source.   Adapted from Shaw and Moreyra 2017.

each mother will be allotted protected time in the group to share her own experiences and takes responsibility for ensuring each member has that time so mothers can be fully present.

Session 1 continues to follow a structure similar to the individual intervention, including reviewing common appearances and behaviors of infants in the NICU, reviewing what mothers can do or are already doing with their infants (at and away from bedside), and introducing the Baby Diary.

In one of our first pilot groups, one mother remarked at the end of the session that she had been using this first session "as a trial run, to see if it is worth my time." She had initially felt nervous about participating in a group with other mothers whom she did not know. "It was strange at first, and then so helpful. I was not that enthusiastic about being a part of a group, [thinking that] I'm going to be on spotlight all the time." She shared that during this first session, she felt instantly connected to other group members and was looking forward to the next session. Soon after this mother shared her sentiments, other group members similarly explained how connected they felt to the group and noted they were looking forward to continuing to participate. The opportunity for connection is the foundational underpinning to Session 1 and continues to be built upon in subsequent sessions.

Lessons Learned

The group facilitator has several opportunities throughout this session to encourage group cohesion. Each mother should have the opportunity to introduce herself and her infant; thus the facilitator must be a careful timekeeper. Varying personalities and levels of comfort come with sharing in a group setting; therefore, the facilitator should encourage each mother to participate while being respectful of individual limits. It would be less helpful for one particular mother to dominate the group because it may discourage others from participating; thus, the facilitator should make a point to include each mother by asking how she may or may not relate to another's experiences, feelings, or thoughts. Knowing that the facilitator is maintaining a balance among group members allows each mother to feel heard, validated, and secure.

SESSION 2: COGNITIVE RESTRUCTURING

To continue promoting group cohesion, Session 2 and all subsequent sessions include regular check-ins with participants to give each mother an opportunity to update the group on the status of her infant and any relevant experiences that occurred between sessions. This also allows members to remain abreast of one another's experiences in the NICU, further enhancing the connectedness among group members. A whiteboard is used to record each mother's responses to the following questions and to signify that each mother's contribution is valuable.

- How is your baby doing today?
- What was one positive experience you had this week with your baby or other family members?
- How did it go with trying out [insert goal set the previous week]? What got in the way?

Mothers are given the opportunity to reflect on their entries in the Visiting Log and Baby Diary (described in Chapter 5). Group facilitators are encouraged to step back and allow mothers to discuss issues among themselves and to connect with one another. Session 2 follows a similar structure to that of the individual intervention. The facilitator identifies and normalizes the stressful reactions of parents to the NICU setting and prompts mothers to share their emotions with each other. The facilitator helps mothers identify their emotions and understand the relationship between events, thoughts, and emotions using the ABC-B Worksheet (i.e., a worksheet detailing the relationship between an activating event, beliefs or thoughts, and consequences or behaviors) and then teaches the techniques of Examining the Evidence, What Would I Tell a Friend?, and Positive Self-Statements. Mothers roleplay with each other to practice each skill. By teaching and learning together, group members forge a sense of competency in themselves as a group and as individuals.

Our experience running these groups has shown how quickly mothers connect with one another. For example, at the end of Session 2, one group elected to exchange telephone numbers and met for lunch the following day in the hospital cafeteria. Mothers initiated this exchange independently and noted they felt as though they had already gained "new friends."

Lessons Learned

This session focuses on teaching mothers about new skills and techniques, ensuring each can leave the session with an understanding of the skills and concepts related to identifying and managing overwhelming thoughts and feelings. Cognitive restructuring is reviewed several times during the session so members can together work through examples of challenging experiences they have each had in the NICU. This allows them to relate to one another's challenges and generates a greater quantity and variety of alternative thoughts they can use when reconceptualizing challenging moments. Inviting mothers to roleplay skills in session can enhance their opportunities to learn and to ask clarifying questions and receive feedback. Roleplaying is a useful tool because mothers practice skills together, build rapport, and clarify their understanding of new skills, which further solidifies learning.

SESSION 3: STRESS, TRIGGERS, AND SELF-CARE

Session 3 sets the stage for preparing mothers to create and share their trauma narratives. The session begins with a check-in and adds a component that will be used in all subsequent sessions: prior to asking about their infants, the facilitator first asks mothers to rate the intensity of their own current emotions. This important aspect highlights that although they may be discussing distressing and overwhelming emotions and experiences, their emotions wax and wane over time, and even the most distressing emotions reduce in intensity.

> How are you feeling? On a scale from 0–10, where 0 is the least distressed and 10 is the most distressed, where would you scale your feelings right now? Keep in mind that distressed can mean any kind of overwhelming emotion like anxiety, sadness, anger, and frustration.

Session 3 continues by reviewing the completed ABC-B Worksheet assigned to mothers for homework after Session 2. One mother is asked to share her homework, and group members are encouraged to assist her if needed. Following this, the physical effects of stress are discussed, and mothers are asked to reflect on where in their bodies they each tend to experience stress (e.g., tightening of their shoulders, clenching their jaw). Mothers are prompted to reflect on activities that reduce stress and increase self-support. Typically, they discuss how difficult it is to find time to care for themselves or to keep the self-care or health routines they may have had prior to the birth of their infant. In one of our groups, one mother invited all group members to her home for lunch to spend some time socializing away from the NICU. The other mothers acknowledged that they would enjoy spending time away from the NICU, yet each briefly reflected on the guilt they would feel about being away from their child's bedside. This became a lead-in to a conversation about relaxation techniques they can use both at bedside and away from the NICU.

The relaxation techniques taught in Session 3 include breathing retraining and Progressive Muscle Relaxation (PMR). Following the PMR exercise, mothers are prompted to re-rate their level of distress on the 0–10 scale. In doing so, they practice awareness of their emotions and the intensity of those emotions and are often able to recognize the utility of relaxation techniques in helping them regulate that intensity.

Finally, perhaps the most powerful component of this session involves discussing the symptoms of posttraumatic stress. We encourage mothers to think about their NICU experiences using the trauma model so they begin to understand their traumatic stress reactions:

> We have talked about the many distressing thoughts and emotions you have experienced in the NICU, and then we worked on tools to deal with those difficulties. For many mothers, the experience in the NICU is very traumatic. It is a series of multiple traumatic events as new things happen to your babies. When we talk about trauma, most people think of soldiers who have been through war. The NICU can be its own kind of war zone, with battles that you are facing every day. Does it make sense to you to think of the experience of your baby's preterm birth and hospitalization as a trauma?

The group facilitator explains the four categories of posttraumatic stress symptoms (i.e., intrusion, avoidance, changes in cognition and mood, arousal and reactivity) previously discussed in Chapter 4. Labeling the NICU experience as a trauma can help mothers better understand their own symptoms and emotional reactions. Most acknowledge that their NICU experiences have been traumatic. They also look forward to sharing this information with their partners. In one group, a mother remarked that she thought she was "going crazy" because her heart rate would suddenly escalate anytime her phone would ring, regardless of who was calling. Another mother explained that she had previously felt the need to downplay her traumatic stress reactions by telling herself, "It's not like I've been to war." She noted that she now felt "relieved" that she could allow herself to think about the NICU as a traumatic experience.

During the wrap-up in Session 3, the group facilitator explains the importance of processing mothers' traumatic experiences and provides the rationale for writing trauma narratives, which will take place in the subsequent session. In our pilot groups, most mothers noted how nervous and anxious they felt when thinking about writing their trauma narratives. The facilitator may remind mothers that the group members will support one another and that they have all learned new coping skills to help them manage their emotions.

Lessons Learned

The group facilitator must understand the nuances of trauma and find ways to explain how trauma may have influenced the mothers' experiences, emotions, cognitions, memories, and engagement with others. One explanation that may help clarify the way trauma can disrupt normative functioning and create distressing symptoms is related to how the brain enjoys and craves order and structure. Group therapists may choose to explain that when an event occurs that is beyond any experience we may have had previously or been prepared for, our minds attempt to fill in the gaps to create order and organize the event. False and incorrect associations may be formed as a result. Thus, after a traumatic event, we may associate that trauma with unexpected things, and seemingly unrelated stimuli may serve as reminders (e.g., a microwave beeping may become associated with monitors beeping in the NICU and thus produce elevated heart rate and flashbacks).

SESSION 4: LOSS AND TRAUMA NARRATIVE

Session 4 focuses on creating the trauma narrative. Mothers are asked during their check-in to rate their current level of distress on the 0–10 scale. This distress rating is referenced later in the session. Mothers often identify feeling more distressed at the start of this session and attribute this to the anticipation of writing their trauma narrative.

Mothers first participate in a deep breathing exercise as taught in the previous session to promote mindfulness and prepare them to engage in the writing process. They should be reminded that distressing and overwhelming emotions may arise as they are writing and encouraged to acknowledge these emotions as they emerge and recognize that the group is a safe place to share their experiences. The facilitator reads a sample trauma narrative aloud (Figure 6–2) to illustrate the amount of sensory detail mothers should include in their narratives and provides a handout of questions to help them write their narratives (Figure 6–3). The handout is divided into three domains: birth experience, NICU experience, and posttraumatic impact. These sections target the most salient traumatic experiences in the NICU and close with reflections on the impact of these experiences. Providing specific instructions also makes it possible for mothers to write a complete narrative (from birth experience to present) that encompasses the full range of emotions, thoughts, and sensory details.

Before they begin writing, mothers are encouraged to participate in an exercise that mentally transports them back to their experiences in the NICU. They are asked to close their eyes and visualize a NICU experience that was particularly challenging and traumatic for them:

Try to put yourself back into this experience and use the present tense to answer these questions in your mind...[pause for 10–15 seconds between each question]

- Whom are you with?
- What emotions do you feel?
- What do you smell?
- What do you see?
- What do you hear?

Now, let's open our eyes and begin writing.

As mothers begin to write their trauma narrative, the facilitator acts as a timekeeper and encourages mothers to spend at least 20 minutes on each section. Mothers should be given an hour to write their narrative. It is crucial that they be encouraged to at least begin writing about each section (birth experience, NICU experience, and posttraumatic impact). At the end of the session, the facilitator collects all the narratives to make copies (originals are returned to the mothers), from which they will highlight selections for mothers to read aloud at the next session. Mothers who are unable to complete their narratives in session are encouraged to continue writing outside of session.

Sample Trauma Narrative

The First Time I Saw My Baby

I don't really remember seeing his whole body, because there were so many people around him. But I said, "I want to see him" to the nurse in the NICU. So, I sat up and I felt like so many barriers between me and him. One of them being my bed. They couldn't bring him to the side of me, they brought him to the foot of the bed. Maybe they wheeled my bed around? No, I think I leaned forward. I must have leaned forward because my bed was in the same position. And he was like at the foot of the bed. And really red. Really red and translucent. I could see all his ribs. And he was so tiny. And they had the bag over his face or his mouth or his nose. And he had this pink, this plastic wrap over him.

But he had his hand out.

His little hand held my finger.

Well, it was such an insignificant and also such an extremely significant moment. Because what I wanted to do was like hold him. Which I couldn't because they had to take him to the NICU and intubate him. And so, it felt so sweet to touch him and it also felt really empty. Because just touching a hand is so insignificant compared to the surface area of his body. Just having his tiny hand wrap around my finger. It was so significant and in a way reminded me how little I could do for him.
Which I felt when they told me I had to deliver.

FIGURE 6–2. **Sample trauma narrative.**
Source.   Adapted from Shaw and Moreyra 2017.

During the last 10 minutes of the session, mothers reflect on the experience of writing their narrative and identify their current level of distress. Most mothers' distress ratings will likely have increased following the trauma narrative activity. The facilitator should validate the difficulty of writing a trauma narrative and acknowledge the possible increase in distress level while also asking mothers to identify what might

Development of the
Trauma Narrative

*Please provide sensory details, including **sights, sounds, smells, thoughts**, and **feelings** throughout. What were you feeling? What were you thinking about?*

TRAUMA NARRATIVE QUESTIONS:

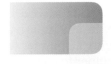

Birth Experience

1. When did you first find out that there was a possibility you might have a premature birth? Do you remember any of the conversations with your doctor?

2. How did you feel when you first found out you were going to deliver early?

3. What do you remember about your birth experience?

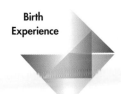

NICU Experience

4. What do you remember about the first time you saw your baby? What were your first thoughts about your baby? What were you feeling? Were you worried? Relieved? Happy? Excited? Scared?

5. Please tell me about the first time you visited your baby in the NICU. What was it like for you? Who was there? Were you surprised/shocked by anything you saw? What were you feeling when you first saw your baby?

6. Please tell me about your experiences since your baby has been here in the hospital, including any difficult or stressful medical events, procedures, or conversations/interactions with nurses or doctors.

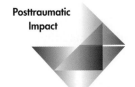

Posttraumatic Impact

7. What impact has this experience had on you and your family?

8. How has this experience affected your view of yourself?

9. How has this experience affected your sense of closeness with other people?

10. How has this experience affected your confidence and ability to handle difficult situations?

FIGURE 6–3. Trauma narrative questions.
Source.   Adapted from Shaw and Moreyra 2017.

---

be keeping their distress level from being the highest it has ever been (i.e., a 10). The facilitator should encourage mothers to practice self-care activities later that day and ask which specific activities mothers might realistically engage in following the session.

Lessons Learned

One of the biggest challenges of the group is helping mothers write a full and detailed account of their trauma experience. In one group, a mother stated that she had completed her narrative with 30 minutes to spare. When such a situation occurs, encourage the mother to continue writing and remind her that avoidance is a core symptom of trauma. Referring back to the previous session, the group facilitator may highlight how, in an effort for self-preservation, overwhelming emotions that arise may be habitually invalidated, avoided, and subdued. They may also emphasize the importance of experiencing those distressing and overwhelming emotions to promote recovery from the traumatic experience and reduce future traumatic stress reactions. Monitor group participants and take note of mothers who may be avoiding the activity, experiencing strong emotions, or writing without emotional expression; this will be important to address in the next session.

Preparation for Session 5

In between Sessions 4 and 5, the facilitator reads each trauma narrative and, depending on group size, identifies three to five themes (feelings or cognitions) common to most if not all of the narratives. The facilitator then selects an excerpt from each mother's narrative that highlights one of those identified themes. For example, in previous groups, some common themes across all narratives were feelings of anger and sadness as well as cognitions related to hopelessness, inadequacy, and hope. These were illustrated by phrases such as, "I couldn't protect my baby," "I don't think I will ever take my baby home," and "I feel stronger having spent time in the NICU." In this example, the facilitator selected an excerpt from one mother's narrative that highlighted anger, an excerpt from another that highlighted sadness, an excerpt from another that highlighted hopelessness, and so on. Each mother should be given the opportunity to read an excerpt of her narrative in session, providing equal time for all participants.

SESSION 5: READING AND PROCESSING TRAUMA NARRATIVES

The principal goal of Session 5 is for the mothers to read selections from their trauma narratives aloud. First, shared themes that emerged in the group's narratives are identified and discussed. Mothers are then asked to read selections of their narratives (preselected by the group facilitator) aloud and encouraged to express and thereby process their emotions while doing so. If a mother reads her narrative with little emotional expression, the facilitator should pause her and ask her to slow down while reading and express the full range of emotions related to her traumatic experience. Following each mother's reading, group members are encouraged to thank the mother for sharing her narrative:

> Thank you so much for sharing with us. This can be very challenging for a mom to share! As a group, let's acknowledge _____ (mother's name) by thanking her for sharing this with us.

Each mother is asked to reflect on her experiences of writing the narrative and sharing it with other mothers. They are also encouraged to reflect on the thoughts and emotions that arise for them while listening to another mother's trauma narrative:

- What was one thing each mother could relate to from the narrative?
- What was one part of another mother's narrative with which each mother could empathize?

This enables mothers to reflect on ways in which their experiences may have been similar and allows for continued exposure to emotions and cognitions often associated with the trauma of being in the NICU and having a preterm delivery.

Although mothers indicated feeling increasingly anxious prior to sharing their narratives, after Session 5 they reported how valuable the experience had been. In some groups, mothers even hugged each other after sharing their narratives as an expression of support. Some offered words of encouragement, such as "You are so brave," and remarked on how they could relate: "I felt the same way" and "I can understand how you feel." Additionally, one mother commented, "I have three successes in my life. The first is my son, the second my marriage, and the third seeking mental health support in the NICU." She further highlighted how important the group was for gaining an understanding of her experiences and establishing support and connection to other mothers.

Session 5 is often the most powerful and emotional session in the treatment intervention and the session we believe has the greatest impact on reducing maternal posttraumatic stress, depression, and anxiety symptoms. The facilitator must emphasize how challenging sharing a trauma narrative can be, while continuing to reference how important it is to process and reduce trauma symptoms. The facilitator should highlight how successful the mothers have been in discussing their distressing memories, experiences, thoughts, and emotions with the group and emphasize that although sharing their trauma narratives was distressing and evoked unpleasant memories and emotions, they were able to tolerate that distress and discomfort and continue to participate in the group.

The final component of Session 5 is introducing the homework assignment of writing a letter to their infant. The hope for this letter is that mothers will think about their infant as a member of the family as opposed to a patient in a hospital. Mothers are given written prompts: describe your baby's time in the NICU, your hopes and wishes for your baby's future, your relationship with your baby, what you have learned about your baby so far, and what strengths your baby has shown you throughout the NICU stay (Figure 6–4).

Lessons Learned

This session requires the group facilitator to contain mothers' expressed feelings while also supporting each mother and the collective group experience. Mothers should be encouraged to express affect as they share their trauma narrative, while also being mindful of how each mother may be responding to sharing and hearing the trauma narratives of other mothers. Mothers should be encouraged to contact the emotions and cognitions they experienced during the traumatic event and be reminded of the ways in which they are able to hold and tolerate distressing emotions without being consumed by them. At the end of the session, the facilitator should remind mothers that they were able to share their trauma narratives without "falling apart," emphasizing that distressing and overwhelming emotions are tolerable and eventually will diminish in intensity.

SESSION 6: PREPARING FOR HOME

The final session begins with a check-in with group members about their experience sharing trauma narratives in the previous session. Group members should be encouraged to share their experience of reading the narrative aloud and review the themes that were present across trauma narratives. If a mother was not present for the previous session, she should be invited to share an excerpt from her own narrative. Mothers may attempt to avoid Session 5 to avoid symptoms of traumatic stress; however, as emphasized in the previous sections, sharing the trauma narrative is vital for reducing posttraumatic stress symptoms.

In reviewing the trauma narrative experience, the facilitator should discuss with mothers how their intensely overwhelming emotions and distressing thoughts and feelings will reduce in intensity over time. By drawing attention to the change in the intensity of their emotions immediately between Sessions 5 and 6, the facilitator can highlight how even the most intense and distressing emotions can only remain at elevated levels for so long before naturally lowering.

In Session 6, the facilitator also encourages mothers to continue to identify the parenting strengths they have established while in the hospital. Mothers may acknowledge how their own knowledge of and relationship with their infant has grown over the past 3 weeks by reflecting on ways they have established connections with their infant and by revisiting what they have learned about their infant's likes, dislikes, and characteristics.

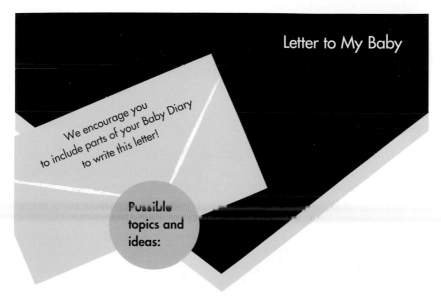

1. Describe your baby's time in the NICU.

2. What do you know about your baby so far?

   a. Which family member do they look like?
   b. Who do they remind you of?
   c. What are their special cues, mannerisms, etc.?
   d. Significance of their name?

3. What do you want your baby to know that you're learned throughout the NICU experience?

4. Describe your relationship with your baby. How has it changed with time?

5. What strengths has your baby shown you throughout their NICU stay?

6. What have you learned about yourself as a parent throughout their NICU stay?

7. What special milestones did you and your baby accomplish that made you proud?

8. What are your hopes and wishes for your baby's future?

FIGURE 6–4. Letter to My Baby handout.

Source.   Adapted from Shaw and Moreyra 2017.

Similar to the individual-format intervention, mothers then discuss overprotective parenting styles and ways in which they, their partners, or their family members have fallen or may fall into these patterns. Finally, they share selected sections from the letters they wrote to their babies (Figure 6–5). The facilitator invites each member to select a brief section of her letter to share with the group and ensures that each mother has sufficient time to share. Mothers then share their reactions to each

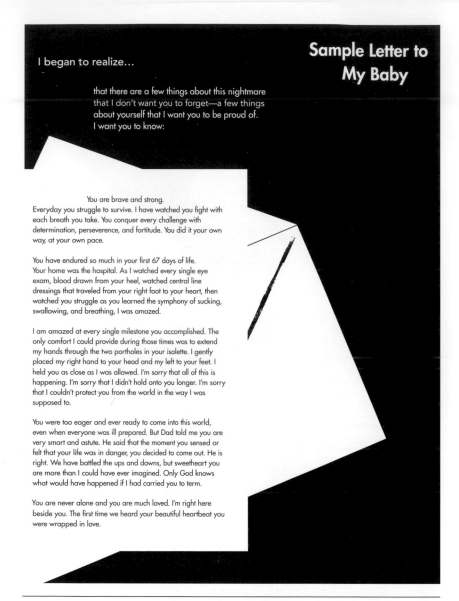

FIGURE 6–5.   **Sample Letter to my Baby handout.**

Source.   Adapted from Shaw and Moreyra 2017.

mother's letter and thank them for sharing. Mothers report enjoying this portion of the session and, in previous groups, have even suggested the group go on longer so each mother can share her entire letter.

In wrapping up, facilitators encourage mothers to read through all of the handouts acquired during the previous 3 weeks to remind themselves about the material covered and the resources they can refer to as they transition home. Mothers are encouraged to continue talking with loved ones or professional providers (e.g., obstetrician/gynecologist, primary care doctor, social worker) about how they are feeling. Finally, members are given graduation certificates indicating successful completion of the group intervention and encouraged to acknowledge what they have noticed about each other's growth and what they appreciate about each member. In previous groups, mothers have enjoyed reflecting on the relationships they have established with group members. One mother noted, "I am leaving this group with not only new friends, but with a new family." Allowing a space for mothers to discuss the relationships established throughout the group process is an important step in saying goodbye and recognizing the relationships forged.

Lessons Learned

Many mothers expressed that although they felt far from thinking about discharge or about setting limits with their child as they grew, they were able to identify the possibility of adopting an overprotective parenting style. Moreover, they discussed recognizing overprotective traits in their partners' parenting style already present while in the NICU. A review of some ways in which the NICU experience may influence parenting styles effectively provides an introduction to vulnerable child syndrome in all but name, initiating reflection on the ways parenting styles can shape or inhibit their baby's development. This is the therapeutic technique of planting a seed, through which mothers are made aware of how their experience of parenting in the NICU can influence their parenting styles long after they have been discharged. It helps mothers recognize that the NICU experience can have a lasting impact on their relationship with their child that can persist well beyond infancy and into childhood and even adolescence.

Conclusions

CHALLENGES OF THE GROUP INTERVENTION

One of the most valuable components of the group also poses one of the greatest challenges in conducting the intervention in the NICU. Having a closed group (in which members start and finish the group at the same time without others joining once it begins) is critical for establishing rapport, trust, and connection among members. These elements create an environment of safety for mothers to share their trauma narratives and resultant emotional experiences. However, a closed-group format presents challenges for initiating groups in a timely manner. Most NICU stays vary in duration, so it may be difficult for multiple mothers to start a group at the same time. Mothers and infants can be admitted to the NICU for various reasons, and not all infants in the NICU were born preterm. Because our intervention is specifically designed to help mothers of preterm infants, only some mothers at any one time are eligible to join a group, which can pose a further challenge to recruitment.

For an intervention so reliant on communication and narrative, issues of language and literacy pose interesting challenges. Literacy proficiency can vary among group members, which may call for inventive approaches to completing a trauma narrative. In our experience, language choice also plays a nuanced role in group sessions. Most of our group participants to date had a language other than English as their native language. This posed challenges but also offered another powerful way in which members related to each other. Although fluent in English, one group member preferred writing in Spanish because she did not want to have to take the time to translate certain words, and writing her narrative in her native language came more easily. The facilitator translated that mother's narrative into English. As a result, the mother was able to write her trauma narrative in what she felt was her most authentic voice while also being able to share it with others. Some mothers may be more comfortable verbalizing their narrative but have challenges with writing it. In this case, a facilitator may step out of the group with the mother and record and transcribe her narrative so she can read it in session. As described throughout this section, there is flexibility for the group facilitator to accommodate each group member's needs.

STRENGTHS OF THE GROUP INTERVENTION

Feedback from mothers who have participated in the group intervention highlights the value of learning skills to identify, understand, and tolerate overwhelming emotions and thoughts following trauma exposure in the NICU. Mothers have noted that the community of support created throughout the group intervention was a particularly valuable component they otherwise would not have had the opportunity to establish. They frequently mention that although they see other families in the NICU, they sometimes feel uncomfortable sharing their experiences in that context. If they did converse with other families, it was solely related to the medical status of their respective infants rather than about their emotional concerns.

Within a 3-week period, mothers learn skills and techniques to improve their ability to manage stress, interactions with others, and emotions and thoughts related to the NICU. They are able to share and focus on information about their infants unrelated to medical status and prognosis. The timing of the group allows mothers in all different stages of the NICU stay to connect and discuss their relationships with their baby, parenting triumphs and difficulties, and ways in which the NICU experience has affected their early parenting experiences. Those who have been in the NICU for several months are still able to connect and relate to mothers who have been in the NICU for several weeks. Mothers whose infants have been in the NICU for a longer period are able to reflect on the changes their infants have shown over time. This provides helpful information to mothers in the group whose infants have only been in the NICU for a short period of time. Regardless of the duration of their NICU stay, and regardless of differences in their infants' current status or health, mothers who participated in the group-based intervention found a space where they could relate to one another's challenges, posttraumatic stress reactions, and various NICU experiences.

References

Akbarian F, Bajoghli H, Haghighi M, et al: The effectiveness of cognitive behavioral therapy with respect to psychological symptoms and recovering autobiographical memory in patients suffering from post-traumatic stress disorder. Neuropsychiatr Dis Treat 11:395–404, 2015

Barrera TL, Mott JM, Hofstein RF, Teng EJ: A meta-analytic review of exposure in group cognitive behavioral therapy for posttraumatic stress disorder. Clin Psychol Rev 33(1):24–32, 2013

Beck JG, Coffey SF: Group cognitive behavioral treatment for PTSD: treatment of motor vehicle accident survivors. Cogn Behav Pract 12(3):267–277, 2005

Beck JG, Coffey SF, Foy DW, et al: Group cognitive behavior therapy for chronic posttraumatic stress disorder: an initial randomized pilot study. Behav Ther 40:82–92, 2009

Beidel DC, Frueh BC, Uhde TW, et al: Multicomponent behavioral treatment for chronic combat-related posttraumatic stress disorder: a randomized controlled trial. J Anxiety Disord 25:224–231, 2011

Bradley RG, Follingstad DR: Group therapy for incarcerated women who experienced interpersonal violence: a pilot study. J Trauma Stress 16:337–340, 2003

Castillo DT, Chee CL, Nason E, et al: Group-delivered cognitive/ exposure therapy for PTSD in women veterans: a randomized controlled trial. Psychol Trauma 8:404–412, 2016

Chard KM: An evaluation of cognitive processing therapy for the treatment of posttraumatic stress disorder related to childhood sexual abuse. J Consult Clin Psychol 73:965–971, 2005

Cohen JA, Mannarino AP: Trauma-focused cognitive behavioural therapy for children and parents. Child Adolesc Ment Health 13(4):158–162, 2008

Department of Veterans Affairs/Department of Defense: VA/DoD Clinical Practice Guideline for the Management of Posttraumatic Stress Disorder and Acute Stress Disorder. Washington, DC, Department of Veterans Affairs/ Department of Defense, 2017. Available at: https://www.healthquality.va.gov/ guidelines/MH/ptsd/VADoDPTSDCPGClinicianSummaryFinal.pdf. Accessed December 4, 2019.

Elwood LS, Mott J, Lohr JM, Galovski TE: Secondary trauma symptoms in clinicians: a critical review of the construct, specificity, and implications for trauma-focused treatment. Clin Psychol Rev 31(1):25–36, 2011

Falsetti SA, Resnick HS, Davis JL: Multiple channel exposure therapy for women with PTSD and comorbid panic attacks. Cogn Behav Ther 37:117–130, 2008

Foa EB: Prolonged exposure therapy: past, present, and future. Depress Anxiety 28(12):1043–1047, 2011

Foa EB, Kozak MJ: Emotional processing of fear: exposure to corrective information. Psychol Bull 99(1):20–35, 1986

Foa EB, Hembree E, Rothbaum BO: Prolonged Exposure Therapy for PTSD: Emotional Processing of Traumatic Experiences Therapist Guide. New York, Oxford University Press, 2007

Foa EB, Keane TM, Friedman MJ, Cohen JA: Effective Treatments for PTSD, 2nd Edition: Practice Guidelines From the International Society for Traumatic Stress Studies. New York, Guilford, 2008

Hariri AR, Bookheimer SY, Mazziotta JC: Modulating emotional responses: effects of a neocortical network on the limbic system. Neuroreport 11(1):43–48, 2000

Hinton DE, Hofmann SG, Rivera E, et al: Culturally adapted CBT (CA-CBT) for Latino women with treatment-resistant PTSD. A pilot study comparing CA-CBT to applied muscle relaxation. Behav Res Ther 49:275–280, 2011

Hollifield M, Sinclair-Lian N, Warner T, et al: Acupuncture for posttraumatic stress disorder: a randomized controlled pilot trial. J Nerv Ment Dis 195:504–513, 2007

Kaminer D: Healing processes in trauma narratives: a review. S Afr J Psychol 36(3):481–499, 2006

Mott JM, Sutherland RJ, Williams W, et al: Patient perspectives on the effectiveness and tolerability of group-based exposure therapy for posttraumatic stress disorder: preliminary self-report findings from 20 veterans. Psychol Trauma 5:453–461, 2013

Nietlisbach G, Maercker A: Effects of social exclusion in trauma survivors with posttraumatic stress disorder. Psychol Trauma 1(4):323–331, 2009

Ozer EJ, Best SR, Lipsey TL, Weiss DS: Predictors of posttraumatic stress disorder and symptoms in adults: a meta-analysis. Psychol Bull 129(1):52–73, 2003

Pennebaker JW: Writing about emotional experiences as a therapeutic process. Psychol Sci 8(3):162–166, 1997

Ready DJ, Thomas KR, Worley V, et al: A field test of group-based exposure therapy with 102 veterans with war-related posttraumatic stress disorder. J Trauma Stress 21:150–157, 2008

Ready DJ, Sylvers P, Worley V, et al: The impact of group-based exposure therapy on the PTSD and depression of 30 combat veterans. Psychol Trauma 4:84–93, 2012

Resick PA, Schnicke MK: Cognitive processing therapy for sexual assault victims. J Consult Clin Psychol 60(5):748–756, 1992

Resick PA, Schuster Wachen J, Dondanville KA, et al: Effect of group vs individual cognitive processing therapy in active-duty military seeking treatment for posttraumatic stress disorder: a randomized clinical trial. JAMA Psychiatry 74(1):28–36, 2017

Roohafza HR, Afshar H, Keshteli AH, et al: What's the role of perceived social support and coping styles in depression and anxiety? J Res Med Sci 19(10):944–949, 2014

Ruzek JI, Riney SJ, Leskin G, et al: Do post-traumatic stress disorder symptoms worsen during trauma focus group treatment? Mil Med 166(10):898–902, 2001

Schauer M, Schauer M, Neuner F, Elbert T: Narrative Exposure Therapy: A Short-Term Treatment for Traumatic Stress Disorders. Göttingen, Germany, Hogrefe, 2011

Schnurr P, Friedman MJ, Foy DW, et al: Randomized trial of trauma-focused group therapy for posttraumatic stress disorder: results from a Department of Veterans Affairs cooperative study. Arch Gen Psychiatry 60(5):481–489, 2003

Schwartze D, Barkowski S, Strauss B, et al: Efficacy of group psychotherapy for posttraumatic stress disorder: systematic review and meta-analysis of randomized controlled trials. Psychother Res 29(4):415–431, 2019

Shaw RJ, Moreyra A: Group Therapy Intervention for Mothers of Premature Infants. Unpublished manual, 2017

Shea MT, McDevitt-Murphy M, Ready DJ, Schnurr PP: Group therapy, in Effective Treatments for PTSD: Practice Guidelines From the International Society for Traumatic Stress Studies, 2nd Edition. New York, Guilford, 2009, pp 306–326

Sloan DM, Feinstein BA, Gallagher MW, et al: Efficacy of group treatment for posttraumatic stress disorder symptoms: a meta-analysis. Psychol Trauma 5:176–183, 2013

Sloan DM, Unger W, Beck JG: Cognitive-behavioral group treatment for veterans diagnosed with PTSD: design of a hybrid efficacy-effectiveness clinical trial. Contemp Clin Trials 47:123–130, 2016

Sloan DM, Beck JG, Sawyer AT: Trauma-focused group therapy, in APA Handbook of Trauma Psychology. Edited by Gold SN. Washington, DC, American Psychological Association, 2017, pp 467–482

Smith ER, Porter KE, Messina MG, et al: Prolonged exposure for PTSD in a veteran group: a pilot effectiveness study. J Anxiety Disord 30:23–27, 2015

Smyth J, True N, Souto J: Effects of writing about traumatic experiences: the necessity for narrative structuring. J Soc Clin Psychol 20(2):161–172, 2001

Taylor S, Fedoroff IC, Koch WJ: Posttraumatic stress disorder due to motor vehicle accidents: patterns and predictors of response to cognitive-behavior therapy, in The International Handbook of Road Traffic Accidents and Psychological Trauma: Current Understanding, Treatment and Law. New York, Elsevier, 1999, pp 353–374

Yalom ID: The Theory and Practice of Group Psychotherapy. New York, Basic Books, 1995

Yalom ID, Leszcz M: The Theory and Practice of Group Psychotherapy, 5th Edition. New York, Basic Books, 2005

CHAPTER 7

Vulnerable Child Syndrome

Margaret K. Hoge, M.D.
LaTrice L. Dowtin, Ph.D., LCPC, NCSP, RPT
Sarah M. Horwitz, Ph.D.
Daniel S. Schechter, M.D.
Richard J. Shaw, M.D.

Vulnerable child syndrome (VCS) is a constellation of symptoms a child experiences as a result overprotective parenting patterns that develop in response to stress from a resolved life-threatening illness or event for their child. In 1964, Green and Solnit, two pediatricians from Yale University School of Medicine, first described the phenomenon of VCS after observing parents' reactions to children who had recovered from a life-threatening illness. These parents commonly sought medical attention for their child for minor or insignificant medical concerns based on anxiety that was disproportionate to the severity of the child's actual physical health. The authors described that, for parents, the "life-threatening incidence remains alive as an experience that attaches itself to many of the growing up experiences" (Green and Solnit 1964, p. 64) for the child, causing a "disturbance in the psycho-social development" of that child (Green and Solnit 1964, p. 58). It was noted that the parents had a heightened sense of the child's vulnerability to poor health outcomes even after the initial life-threatening condition had resolved.

Further research notes that increased parental perception of child vulnerability (PPCV) was often not consistent with the level of medical vulnerability assigned by the medical team (De Ocampo et al. 2003; Malin et al. 2019). This increased PPCV is hypothesized to cause patterns of overprotective parenting that include parental difficulties with separation, failure to set age-appropriate limits, and an excessive focus on bodily complaints often associated with greater health care use (Green and Solnit 1964). Furthermore, research supports the consistency of these maladaptive parental patterns in the development of VCS and adds that parents often lack confidence in their own parenting skills (Estroff et al. 1994). Children with a diagnosis of VCS raised by parents with overprotective parenting behaviors were noted to have increased behavioral problems, delays in psychomotor developmental milestones at 1 year of age, aggressive behavior, anxiety, or depression and a continued belief in their own medical vulnerability compared with others (Allen et al. 2004; De Ocampo et al. 2003; Estroff et al. 1994). Research evaluating the extent of VCS suggests it is a complex interaction of parent and child factors. VCS is defined in the literature as being present when the following three criteria are met (Forsyth 2009; Figure 7–1):

1. The child experienced a serious or life-threatening illness that has now resolved.
2. A parent of the child has a heightened PPCV to future illness and poor health outcomes, which results in a pattern of overprotective parenting behaviors.
3. There are adverse behavioral, development, and health outcomes for the child.

Numerous authors have published on the topic of VCS since the first description of 25 cases by Green and Solnit (1964), supporting the presence of this common reaction in parents of children with resolved serious and life-threatening illness.

Prevalence

Limited large population studies have been published on the prevalence of VCS. Two studies of all pediatric patients in the general population suggested that 10%–27% of parents had heightened PPCV and that 1.8% of those parents met all three criteria for VCS, including changes in child outcomes (Forsyth 2009; Levy 1980). However, rates of VCS are expected to increase in populations with serious and life-threatening illness, for example, in pediatric subspecialties or intensive care units.

A particular population of interest and at high risk for VCS development is families in the NICU, where there is a higher prevalence of trau-

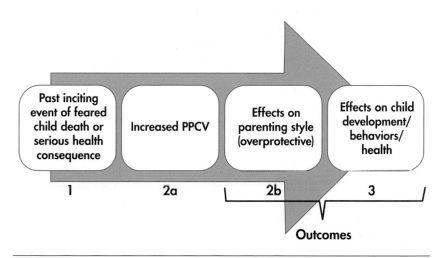

FIGURE 7–1. **Summary course of vulnerable child syndrome (VCS).**

Numbered elements are necessary components for the definition of VCS according to For-syth (2009): 1) a past health event for the child, 2) increased parental perceptions of child vulnerability (PPCV) and effects on the parenting style, and 3) effects on the child. The components of VCS are listed in order of temporal occurrence to depict the progression of a reaction from the parent that later affects parenting behaviors and the child's outcomes. *Source.* Adapted from Hoge and Shaw 2019.

matic or life-threatening illness as well as a high likelihood of survival, given advancements in medical care. In light of the impact of parenting on child development, it is important to be aware of how alterations in PPCV might affect the well-being of the child.

Literature suggests that rates of PPCV and VCS are higher in the NICU population. In one study, 39 parents of now-healthy formerly premature children had higher PPCV scores (27.5%) than 41 parents of healthy-term infants (2.8%). Of 10 parents of formerly premature infants with current health or developmental problems, 25% had higher PPCV scores (Perrin et al. 1989). Another study that included 50 mothers of prematurely born (median gestational age 30 weeks) former NICU infants who were now preschool age documented that 64% of parents had high PPCV on the Child Vulnerability Scale (CVS); furthermore, two-thirds of these parents were more likely to report that their child had behavioral problems such as aggression and poor socialization (Estroff et al. 1994). In a separate study, Culley et al. (1989) demonstrated that about 28% of parents of formerly premature infants with a birth weight <1,500 g and now healthy children had higher PPCV scores. This would suggest that of those parents with high PPCV, 66% have children with the full spectrum of VCS.

Of importance is the finding that, in spite of improved survival and health outcomes (Estroff et al. 1994; Perrin et al. 1989), parents still have a high perception of vulnerability regarding their child. This imbalance of PPCV versus the actual health status of the NICU infant was described in a study by Malin et al. (2019) in which parents were asked to state their perceptions of sickness and were scored against objective measures of illness through medical records. The study found that 44%–47% of parents disagreed with nurses and doctors on the "sickness" rating of their infants, stating that the child was ill when the nurses and doctors said they were well, suggesting that parents' perceptions of their NICU infants were much worse than the perceptions of their care providers. The imbalance of PPCV in NICU populations puts these infants at further risk for development of VCS compared with the general population.

Etiology

Various studies and theoretical models have been suggested to describe risk factors thought to be implicated in development of VCS. Maternal, child, and environmental factors are all potential contributors. Green and Solnit (1964) first postulated that VCS developed in parents who continued to maintain perceptions of their child's vulnerability even after their child's illness resolved. Looking further into altered parenting behaviors specific to parents of infants born preterm, Miles et al. (1998) drew attention to the psychological stress of having a premature infant and the challenges it causes parents who are trying to navigate parenting a premature infant in the NICU and beyond. The authors noted that parents had particular difficulty with child behavioral management, such as discipline and limit setting; feeling they must be especially protective of their child; and ongoing fear for the child's well-being, which mothers attributed to their child having survived prematurity (Miles et al. 1998). These difficulties have been compared with patterns of overprotective parenting seen in childhood cancer (Miles and Holditch-Davis 1995).

Lieberman's (1997) work with parents and infants who have experienced traumatic events supports that parent–child attachment and child outcomes are influenced by both parental experiences and parents' unconscious representations of their child. Although the NICU experience may be a relatively short period of time in the child's overall life, the parents can be left with a lasting traumatic impression of their child that begins to form their internal working model of the child, or how the parents see the child (Zeanah et al. 1994). This directly impacts how they interact with and care for the child.

Cohen et al. (2008) looked further into the role of trauma for parents with or without histories of substance abuse and depression. In a study of 176 mothers from a low socioeconomic minority group in New York City, they found that when controlling for substance abuse and depression, cumulative trauma exposure was associated with higher negative parenting behaviors such as punitive practices, abuse potential, parent dissatisfaction, and psychological and physical aggression. This suggests that individual trauma exposure highly impacts a variety of parenting behaviors.

The role of trauma in parental perceptions has further been described by Schechter et al. (2015). They reported that parents can often project inward opinions on their child, ranging from positive to negative. When these projections differ from the child's age-appropriate abilities, such as a child who is "stubborn" or "hurtful to others," an entrenched view of the parents may develop and limit the child's evolving sense of self and relationships. These altered perceptions happen more often in trauma-exposed parents and are often a response to past trauma that is projected onto the child. The "caregiver's inability to perceive, reflect on, and appropriately respond to distressed infant states" may further the misperception of the child (Schechter et al. 2015, p. 3). To further test this concept, Schechter et al. (2015) studied a group of 59 mothers to determine if those with PTSD related to violence had more negative attributions for their children than a control group of mothers without PTSD. They also hypothesized that the PTSD group would have a greater reduction in negative perceptions of the child following a three-part video intervention that focused on observing positive and negative parent–child interactions and reviewing them with the interventionist. The researchers found that negative perceptions of child and self were more present in mothers with PTSD and that the video intervention did allow for a decrease in negativity toward the child but not toward the self (Schechter et al. 2006, 2015). This research suggests an important link between parental trauma and altered parental perceptions.

Allen et al. (2004) examined PPCV in a NICU-specific population to identify factors present at NICU discharge that may predict high PPCV. They also studied the relationship between timing and severity of PPCV and predictions of poor developmental outcomes in the child at 1 year of age. The study population included parents of infants born at a gestational age of ≤32 weeks who had bronchopulmonary dysplasia (BPD) at 36 weeks. At discharge, parents completed questionnaires assessing anxiety, depression, impact on family, life orientation, social support, and general health of the infant. When their child reached 1 year of age, parents completed questionnaires to assess PPCV using the 16-item Vulnerable Child Scale (Perrin et al. 1989) and behavioral outcomes for their child using the Bayley Scale of Infant Development (Bayley 1993) and Vineland Adaptive Behavior Scale (Sparrow et al. 1984). In the first analysis, a correlation was found between high PPCV scores and several factors including hospitalization length, maternal anxiety and depression, high impact of illness on the family, and low maternal optimism, life satisfaction, and social support. However, after a linear regression model was completed, only maternal anxiety remained a statistically significant predictor. Furthermore, higher PPCV scores were associated with more psychomotor developmental delay at 1 year of life, but no difference was found in cognitive development on the Bayley Scale.

To further elucidate a theoretical model of VCS development in neonatal populations, Horwitz et al. (2015b) illustrated the relationship between VCS and parental responses to the NICU admission related to experiences of parental trauma. The proposed model suggested a complex interaction of parent and child demographics, parents' psychological response to the trauma of the child's life-threatening illness, and the behavioral reactions of the parents (Figure 7–2). The population used to create the theoretical model included 105 mothers of infants born between 25 and 34 weeks' gestation who had a birth weight >600 g, had no developmental abnormalities or were awaiting cardiac surgery, and a had high likelihood of survival. Mothers had to qualify for symptoms of depression, anxiety, or acute stress disorder to participate in the study. In a multiregression model, the authors assessed all risk factors and their relation to PPCV scores as measured by the Vulnerable Baby Scale when the children reached 6 months of age. Horwitz et al.'s (2015b) multiregression model demonstrated that the most influential factors for the development of VCS were 1) a mother having a positive past psychological history, such as mental health disorders or exposure to trauma; 2) maladaptive maternal coping styles, such as behavioral disengagement, denial, self-blame, self-distraction, substance use, and venting; and 3) maternal responses of depression, anxiety, and trauma to the stress of the child's illness. They found that if the mother had high social support, this mediated the effects of maladaptive maternal coping styles. Interestingly, the medical severity of the infant's condition did not significantly predict PPCV scores. These findings are important given that depression, anxiety, and PTSD are highly prevalent among NICU parents, more so than in parents of healthy-term infants (Horwitz et al. 2015b; Keesara and Kim 2018; Pace et al. 2016; Shaw et al. 2006, 2013). Malin et al. (2019) have also found that parents' perceptions of illness and vulnerability of the child contributed to higher rates of PTSD.

Much still needs to be learned about the development of VCS and why some families progress to the full spectrum of VCS, with child developmental delays and problems, whereas other families do not. Of note, most literature on the subject investigates maternal characteristics and PPCV scores but not paternal characteristics. No studies have specifically looked at the role of fathers with respect to the development of VCS.

Implications of Vulnerable Child Syndrome: Relevance and Child Outcomes

The impact of maternal perception of infant and child vulnerability on child outcomes has been well documented. Although this is still an area

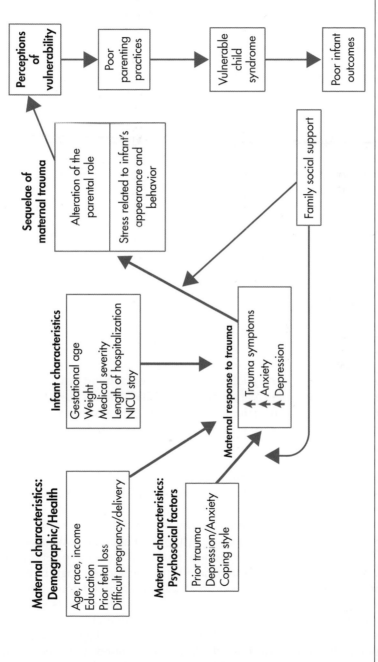

FIGURE 7–2. **Horwitz model for development of vulnerable child syndrome in the NICU.**

Source. Horwitz SM, Storfer-Isser A, Kerker BD, et al: "A Model for the Development of Mothers' Perceived Vulnerability of Preterm Infants." *Journal of Developmental and Behavioral Pediatrics* 36(5):371, 2015. Reprinted with permission from Wolters Kluwer Health, Inc.

of ongoing discovery and research, current literature supports that high PPCV may have sequelae beyond the phenomena of poor school performance, illness, and anxiety originally described by Green and Solnit in 1964. Increased PPCV may affect the child's social, cognitive, and emotional development. Other effects include delays in psychomotor and speech development, aggressive behaviors, poor socialization, school performance problems, "hypochondriac mentality," and high health care utilization (Allen et al. 2004; Estroff et al. 1994; Leslie and Boyce 1996). This is thought to happen as a consequence of altered parenting behaviors from increased PPCV (Estroff et al. 1994; Green and Solnit 1964).

ALTERED PARENTING PRACTICES

Research has shown increased PPCV can manifest in certain parenting behaviors. Parents exhibit difficulty separating from their child, have trouble setting age-appropriate boundaries, are overly concerned with the child's bodily complaints and symptoms (i.e., coughs and abdominal pain), and have low parenting confidence (Estroff et al. 1994; Green and Solnit 1964; Leslie and Boyce 1996). These types of altered parenting behaviors are thought to lead to child outcomes seen in VCS.

DEVELOPMENTAL OUTCOMES

Parents who have a distorted or disengaged internal working model of their child are more likely to have a child with an insecure or disorganized attachment style, developmental challenges, and behavioral difficulties (Benoit et al. 1997). Differences in development outcomes may also arise as a consequence of heightened PPCV. Allen et al. (2004) studied 116 formerly premature infants who were <32 weeks' gestational age at birth and still required oxygen at 36 weeks' corrected age. They compared the neurodevelopmental outcomes at 1 year adjusted age of children whose parents had heightened PPCV with those whose parents had no heightened PPCV. Children of parents with heightened PPCV had a significant psychomotor delay and adaptive developmental delay (communication, socialization, motor skills, and daily living skills) at 1 year adjusted age as measured by the Bayley Scales of Infant Development (Bayley 1993) and Vineland Adaptive Behavior Scale (Sparrow et al. 1984) compared with those whose parents did not have heightened PPCV. Allen et al. (2004) did not find a difference on the cognitive component of the Bayley scale. Greene et al. (2017) examined neurodevelopment outcomes of toddlers born with very low birth weights (VLBWs) when measuring maternal perceptions of child vulnerability. Their study included 69 mothers and assessed infants at corrected ages of 4 months and 20 months and found that PPCV was associated with poorer language performance for their children at 20 months.

BEHAVIORAL DIFFICULTIES

De Ocampo et al. (2003) evaluated 90 infants ages 20–81 months' post-menstrual age who had been born preterm and were being followed at a NICU high-risk clinic. They measured the infants' behavior with the Child Behavioral Checklist (CBCL; Achenbach 1991) and used a multivariate regression analysis to assess factors associated with the CBCL scores, including neonatal medical problems, PPCV, child developmental quotient (DQ) or intelligence quotient (IQ), and parent demographics. PPCV scores were found to be the major predictor of child behaviors and accounted for 13% of the variance. Children of parents with higher PPCV scores also had increased somatic complaints, anxiety, depression, and aggressive behaviors. Younger children (≤36 months) had increased somatic complaints, aggressive behavior, and other behavioral problems. Children older than 36 months were found to have higher rates of anxiety and depression.

HEALTH CARE UTILIZATION

PPCV is associated with greater use of resources and a higher number of medical care visits. Chambers et al. (2011) looked at PPCV scores and the frequency of emergency department (ED) visits in 351 parents of children brought to the ED with nonurgent complaints. Parents with heightened PPCV measured by the CVS had significantly higher ED visits and hospitalization occurrences and higher rates of child mental health problems and developmental concerns. Higher rates of unnecessary health care utilization in parents with heightened PPCV suggest that VCS may place a significant financial burden on the family and the health care system. No existing studies document the medical cost of VCS on the health care system.

Assessment

Interest in the construct and impact of VCS has led to the development of instruments to assess its presence in parents and children. Given that VCS was originally observed in older children (Green and Solnit 1964), scales were originally developed with that group in mind. As evidence built to suggest the importance of VCS in at-risk younger populations, such as infants in the NICU, a scale for younger children was developed. Six variations of the scales have now been produced. In this chapter, we describe and discuss the most frequently used scales in the literature. To understand the strengths and limitations of these scales, it is important to know that to a large degree they describe parents' behaviors and perceptions and thus more accurately measure the construct of PPCV. In fact, these scales do not, to any significant degree, measure the child outcome criteria used by Green and Solnit (1964) in their original description of VCS. Implicit in the design of the existing scales is the hypothesis that PPCV leads to changes in parenting behaviors that then result in VCS. In addition, existing scales show elevated scores for children with true medical vulnerability as well as for children who are not medically vulnerable but whose parents have increased PPCV.

FORSYTH'S CHILD VULNERABILITY SCALE

Forsyth (1987) first developed the CVS as a research tool to identify vulnerable children. This scale is referred to as "Forsyth's CVS" for the remainder of this chapter (Table 7–1). Forsyth's CVS had 12 questions and was modified in 1991 by Forsyth and Canny to have only 10 questions. However, neither instrument was ever validated. The purpose of Forsyth's CVS was to identify families at risk of developing VCS by identifying parents with high PPCV scores and children who were viewed by their parents as being vulnerable. The items of the scale were chosen by the authors from both literature reviews and clinical experience and were considered to be consistent with the manifestations of VCS. Forsyth's CVS consists of 12 self-report questions answered by parents. It is scored on a Likert scale ranging from 1 to 5, with lower scores suggesting higher perception of vulnerability. Efforts were made to demonstrate the validity of the CVS; however, this work has been complicated because no other gold-standard scales or measures with which to compare it are available. In 1999, Thomasgard and Metz further validated the content validity of Forsyth's Revised CVS by confirming that high total scores on the scale are significantly correlated with the following parental concepts: "general concerns about the child's health, a previous serious illness for the child, a fear that the child might die, and difficulty setting limits on the child's behavior," (p. 348) all of which are components of the aforementioned VCS.

FORSYTH'S REVISED CHILD VULNERABILITY SCALE

In 1996, Forsyth and colleagues created a revised version of Forsyth's CVS (referred to here as "Forsyth's Revised CVS"). As part of a larger study, data were gathered to validate the original Forsyth's CVS by measuring scores of truly vulnerable children against those of children without medical problems. Forsyth et al. (1996) enrolled 1,095 children ages 4–8 years from a local pediatrician's office who were rated by an expert panel as either truly medically vulnerable (168 qualifying conditions) or not medically vulnerable. Each parent then completed Forsyth's CVS and a CBCL to assess behavioral problems. The CBCL and presence or

---

Table 7–1.   Forsyth's Child Vulnerability Scale

Each item scored 1–5: 1=Strongly Agree, 2=Agree, 3=Do Not Agree or Disagree, 4=Disagree, 5=Strongly Disagree

Item

1. In general my child seems less healthy than other children.

2. I often think about calling the doctor about my child.

3. I often have to keep my child indoors because of health reasons.

4. My child gets more colds than other children I know.

5. When there is something going around my child usually catches it.

6. I get concerned about circles under my child's eyes.

7. Sometimes I get concerned that my child doesn't look as healthy as s/he should.

8. I often check on my child at night to make sure that s/he is okay.

9. My child seems to have more accidents and injuries than other children.

10. My child often gets stomach pains or other types of pains.

11.* My child seems to have as much energy as other children.

12.* My child usually has a healthy appetite.

---

*Items 11 and 12 are reverse scored.
Source.   Forsyth BWC, Horwitz S, Leventhal JM, et al: "The Child Vulnerability Scale: An Instrument to Measure Parental Perceptions of Child Vulnerability." *Journal of Pediatric Psychology* 21(1):97, 1996. Reprinted with permission from Oxford University Press, 1996.

absence of medical problems were used as measures to assess the validity of Forsyth's CVS scores for parents of medically vulnerable versus not medically vulnerable children, with the hypothesis that truly medically vulnerable children would have higher CBCL and CVS scores. Results were used to develop a cutoff score that could be used as an index of the presence of significant PPCV scores. Forsyth et al. (1996) also determined that some of the items from the original Forsyth's CVS had poor association with two major variables for PPCV (a child with a medical condition and a parent's prior fear of the child dying). These two questions were eliminated in the revision. Forsyth's Revised CVS has eight questions and uses a Likert scale ranging from 0 to 3, with a maximum possible score of 24 (Table 7–2). Higher scores suggest a higher PPCV, and a cutoff score of ≥10 was used to determine significant PPCV. Questions in the modified scale are phrased to be more appropriate for older children. Forsyth's Revised CVS is now the most widely used scale in VCS literature and has been used for parents of children ages 6 months to 8 years.

Table 7–2.   Forsyth's Revised Child Vulnerability Scale

Each item scored 0–3: 0=Definitely False, 1=Mostly False, 2=Mostly True, 3= Definitely True

Item

1. My child gets more colds than other children I know.
2. I often think about calling the doctor about my child.
3. When there is something going around my child usually catches it.
4. In general, my child seems less healthy than other children.
5. I often have to keep my child indoors because of health reasons.
6. Sometimes I get concerned that my child doesn't look as healthy as s/he should.
7. I get concerned about circles under my child's eyes.
8. I often check on my child at night to make sure s/he is okay.

Source.   Forsyth BWC, Horwitz S, Leventhal JM, et al: "The Child Vulnerability Scale: An Instrument to Measure Parental Perceptions of Child Vulnerability." *Journal of Pediatric Psychology* 21(1):97, 1996. Reprinted with permission from Oxford University Press, 1996.

PERRIN'S VULNERABLE CHILD SCALE

Perrin et al. (1989) developed and validated their own Vulnerable Child Scale, which expanded on the 12 questions in Forsyth's original CVS and contains 16 questions scored on a Likert scale of 1–4, with a total score ranging from 16 to 64. Lower scores indicate a higher PPCV. The scale was validated against the Personality Inventory for Children (Wirt et al. 1982). This scale deserves mention; however, it is not as widely used in literature as Forsyth's Revised CVS.

VULNERABLE BABY SCALE

In 2005, Kerruish and colleagues developed the Vulnerable Baby Scale for infants and younger children, given that the question structure of Forsyth's CVS was geared more toward toddlers and older children (Table 7–3). They modified the original 12-question Forsyth's CVS with questions more suitable for infants. The scale has items focusing on four areas: 1) degree of protectiveness, 2) parental readiness for separation, 3) parental concern for infant health, and 4) frequency of nonroutine health care use. Parents of infants in three different groups were asked to participate. The groups differed by infant medical problems and were classified as medically fragile infants (diaphragmatic hernia, exchange transfusions for hemolytic disease, apnea at 35 weeks' gestational age, or respiratory distress at 36 weeks gestational age), infants requiring only phototherapy for jaundice, and healthy full-term infants. A total of 75 families were enrolled: 17 medically fragile infants, 19 jaundiced in-

Table 7–3.   Vulnerable Baby Scale

1. I generally check on my baby while he/she is asleep at night:

1	2	3	4	5
Not at all		1–2 times each night		Frequently

2.* If baby was awake and playing, I would leave them unattended and out of ear shot for:

1	2	3	4	5
Not at all		About 15 minutes		>1 hour

3.* If a friend came to visit and they had a cold, I would:

1	2	3	4	5
Not allow them in		Allow in but not hold baby		Ask them in and not restrict

4.* My baby seems to get stomach pains or other pains:

1	2	3	4	5
All the time				Not at all

5.* I am concerned that my baby is not as healthy as he/she should be:

1	2	3	4	5
Always				Not concerned

6.* In general, when I compare my baby's health to that of other children the same age I think he/she is:

1	2	3	4	5
Less healthy				More healthy

7.* I find myself worrying that my baby may become seriously ill:

1	2	3	4	5
All the time				Not at all

8.* I worry about cot death (SIDS):

1	2	3	4	5
All the time				Not at all

9.* If you left baby with someone else would you make contact with them while you were away?

1	2	3	4	5
Yes, definitely				No, not at all

Table 7–3.	Vulnerable Baby Scale *(continued)*

10. In the last 2 weeks I have contacted a health professional after hours or emergency doctors about my baby:

1	2	3	4	5
Not at all		About once a week		Daily or more

*Items 2–9 are reverse scored.

Source.   Kerruish NJ, Settle K, Campbell-Stokes P, Taylor BJ: Vulnerable Baby Scale: Development and Piloting of a Questionnaire to Measure Maternal Perceptions of Their Baby's Vulnerability. *Journal of Paediatrics and Child Health*?41(8):419–423, 2005. Reprinted with permission from John Wiley and Sons.

fants, and 39 healthy full-term infants. Parents completed the new Vulnerable Baby Scale as well as the State-Trait Anxiety Scale (Spielberger et al. 1983) and the Edinburgh Postnatal Depression Scale (Boyce et al. 1993) when their infants were 12 weeks of age. Statistical analysis examined the differences in mean scores on the Vulnerable Baby Scale in the different groups and their relation to parental anxiety and depression and demographic variables. Due to statistical correlation with medical fragility and PPCV of 0.3–0.7, 10 total questions were included in the final scale. The final version of the Vulnerable Baby Scale has 10 questions and is scored on a 1–5 Likert scale, with a maximum score of 50. A score of ≥27 is considered to indicate high and clinically significant PPCV.

Commentary on Existing Scales

Our own review of the literature suggests that there is confusion about the terminology and theoretical bases of the scales used to measure VCS. Although both Forsyth's Revised CVS and the Vulnerable Baby Scale purport to measure VCS, they more accurately measure PPCV. In addition, in their original design, no explicit description was given of a theoretical model to explain how VCS was related to PPCV. In reality, the items in the scales measure different categories of parenting responses to a medically ill or fragile child. Closer analysis demonstrates that both scales include items assessing one of three domains of parental response to the child's experience: 1) parental perceptions of their child's health; 2) parental anxieties and other feelings about their child's health and safety; and 3) habitual parenting behaviors.

PARENTAL THOUGHTS AND PERCEPTIONS

The thoughts and perceptions domain involves questions about parents' negative *thoughts* or *perceptions* regarding their child's health and well-being. Perceptions and thoughts can be understood as parents' internal dialogues, such as "In general, my child seems less healthy than other children" from Forsyth's Revised CVS and "My baby seems to get stomach pains or other pains" from the Vulnerable Baby Scale.

PARENTAL FEELINGS AND EMOTIONS

The emotions and feelings domain involves questions about parents' *feelings* or *emotions* related to their child, including guilt, fear, anxiety, or sadness. Feelings and emotions are distinct from thoughts or perceptions; they are usually reactions to a thought or perception and are easily recognizable in body language and facial expressions. Examples in the scales include items such as "I get *concerned* about circles under my child's eyes" from Forsyth's Revised CVS and "I find myself *worrying* that my baby may become seriously ill" from the Vulnerable Baby Scale.

PARENTAL BEHAVIORS

The parent behavior domain assesses parenting behaviors that develop in response to these thoughts and emotions, such as overprotective habits or failure to set appropriate limits. Examples include questions such as "I often have to keep my child indoors because of health reasons" from Forsyth's Revised CVS and "I generally check on my baby while he/she is asleep at night" from the Vulnerable Baby Scale.

These scales have no outcome questions assessing child behaviors and development, which is one of the three necessary criteria for VCS. Therefore, they cannot be used to measure VCS, only PPCV, a construct hypothesized to be associated with development of VCS. Closer analysis of the existing scales using this classification shows that distribution of questions across these three categories is not balanced. For example, Forsyth's Revised CVS has eight questions: four focused on parenting perceptions (e.g., "In general my child seems less healthy than other children"), two on parental emotions (e.g., "I get concerned about circles under my child's eyes"), and two on parenting behaviors (e.g., "I often have to keep my child indoors because of health reasons"). By contrast, the Vulnerable Baby Scale has 10 questions, two focused on parental perceptions (e.g., "In general when I compare my baby's health to that of another child the same age, I think my child is less/more healthy"), two on parental emotions (e.g., "I find myself worrying that my baby may become seriously ill"), and five on parenting behaviors (e.g., "I generally check on my baby while he/she is asleep at night"). Each scale generates a single score used to assess the presence and severity of VCS.

The existing scales raise additional questions. Research has found a positive correlation between scores on Forsyth's Revised CVS and the Vulnerable Baby Scale and health care use. However, given that some items on the Vulnerable Baby Scale are direct measures of health care use (e.g., "In the last 2 weeks I have contacted a health professional about my baby"), the relationship between these scores and outcomes would inevitably be positive. This has the potential to skew results and research conclusions based on use of these scales. Important questions remain about whether VCS should be defined based on parenting practices (i.e., problems setting age-appropriate limits and rules for the child, problems with separation from the child, or overindulgent parenting) or if the child must also demonstrate specific negative behaviors, such as psychosocial problems or poor academic outcomes, for a diagnosis of VCS.

Trauma-Based Model of Vulnerable Child Syndrome

DEVELOPMENT

Recently, researchers have postulated a trauma model to explain aspects of VCS (Horwitz et al. 2015b). Parental trauma related to the child's premature birth, along with fears about the child's survival or well-being, commonly lead to symptoms of PTSD, including intrusive fears about the child's health. Benign physical signs and symptoms in the child may trigger recurrent and automatic feelings and anxiety in the parents and cause them to engage in parenting behaviors that over time result in symptoms of VCS (see Figure 7–2).

In adopting a trauma model to explain VCS in parents of premature infants, two primary emotions are at play. The infant's premature birth and the frequently stressful and unpredictable course of the NICU experience trigger feelings of *parental anxiety* about the child's medical well-being. Automatic negative thoughts, such as "Something bad will happen" or "My child is weak and fragile," lead to worry or fear. In response, parents may develop overprotective parenting behaviors. Feelings of *parental guilt*, often triggered by the mother's usually irrational belief that she somehow caused the premature birth, may lead to "guilty" parents engaging in patterns of permissive or overindulgent parenting to "make up" for the trauma they "caused," such as failing to set appropriate limits as the child grows, much as had been described by Cohen et al. (2008) in relation to mothers who had been traumatized before their pregnancy and the birth of the child. The combination of overprotective and overly permissive parenting sets the child up to develop VCS.

MEASUREMENT

The development of a trauma-based conceptualization of VCS lends itself to a revised approach to the measurement of VCS. Given that two of the principal existing VCS scales tend to ask questions that fall into the three domains of cognitive behavioral therapy (CBT; thoughts, feelings,

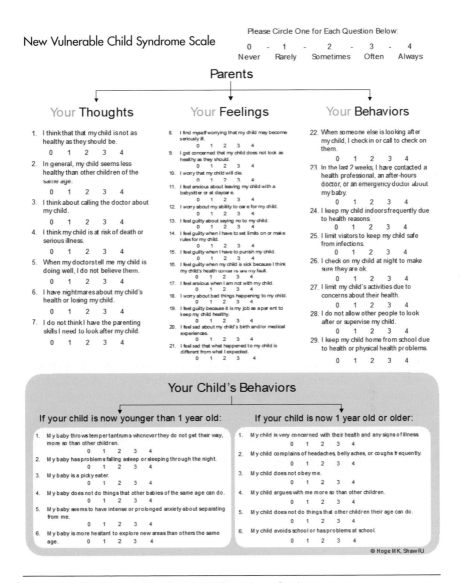

FIGURE 7–3.   **New Vulnerable Child Syndrome Scale.**
Source.   Adapted from Hoge and Shaw 2019.

and behaviors), we propose a revised version of the Vulnerable Child Scale built around these three principles (Figure 7–3).

The questionnaire is divided into two sections, one directed at parent's thoughts, feelings, and behaviors and another at the child's behaviors. PPCV is assessed in the category of "parental thoughts" about the health and well-being of their child and measured with questions 1–7. "Parental feelings" that develop in response to PPCV are measured with questions 8–21. "Parenting behaviors" that develop in response to PPCV and parental feelings are measured with questions 22–29. To assess VCS, a section on child behaviors is included in which questions are tailored to the chronological age of the child. Parents respond only to the section that is relevant to their child's age. Efforts are under way to assess the validity of this revised scale.

Treatment

Green and Solnit (1964) proposed that it might be possible to intervene in VCS once the link between PPCV and a past traumatic event was identified by the parents. However, research on interventions for VCS is lacking. Horwitz et al. (2015a) reported data from a randomized controlled study of 105 parents of premature infants randomly assigned to receive six to nine sessions of trauma-focused cognitive behavioral therapy (TF-CBT) versus receiving education on the developmental needs of the infants and parental support groups during the first 5 weeks of admission (Shaw et al. 2013, 2014). Vulnerable Baby Scale scores from enrollment to the end of the study when the children reached 6 months of age showed a trend but no statistically significant difference between the groups. The authors viewed the timing of the intervention (too early in a child's life) as one possible reason for the negative findings. Efforts to address parenting behaviors using a trauma-based CBT model may need to be made at a later developmental stage when the child is engaging in behaviors that might trigger overprotective or overindulgent parenting.

Manualized Intervention to Prevent VCS in Premature Infants

Using our developmental trauma-based model of VCS, we have created a five-session manualized intervention to prevent VCS in medically fragile preterm infants. The manual is based on principles of TF-CBT sessions and is available in both English and Spanish. Timing of the sessions was determined based upon research suggesting that early treatments in the NICU course are ineffective (Horwitz et al. 2015b). Past research has suggested that parent mental health symptoms peak when the child is 2 weeks of age but decrease toward the child's discharge. This makes the time prior to discharge from the NICU a good time to start the therapy because the initial traumatic events have subsided and infants are in a well-enough state that the parents may start preparing for discharge to home (Pace et al. 2016). Parents receive three sessions, once weekly, in the NICU, starting when their infant has reached 34 weeks' gestational age, when most premature infants are stable clinically and survival is no longer in question. The subsequent two sessions occur in the long-term follow-up clinic 1 and 2 months after discharge from the NICU. Sessions are scheduled at this time to reinforce concepts based on CBT principles that were taught in the NICU, rather than relying on NICU staff. During the two outpatient sessions, parents learn age-appropriate expectations for their prematurely born infants. Parents also start to develop realistic expectations as well as positive parenting responses and skills that are developmentally appropriate for their child's corrected age. This helps parents learn to avoid negative parenting patterns that may be connected to past traumatic experiences in the NICU and in turn may contribute to the development of VCS (Table 7–4).

SESSION 1: PARENTS' NICU EXPERIENCE AND STRESS MANAGEMENT

The content of Session 1, which is adapted from the Individual Treatment Intervention for Mothers of Premature Infants (see Chapter 5), focuses primarily on helping parents understand their NICU experience, build rapport with the therapist, gain stress education, and learn self-care techniques to help them manage stress. Parents are asked to recount their memories of the NICU, both positive and negative. They are encouraged to remember a stressful time in the NICU and how their body felt during that moment. Parents are educated about the CBT model of feelings and thoughts and how their body's physical responses are interconnected. They learn to recognize signs of stress by first recognizing their body's response to stress, for example, tightened muscles, headaches, and lack of sleep, and then taught techniques on how to relieve stress by altering their body's response as demonstrated in the Stress Triangle (see Chapter 5) using techniques that include deep breathing, muscle relaxation, and infant massage. Each parent is given goals at the end of the session that include practicing these techniques prior to the next session.

SESSION 2: TRAUMA PSYCHOEDUCATION AND COGNITIVE RESTRUCTURING

Session 2 in the NICU focuses on trauma education as well as the introduction of thought retraining exercises. The notion that having a child in the NICU is a traumatic experience is explored with the parents. Parents are taught to recognize signs and symptoms of traumatic stress and asked to consider whether they have been experiencing any of these symptoms. Parents learn how symptoms of traumatic stress can automatically affect their thoughts, feelings, and behaviors in response to future events, often in a negative way, and learn cognitive restructuring as previously described (see Chapter 5).

Table 7–4.   Treatment manual session content and timing

Session and Timing	Location	Content
Session 1: 34 weeks' gestational age	NICU	Introduction to the treatment
		Build rapport
		Psychoeducation and normalization of the typical NICU parent experience
Session 2: 35 weeks' gestational age	NICU	Psychoeducation about psychological trauma and PTSD
		Cognitive restructuring
		Examining the Evidence
		What Would I Tell a Friend?/Positive Self-Statements
Session 3: 36 weeks' gestational age	NICU	Education about VCS
		Debunking the myths
		Reinforcement about infant massage, PMR, breathing, and journaling
		Preparation for discharge
Session 4: 1 month post discharge	Outpatient follow-up clinic	Check in about progress since discharge
		Re-education about VCS
		Debunking the myths (for 3- to 5-month-old infants)
		Reinforcement about infant massage, PMR, breathing, and journaling
Session 5: 2 months post discharge	Outpatient follow-up clinic	Check in about progress since discharge
		Re-education about VCS
		Debunking the myths (for 4- to 6-month-old infants)
		Reinforcement about infant massage, PMR, breathing, and journaling
		Discussion and wrap up

PMR=Progressive Muscle Relaxation; VCS=vulnerable child syndrome

SESSION 3: VCS EDUCATION AND PREPARING FOR HOME

Session 3 is the last session scheduled to take place in the NICU. Session content includes education about VCS and how to use the skills learned in past sessions, such as the ABC-B Worksheet and Examining the Evidence exercise, to evaluate hypothetical events that might concern parents after their infant has been discharged from the NICU. In the VCS education component, parents learn that traumatic experiences, such as having a child born prematurely and having a child in the NICU, can influence how they automatically think, feel, and act toward that child, even as the child recovers from the trauma of those experiences as well. Parents also learn how overprotective parenting responses may occur in response to triggers that remind them of their child's traumatic birth and hospitalization. Parents are educated on the potential negative impact this may have on their child's development. To describe common aspects of VCS, the VCS triangle is used to illustrate the principles (Figure 7–4).

After learning about VCS, the parents choose one or two examples of common scenarios that they anticipate may create anxiety for them after discharge (Figure 7–5). These scenarios are used as examples to practice using both the ABC-B Worksheet and Examining the Evidence skills to work through anxieties and prevent unwanted VCS. Parents learn about the differences between premature and full-term infants to dispel common parenting myths and anxieties. Using the ABC-B Worksheet and Examining the Evidence techniques, parents learn to recognize their automatic initial negative and unhelpful thoughts, feelings, and actions. They then review the current situation to reinterpret their infant's behavior and devise an alternative sequence of more adaptive and helpful thoughts, feelings, and parenting responses. Handouts for each scenario are provided to illustrate the common automatic thoughts, feelings, and actions that parents have and experience in response to these situations.

For example, if the parent chose the scenario "My baby gets a cough," they would first complete the ABC-B Worksheet to understand their initial thoughts, feelings, and actions. The parent's potential first thought—"My baby is small, weak, and fragile and something bad might happen (my child might die)"—may lead them to feel anxious, which not unreasonably might lead them to take their child to the doctor or ED. However, the therapist intervenes by showing the parent how much greater resilience their child has compared with their situation in the NICU and that a cough at 6 months is different from a cough at 6 weeks of age. Using this new information, parents are led through an exercise of Examining the Evidence and encouraged to list all examples of evidence both for and against the thought that their child's health is at risk. They are guided toward appreciating that the evidence supports the child's resilience. Some examples of evidence in favor of the child's resilience could be "my baby is getting stronger and growing," "my baby is not struggling to breathe," "my baby has had a cough before and has been okay." Parents are then guided to come up with an alternative thought, based on evidence, that the child is not at high risk and that they do not need to feel so anxious and perhaps could call the advice nurse rather than going to the ED. Handouts specific to the scenario are used to illustrate

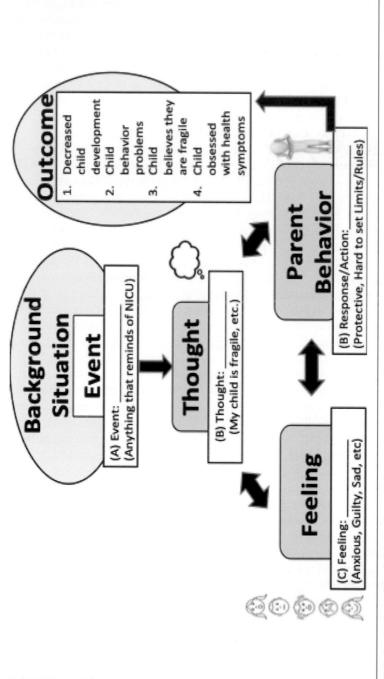

FIGURE 7–4. **Vulnerable child syndrome triangle.**

Source. Adapted from Hoge and Shaw 2019.

Things that make me worried:				
1	2	3	4	5
Baby sleeping without monitors	Baby is crying a lot and I don't know why	Baby throws up	Someone wants to visit my baby and I am worried my baby will get sick.	I am worried to let someone else care for my baby and leave my baby.

Common events for babies around NICU discharge

FIGURE 7–5. **Common concerns for parents of premature infants around NICU discharge.**

Source. Adapted from Hoge and Shaw 2019.

common automatic first thoughts, feelings, and actions, with evidence for or against each point to support discussion (Figure 7–6).

SESSION 4: VCS AT AGE 1–3 MONTHS

Session 4 takes place at the infant's follow-up clinic appointment approximately 1 month after NICU discharge. By this time, parents will have had the opportunity to encounter common and predictably stressful parenting moments and hopefully have applied some of the skills taught to them in the first three sessions. Parents are asked to recount how the time at home has been with their infant during both good and stressful times. Session 4 includes a brief review of the content from all the other sessions, reinforcing the concepts of stress and trauma and how they are related to the development of VCS. A comprehensive review of VCS and its presentation in older infants is completed with the assistance of the VCS triangle that was used in Session 3. The ABC-B Worksheet and Examining the Evidence techniques are also briefly reviewed.

After the review is completed, parents go through a list of scenarios that are commonly concerning to parents of prematurely born children at this time of their life (Figure 7–7). Parents select one or two scenarios and then work with the therapist on how to address their anxieties and potential responses using their ABC-B Worksheet and Examining the Evidence skills. Those skills are practiced by the parents for each chosen scenario, with guidance from the therapist. After the parents go through the scenario on their own, handouts for each scenario are provided to illustrate the common automatic thoughts, feelings, and actions parents have in response to these situations and how to use their learned skills. Finally, parents are taught how to calculate their child's corrected age in order to better base their expectations for the child. They are also taught additional skills that are age-appropriate for their child to help them continue to develop positive parenting habits prior to the following session.

SESSION 5: VCS AT AGE 4–6 MONTHS

Session 5 is scheduled 1 month after Session 4, or 2 months following discharge from the NICU. By this age, the child will have developed further and may be manifesting behaviors that require more parental firmness and limit setting, which may be challenging for a parent in the context of VCS (e.g., sleep training). Session 5 includes another brief review of the content from all the previous sessions, including a review of the trauma model, VCS, and the ABC-B Worksheet and Examining the Evidence exercise. Parents then recount a list of common scenarios that create anxiety for parents with children of their own child's age (Figure 7–8). Parents choose one or two scenarios from the list and approach them using the same methods described in Session 4. They are taught the importance of

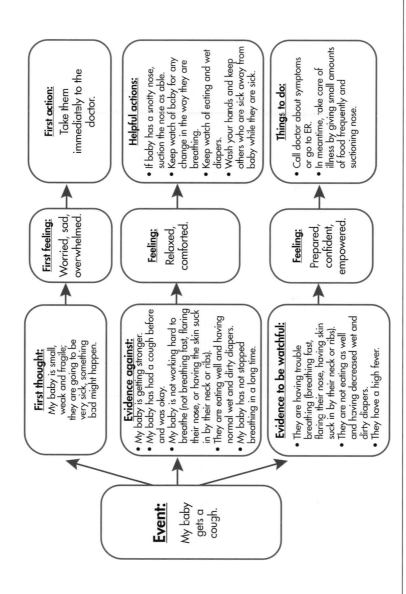

FIGURE 7–6. **Handout scenario specific event.**

Source. Adapted from Hoge and Shaw 2019.

Common events:

	1	2	3	4	5	6	7
Common worries for NICU babies at home, age 3–6 months (1–4 months corrected age)	My baby cries during the night.	My baby is having trouble learning something new.	I don't know if my baby's growth and eating are good enough.	My baby gets a cough.	Someone wants to visit my baby and I am worried my baby will get sick.	I am worried to let someone else care for my baby or leave my baby.	I don't have the NICU staff to help me take care of my baby.

FIGURE 7–7. **Common concerns of parents of infants at age 3–6 months.**

Source. Adapted from Hoge and Shaw 2019.

Common events:

1	2	3	4	5	6	7
My child is having temper tantrums.	My child is having trouble learning something new.	My child is a picky eater.	My child gets a cough or cold.	My child wants to play with new friends.	I am worried to let my child go to daycare.	I have to punish my child or set rules for my child.

Common worries for NICU babies at home, age 7–12 months (5–10 months corrected age)

FIGURE 7–8. Common concerns of parents of infants at age 7–12 months.

Source. Adapted from Hoge and Shaw 2019.

setting age-appropriate limits and being vigilant about the potential for overprotective or indulgent parenting. At this visit, parents also learn about sleeping routines and infant self-soothing techniques during sleep as well as parenting skills to create positive future parenting practices.

Future Directions

VCS is a multifaceted phenomenon and has many ramifications for parents, children, and the health care system at large. Despite the best efforts of providers to ensure good outcomes for premature infants, these may easily be complicated in families with PPCV and VCS. Faulty perceptions of vulnerability have the potential to result in negative consequences for the child, including parental concerns or illness anxiety, interference with development, and other mental health concerns. Given the increased prevalence of VCS in families of premature infants, it is important to pay attention to developing support, resources, and interventions for parents in the NICU to minimize these risks.

To accomplish these goals, it is necessary first to have a sound conceptual model of PPCV and VCS. The trauma-based view of VCS is one such model that lends itself to understanding potential risk factors as well as suggesting ways to intervene. In particular, techniques based on principles of CBT, which has been used in multiple settings, seem applicable in the context of the NICU environment. The trauma model is also useful in helping refine our methods of measurement and assessment, as suggested in our New Revised Vulnerable Child Scale, which could be used to screen for risk factors and track the response to treatment.

We have proposed a short, cost-effective five-session CBT intervention designed to both prevent and reduce PPCV that has the potential to reduce the future risk of VCS. Efforts are under way to evaluate the feasibility and effectiveness of this intervention. The Preventing Vulnerable Child Syndrome in the NICU with Cognitive Behavioral Therapy Trial (PreVNT; Hoge et al. 2019) assesses the utility of a CBT manual-based intervention consisting of five sessions aimed at the prevention of VCS in families of NICU infants born at <31 weeks' gestation. PreVNT incorporates the New Vulnerable Child Syndrome Scale to compare it with the existing Vulnerable Baby Scale and Forsyth's Revised CVS.

More research is needed in this area to guide standards of care. The expanding focus on family-centered models of care is encouraging, as is the growing understanding of the importance of incorporating bonding, mental health, and parental perceptions of the child into holistic NICU care. Focusing on interventions in these areas gives hope for other novel ways of improving outcomes for children and parents in the NICU.

References

Achenbach TM: Manual for the Child Behavior Checklist 4–18. Burlington, VT, University of Vermont, 1991

Allen EC, Manuel JC, Legault C, et al: Perception of child vulnerability among mothers of former premature infants. Pediatrics 113(2):267–273, 2004

Bayley N: Bayley Scales of Infant Development: Manual. New York, Psychological Corporation, 1993

Benoit D, Zeanah CH, Parker KCH, et al: Working model of the child interview: infant clinical related to maternal perceptions. Infant Ment Health J 18(1):107–121, 1997

Boyce P, Stubbs J, Todd A: The Edinburgh Postnatal Depression Scale. validation for an Australian sample. Aust NZ J Psychiatry 27(3):472–476, 1993

Chambers PL, Mahabee-Gittens EM, Leonard AC: Vulnerable child syndrome, parental perception of child vulnerability, and emergency department usage. Pediatr Emerg Care 27(11):1009, 2011

Cohen LR, Hien DA, Batchelder S: The impact of cumulative maternal trauma and diagnosis on parenting behavior. Child Maltreatment 13(1):27–28, 2008

Culley BS, Perrin EC, Jordan Chaberski M: Parental perceptions of vulnerability of formerly premature infants. J Pediatr Health Care 3(5):237–245, 1989

De Ocampo AC, Macias MM, et al: Caretaker perception of child vulnerability predicts behavior problems in NICU graduates. Child Psychiatry Hum Dev 34(2):83–96, 2003

Estroff DB, Yando R, Burke K, Synder D: Perceptions of preschoolers' vulnerability by mothers who had delivered preterm. J Pediatr Psychol 19(6):709–721, 1994

Forsyth BWC: Mothers' perceptions of their children's vulnerability after hospitalization for infection (abstract). Am J Dis Child 141:377, 1987

Forsyth BWC: Early health crises and vulnerable children. J Dev Behav Pediatr 4:337–342, 2009

Forsyth BWC, Canny PF: Perceptions of vulnerability 3½ years after problems of feeding and crying behavior in early infancy. Pediatr 88(4):757–763, 1991

Forsyth BWC, Horwitz SM, Leventhal JM, et al: The Child Vulnerability Scale: an instrument to measure parental perceptions of child vulnerability. J Pediatr Psychol 21(1):89–101, 1996

Green M, Solnit AJ: Reactions to the threatened loss of a child: a vulnerable child syndrome: pediatric management of the dying child. Pediatr 34(1):58–66, 1964

Greene MM, Rossman B, Meier P, Patra K: Parental perception of child vulnerability among mothers of very low birth weight infants: psychological predictors and neurodevelopmental sequelae at 2 years. J Perinatol 37(4):454–460, 2017

Hoge MK, Heyne ET, De Freitas Nicholson T, et al: Preventing Vulnerable Child Syndrome in the NICU With Cognitive Behavioral Therapy (PreVNT Trial) (PreVNT) (Clinicaltrials.gov Identifier NCT03906435), 2019. Available at: https://clinicaltrials.gov/ct2/show/NCT03906435. Accessed June 18,2020.

Hoge MK, Shaw RJ: PreVNT Treatment Manual. Unpublished, 2019

Horwitz SM, Leibovitz A, Lilo E, et al: Does an intervention to reduce maternal anxiety, depression and trauma also improve mothers' perceptions of their preterm infants' vulnerability? Infant Ment Health J 36(1):42–52, 2015a

Horwitz SM, Storfer-Isser A, Kerker BD, et al: A model for the development of mothers' perceived vulnerability of preterm infants. J Dev Behav Pediatr 36(5):371, 2015b

Keesara S, Kim JJ: Outcomes of universal perinatal mood screening in the obstetric and pediatric setting. NeoReviews 19(3):152–159, 2018

Kerruish NJ, Settle K, Campbell-Stokes P, Taylor BJ: Vulnerable baby scale: development and piloting of a questionnaire to measure maternal perceptions of their baby's vulnerability. J Paediatr Child Health 41(8):419–423, 2005

Leslie LK, Boyce WT: Consultation with the specialist: the vulnerable child. Pediatr Rev 17(9):323, 1996

Levy JC: Vulnerable children: parent's perspectives and the use of medical care. Pediatrics 65:956–963, 1980

Lieberman AF: Toddler's internalization of maternal attributions as a factor in quality attachment, in Attachment and Psychopathology. Edited by Atkinson L, Zucker KJ. New York, Guilford, 1997, pp 277–291

Malin KJ, Johnson TS, McAndrew S, Westerdahl J, et al: Infant illness severity and perinatal post-traumatic stress disorder after discharge from the neonatal intensive care unit. Early Hum Dev 140:104930, 2019

Miles MS, Holditch-Davis D: Compensatory parenting: how mothers describe parenting their 3-year-old, prematurely born children. J Pediatr Nurs 10(4):243–253, 1995

Miles MS, Holditch-Davis D, Shepherd H: Maternal concerns about parenting: prematurely born children. MCN Am J Matern Child Nurs 23(2):70–75, 1998

Pace CC, Spittle AJ, Molesworth CM, et al: Evolution of depression and anxiety symptoms in parents of very preterm infants during the newborn period. JAMA Pediatr 170(9):863–870, 2016

Perrin EC, West PD, Culley BS: Is my child normal yet? Correlates of vulnerability. Pediatrics 83(3):355–363, 1989

Schechter DS, Myers MM, Brunelli SA, et al: Traumatized mothers can change their minds about their toddlers: understanding how a novel use of videofeedback supports positive change of maternal attributions. Infant Ment Health J 27(5):429–447, 2006

Schechter DS, Moser DA, Reliford A, et al: Negative and distorted attributions towards child, self, and primary attachment figure among posttraumatically stressed mothers: what changes with Clinician Assisted Videofeedback Exposure Sessions (CAVES). Child Psychiatry Hum Dev 46(1):10–20, 2015

Shaw RJ, Deblois T, Ikuta L, Ginzburg K: Acute stress disorder among parents of infants in the neonatal intensive care nursery. Psychosomatics 47(3):206–212, 2006

Shaw RJ, St John N, Lilo EA, Jo B: Prevention of traumatic stress in mothers with preterm infants: a randomized controlled trial. Pediatr 132(4):e886–e894, 2013

Shaw RJ, Lilo EA, Storfer-Isser A, et al: Screening for symptoms of postpartum traumatic stress in a sample of mothers with preterm infants. Issues Ment Health Nurs 35(3):198–207, 2014

Sparrow SS, Balla D, Cicchetti DV: Survey: Vineland Adaptive Behavior Scales. Circle Pines, MN, American Guidance Service, 1984

Spielberger CD, Gorsuch RL, Lushene PR, et al: Manual for the State-Trait Anxiety Inventory (Form Y). Palo Alto, CA, Consulting Psychologists Press, 1983

Thomasgard M, Metz WP: Parent–child relationship disorders: what do the Child Vulnerability Scale and the Parent Protection Scale measure? Clin Pediatr 38(6):347–356, 1999

Wirt RD, Lachar D, Klinedienst JK, et al: Personality Inventory for Children, Revised Format. Los Angeles, CA, Western Psychological Services, 1982

Zeanah CH (ed): Handbook of Infant Mental Health. New York, Guilford, 2018

Zeanah CH, Benoit D, Hirshberg L, et al: Mothers' representations of their infants are concordant with infant attachment classifications. Developmental Issues in Psychiatry and Psychology 1:9–18, 1994

CHAPTER 8

Implementing the Evidence-Based Intervention to Address Psychological Distress in Women With Premature Infants

Sarah M. Horwitz, Ph.D.

LaTrice L. Dowtin, Ph.D., LCPC, NCSP, RPT

Emily A. Lilo, Ph.D., M.P.H.

The introduction of evidence-based or evidence-informed practices into routine health care has been the focus of considerable investigation in the past two decades. The Institute of Medicine's 2001 seminal work *Crossing the Quality Chasm: A New Health System for the 21st Century* pointed out that health care fails to translate knowledge into routine practice and that, on average, it takes 17 years for scientific advances to be translated into routine health care practices. Numerous models describing implementation challenges and facilitators exist (Aarons et al. 2011a; Damschroder et al. 2009; Greenhalgh et al. 2004), and attending to the key driving elements in these models will facilitate the uptake of the intervention to reduce anxiety, depression, and trauma in mothers who deliver preterm infants.

Given that the adoption of a new evidence-based intervention is usually a practice-specific decision, focusing on what Aarons et al. (2011a) called the "inner context" of the active implementation phase may make adoption of this intervention in NICUs easier and more successful. Aarons et al. (2011a) postulated that three broad categories of features are important for implementation: organizational structure, innovation/values fit, and individual adopter characteristics. Given that NICUs are often centralized, understanding who makes the decisions and ensuring the decision-makers support adoption of the intervention for mothers is critical, as is understanding whether the NICU is ready for change and whether its procedures can be modified to support changes, such as screening, that are necessary to implement the program. Similarly, assessing staff interest and the ability to modify workloads to make time for the intervention are critical, as are staff attitudes and beliefs about the intervention, self-efficacy with respect to capacity to implement it, and personal attributes (Damschroder et al. 2009). For example, in one large-scale effort to train community mental health clinic providers in delivery of an evidence-informed practice, a major impediment to implementation was the providers' lack of technology skills, especially among older providers. The training had to be modified considerably to prevent dropout and facilitate implementation (Olin et al. 2016).

Implementation Experiences at Lucile Packard Children's Hospital

ENGAGEMENT OF LEADERSHIP

Our experience implementing the individual intervention for mothers in the NICU at the Lucile Packard Children's Hospital (LPCH) showed us the importance of these key features for successful implementation. Prior to submitting a proposal to the National Institute of Mental Health for funding to conduct a clinical trial establishing the effectiveness of the intervention, investigators confirmed the interest of both the current and past neonatology chiefs. Having supportive, interested leadership was critical for successful implementation of the intervention, as had been repeatedly documented in the literature. Aarons and colleagues, in a series of studies, found that transformational leadership facilitates evidence-based practice implementation efforts, predicts sustainment of evidence-based practices, and is particularly important during times of change (Aarons and Sommerfeld 2012; Aarons et al. 2011b, 2016). To sustain an evidence-based practice, having frontline leaders who champion the practice and provide practical support appears to be essential (Aarons et al. 2016), as is the availability of opinion leaders—people who are respected, enthusiastic about the intervention, and actively promote it (Rogers 2003). For our intervention, the NICU attending physicians adopted this role in several important ways, including obtaining NICU staff buy-in for establishment of the individual intervention as well as freeing up financial and other logistical resources without which the program would not have been possible. During the research phase, attending physician support in the form of assistance with publicizing and recruiting parents for the study played a key role not only with respect to parent participation but also in helping shift the NICU culture toward recognizing the importance of maternal psychological adjustment.

ENGAGEMENT OF ANCILLARY STAFF

After receiving funding, we met with the nursing, developmental, and social work staffs to describe the project and welcome the participation of anyone interested either in the development of study-related materials or in delivering the actual intervention. The nursing staff was enthusiastic about the intervention, citing the psychological needs of mothers that they constantly observed. Several members of the nursing staff met with us to review the content of the psychological intervention and develop the educational materials to be distributed to the comparison group. This enthusiasm was invaluable for ensuring that both the intervention and the related study educational materials contained important information, that eligible women received notice of the study, and that eligible women gave study participation full consideration. Like the nursing staff, the developmental intervention specialists were extremely helpful. In fact, one of the specialists became a member of the study team and designed the initial session of the intervention.

The members of the social work staff, although supportive, were less involved initially, largely due to their role in the NICU. The amount of instrumental support they supplied to families left little time in their schedules for therapeutic activities. There was one exception: a member of the social work staff volunteered to be trained as an interventionist and remained a study team member until she left Stanford. Over the course of the study, as positive impacts on mothers were observed, the social work staff became key proponents of the individual intervention. Social work buy-in was also enhanced by our decision to set up our screening program prior to the group therapy intervention. The large percentage of parents, both mothers and fathers, who screened positive on measures of depression, anxiety, and trauma helped raise awareness of the nature and extent of parental psychological distress and helped convince all staff of the value of the proposed intervention.

One potential risk when implementing an intervention of this nature in a NICU is of the social work staff feeling that their primary role in providing psychological support to the parents is being usurped. Cognizant of these issues, our team worked actively to include social workers in the screening process, offered them the opportunity to receive training and participate as therapists in the intervention, and established a regular meeting to discuss individual parent participants.

Secondary Traumatization and Staff Support

Establishing a new program in the NICU requires support and facilitation from staff. Specifically, involvement of NICU staff is critical to ensure the successful implementation of any new program, given that new programs and practices often require shifting or changing responsibilities. However, NICU staff members already have stressful jobs and are at increased risk of secondary traumatization or incidental contact with individuals who have experienced a traumatic event (Peebles-Kleiger 2000). Therefore, before enlisting their active involvement in recruiting patients for a mental health program, it is important to consider their psychosocial needs. Secondary traumatic stress (STS), PTSD, compassion fatigue, and burnout may present as a result of their call to care for the most vulnerable infants and their families. Many professionals, including those in the mental health and medical fields, are repeatedly indirectly exposed to traumatic events (Meadors et al. 2010). Exploring opportunities and options to provide support and care for staff is important for implementing a NICU-based program to alleviate mental health challenges for parents.

SECONDARY TRAUMATIC STRESS

STS typically occurs in professionals who develop adverse symptoms related to caring for trauma survivors or learning about significant traumatic events (Peebles-Kleiger 2000). STS is similar in nature to PTSD and includes symptoms of hyperarousal, avoidance, and intrusive thoughts (American Psychiatric Association 2013), with the exception that the person does not directly experience the traumatic event (Bride 2007). Seminal work on STS outlines previous trauma exposure and unresolved and similar trauma by the staff person and difficulty managing the trauma of child survivors as factors that contribute to the likelihood a provider will develop STS (Figley 1995). Joinson (1992) used *compassion fatigue* to describe nurses' emotional states related to their job functions and directly related it to the loss of empathy or decreased capacity for empathy. Figley (1995) suggested this term be used in place of STS in an effort to find terminology that was more acceptable to providers and perhaps less stigmatizing. However, research suggests that some of the common measures used to capture the prevalence of STS and compassion fatigue may in fact be measuring distinct features (Meadors et al. 2010).

COMPASSION FATIGUE

Compassion fatigue develops as a result of having a caseload with a high number of trauma cases and is more likely to affect health care providers who have an increased capacity for empathy (Figley 1995). Although STS and compassion fatigue are closely related to repeated secondary exposure to traumatic events, there is some disagreement in the literature regarding whether empathy needs to be present for STS, whereas empathy is part of the definition of compassion fatigue (Meadors et al. 2010; White 2006). Similarly, a study using the Impact of Events Scale, the Professional Quality of Life Scale, and the Secondary Traumatic Stress Scale (Meadors et al. 2010) to determine unique differences between STS and compassion fatigue found significant differences among health care providers in high-trauma settings, including the NICU.

BURNOUT

Burnout encapsulates the environmental factors that exist for health care providers exposed to secondary trauma. Jenkins and Baird (2002) defined *burnout* as a "defensive response to prolonged occupational exposure to demanding interpersonal situations that produce psychological strain and provide inadequate support" (p. 424). Thus, although a provider may not have symptoms of STS or compassion fatigue, he or she may experience burnout when the NICU setting lacks appropriate structure, policies, and supports for staff. Most commonly, burnout is assessed using three concepts on the Maslach Burnout Inventory (MBI; Maslach et al. 1986): 1) emotional exhaustion, 2) depersonalization, and 3) personal accomplishment (feeling a lack of accomplishment and success at work). Studies on NICU staff burnout, with a particular focus on NICU nursing staff, have used the MBI and found that as levels of burnout among NICU staff increase, general quality of life decreases (Aytekin et al. 2013). Many NICU nurses score in the moderate range for burnout in the areas of emotional exhaustion and personal accomplishment and have lower levels of depersonalization (Aytekin et al. 2013).

Similarly, a statistically significant relationship exists between burnout and compassion fatigue such that as the former increases, the latter increases and can lead to poor job satisfaction (Meadors et al. 2010). Prevalence rates for burnout among NICU staff are high. A recent study conducted across 41 NICUs assessed staff ($N=1,934$) perceptions of burnout and found that 26.7% of participants reported burnout above clinical cutoffs (Tawfik et al. 2017). The highest burnout rates have been found among NICU staff with high new-patient caseloads and electronic health record systems. Challenges with hospital administration (Tawfik et al. 2017), staff feeling undervalued, and numerous incidents of moral distress (Wagner 2015) have also been documented as characteristics contributing to symptoms of posttraumatic stress, compassion fatigue, and burnout among NICU staff.

IMPACT ON INFANTS AND FAMILIES

NICU infants and their families are also adversely affected when burnout occurs among NICU staff. Burnout has been correlated with poor NICU safety culture and parental dissatisfaction (Dessy 2009; Profit et al. 2014), which is in direct conflict with the recommendation to support family-centered and family-integrated care in the NICU. Van Mol et al. (2015) conducted a systematic review of studies examining secondary traumatization among intensive care unit staff. Researchers reviewed studies reporting prevalence rates of and intervention approaches for secondary trauma symptoms (i.e., burnout, compassion fatigue, STS, and vicarious trauma) from 1992 to 2014. They identified 1,623 publications, of which 40 met the criteria for review. The authors found that the reported rates of compassion fatigue ranged from 7.3% to 40%, STS from 0% to 38.5%, and burnout from 0% to 70.1%. Intervention techniques were outlined to include modifications in NICU staff work schedules, psychoeducation on emotion regulation, focus on improving communication skills among NICU team members, and the inclusion of mindfulness and relaxation-based teachings. We conducted an analysis of semistructured maternal narratives about pregnancy, birth, and NICU experiences and found that many mothers reported experiencing negative interactions with the care teams that caused them to feel disenfranchised, despite being at hospitals that claimed to engage in family-centered care. Those who reported more positive interactions with the care teams felt more empowered and engaged in their infant's care (Lilo et al. 2016). The impact these interactions have on families can affect mother–child bonding and family/staff interactions in the NICU as well as the mental health and well-being of providers, making an even stronger case for the need to address symptoms of burnout, compassion fatigue, and STS.

PSYCHOSOCIAL SUPPORT FOR NICU STAFF

As suggested in the literature, defining and exploring secondary traumatization among NICU staff is not enough to reduce symptoms or increase job satisfaction. Thus, we examined the needs of our NICU staff through conversations with social workers, neonatologists, a neonatal nurse practitioner, and a nurse manager/patient care manager. We learned that psychosocial support for NICU nurses and fellows was both needed and welcomed. Our meetings helped us establish clear considerations prior to moving forward with a support group designed to decrease symptoms of secondary traumatization (Table 8–1).

IMPLEMENTATION OF A NICU STAFF SUPPORT GROUP

After gaining approval and buy-in from the NICU team, we designed a preliminary six-session, 30-minute rotating intervention. On the basis of our research and nursing staff input, we identified six topics (Table 8–2).

Table 8–1.   Considerations for implementing a NICU staff support group

Types of shifts	12-hour shifts provide unique staffing needs in terms of breaks and days away from the unit.
Scheduling flexibility and inclusion	Most NICU mental health professionals work traditional day-shift hours, which may leave night-shift nurses unsupported.
	Break and float nurses often move between the NICU and intermediate care nursery.
Session length	Traditional support groups are 90 minutes in length; however, meetings of that length are not feasible for NICU staff during working hours
Confidentiality	Depending on the level of integration for the NICU mental health professionals, staff may not feel comfortable discussing emotionally sensitive topics.

An important factor to consider for each session was ensuring nurses felt they were given an opportunity to talk about cases and recent events that were pressing and relevant to them rather than attending a group that was solely didactic. This proved to be challenging given the length of the sessions. At times when we had prepared topics, we allowed a nurse to present a case or concern and then applied a didactic strategy, if appropriate.

Through hosting these meetings, we identified a minimum of seven questions for NICU mental health professionals to ask themselves and their team prior to implementing a staff support group. We recommend these questions be used to help evaluate the ongoing needs of the support group (Table 8–3). We also have included issues to consider when developing NICU staff support groups (Table 8–4).

Treatment Fidelity

In addition to leadership and staff buy-in, implementing a successful program to decrease anxiety, depression, and trauma in women who deliver their infant prematurely requires being able to identify women who would benefit from the intervention, train staff to implement it with fidelity, and consistently monitor delivery of the intervention for evidence of program "drift." Drift occurs when the individuals who deliver an intervention move away from the intervention as it was designed, either in therapeutic content or means of delivery (Waller and Turner 2016). The effectiveness of evidence-based interventions depends on their being delivered in the manner in which they were tested. This is often in con-

Table 8–2.   Support group session topics and descriptions

Topic	Session description
Identifying emotions and what to do with them	Psychoeducation on how thoughts, feelings, and physiological sensations are interconnected; teaches select mindfulness and relaxation strategies.
Navigating signs of burnout	Psychoeducation on signs and symptoms of burnout; discusses the bidirectional influence of stress on home and work environments.
Exploring boundary setting in personal and professional environments	Discussion of the impact of social media on professional and personal relationships; attendees practice phrasing to use to decline friend requests and parental blogs about NICU patients.
Repairing relationships at bedside	Discussion of working with NICU parents and other NICU staff following challenging events and conversations.
General mental health and well-being	Discussion of mental health hygiene to encourage regular breaks from work, including using paid time off.
Open reflection and sensitive case reflections	Session starts with a selected relaxation strategy, then a nurse is encouraged to discuss a distressing case or recent event; group reflects on the case with the support of the facilitator(s).

flict with therapeutic training that emphasizes tailoring the content and mode of delivery to an individual's specific needs. Garland et al. (2010), in a study that coded video recordings of actual therapeutic sessions, found that half of the therapeutic sessions did not deliver any therapeutic strategy at high intensity and that many strategies consistent with evidence-based care for the condition under study were infrequently used.

Screening

In recent literature, universal screening in medical settings for parental mental health distress, specifically for trauma and depression among women, has been widely discussed, and recommendations for screening have been developed by professional organizations such as the American College of Obstetricians and Gynecologists (2010), the American Academy of Pediatrics (Earls et al. 2019), and the American College of Nurse-Midwives (2003, 2013). Although not all organizations agree on the timing, number of screening measures to use, or specificity of screening measures, many medical agencies urge hospitals to either consider or implement screening programs (Hynan et al. 2013). Because NICU par-

Table 8–3.   Guiding questions for implementation and evaluation

Approvals	Which entities can give permission for the implementation of this support group?
Funding	Is there any available funding to cover NICU staff for extended breaks away to attend the support group?
Service duplication	Are there any similar services offered in the hospital that may be underutilized?
Timing	What times of day and night should the sessions occur, when considering major transitions for the families and NICU staff?
Location	Does the same meeting place make sense for both day- and night-shift sessions?
Topics	Does your proposed session outline allow NICU staff to feel included and listened to?
Advertising	Has enough effort been put in place for NICU staff to know when, where, and what will be discussed?
Feedback	Is there a system for accepting either direct or anonymous feedback for session attendees?

ents are at a higher risk for psychological distress than parents of infants without intensive medical needs, the discussion of NICU parental mental health screening has gained support when considering family-centered care and NICU psychosocial care (Hynan et al. 2013).

Initiating a screening program requires decisions regarding when to screen, who to screen, who will be responsible for screening, and, most importantly, what follow-up services will be offered based on the screening results. In the randomized trial establishing the effectiveness of this intervention, strict eligibility criteria were necessary. Women had to be >18 years of age and their infants had to weigh >600 g, be born at or transferred to one of the four participating NICUs within 1 week of delivery, and be 25–34 weeks' gestational age. Mothers of infants who had developmental abnormalities, were awaiting cardiac surgery, or had been assessed as unlikely to survive were excluded (Shaw et al. 2013). The maternal age restriction need not apply when implementing this program in routine-care settings because informed consent would not be necessary if the intervention were part of routine care. However, programs instituting this intervention may want to consider the restrictions on the infants used in the clinical trial because, although effective for lessening symptoms of anxiety, depression, and trauma, the intervention is not designed to treat grief from the loss of an infant.

Assuming a program does not institute universal screening, a systematic way to identify women who are eligible screening is needed, such as

Table 8–4.   Screening measures

Measure	Number of Items	Completion time	Sensitivity/ specificity	Cost
Depression				
Edinburgh Postnatal Depression Scale	10	<5 minutes	59%–100%/ 49%–100%	Free
Patient Health Questionnaire	9	<5 minutes	75%/90%	Free
Beck Depression Inventory–II	21	5–10 minutes	56%–57%/ 97%–100%	Available for purchase in English and Spanish
Anxiety				
Beck Anxiety Inventory	21	5–10 minutes	75%/74%	Available for purchase in English and Spanish
Quality of Life in Neurological Disorders, Anxiety Short Form	8	<5 minutes		Free
PTSD				
Perinatal PTSD Questionnaire	14	5–10 minutes	82%/90%	Free
PTSD Checklist for DSM-5	20	5–10 minutes	80%/80.7%	Free

admission logs, as is a systematic procedure for doing so, such as review-ing the log at a set time each day. Importantly, a standardized approach must be taken to informing mothers about the intervention, securing their participation, administering the screening instruments, and scor-ing the instruments. In the randomized trial, we used three short and easy-to-score instruments: the Beck Anxiety Inventory (Beck and Steer 1993), the Beck Depression Inventory–II (Beck et al. 1996), and the Stan-ford Acute Stress Reaction Questionnaire (Shaw et al. 2013). Although administered by study staff in the randomized trial, these instruments could easily be programmed into a handheld electronic device, and scor-ing could be done electronically. We recommend women scoring above the clinical cutoffs on any instrument (depression ≥20; anxiety ≥16; stress ≥3 for required questions in two or more symptom categories) be offered the intervention. If women do not meet the symptom criteria, providing them with psychoeducational materials that cover the topics in the intervention would be good clinical practice, as would informing them that, if they begin to experience any of the symptoms asked about, they should report their symptoms to the people in charge of screening to prompt rescreening. This would also align with the general recommendation that NICU parents who screen below clinical levels at the first time point be screened again before discharge and provided with appropriate feedback and referrals as needed (Hynan et al. 2013). These procedures should also be used with women who screen positive but refuse the intervention. Furthermore, for women who are uninterested in being screened, giving them the psychoeducational materials and letting them know that if they want to be screened in the future they can contact the people responsible for screening would likewise be good clinical practice.

Often, changes to screening programs need to be implemented to best support the needs of parents. We considered several common screening tools when implementing the universal screening program (Table 8–4). We wanted tools that balanced time efficiency, cost, sensitivity, and specificity. We ultimately chose the Perinatal Posttraumatic Stress Disorder Questionnaire (Demier et al. 1996), Patient Health Questionnaire–9 (Kroenke et al. 2001), and Quality of Life in Neurological Disorders–Adult Anxiety Short (Cella et al. 2012) in both English and Spanish. More detail about changes to this screening program to be more sensitive to the needs of NICU fathers was discussed in Chapter 3 earlier in this book.

As we developed the group therapy intervention program, with the goal of creating a social network to reduce feelings of isolation in mothers of preterm infants, we found it important to be inclusive of mothers regardless of their clinical cutoff. To this end, we added a self-referral arm to our recruitment efforts. At present, our NICU social work and psychology services perform universal screening for all NICU parents at 2 weeks postpartum. NICU mothers who speak languages other than English are screened using the English measures while an interpreter helps navigate cultural nuances. Mothers who screen positively on any of our three measures are eligible for a range of clinical interventions. Although all mothers of preterm infants are screened, they are informed about the group therapy intervention and invited to participate regardless of their screening results. Thus, although clinical results may not suggest they need further psychological interventions, mothers can elect to participate if they think joining the group may be helpful for them.

In addition to establishing eligibility and a system for screening, practitioners must attend to two other important issues. First, the materials for this screening and intervention program are only available in English and Spanish. If a significant portion of the patient population speaks another language, it will be necessary to have both the screening instruments and the intervention materials translated into that language and culturally adapted and the results delivered with the aid of a spoken language interpreter. Given that the screening instruments and intervention protocol were only tested in two languages, the translated materials may not be effective because even if the materials are accurately translated, the concepts may have different meanings (Brown et al. 2014; Waheed et al. 2015).

Second, some cultural groups may not be comfortable with either the screening instruments or the intervention. Lower use of mental health services and lower participation in mental health services research by ethnic minorities are well documented (Brown et al. 2014; LeCook et al. 2019; Shavers-Hornaday et al. 1997; Waheed et al. 2015). There are numerous reasons for the lack of use of mental health services, including distrust of the medical system, cultural beliefs, stigma, explanatory models of disease, and religious beliefs (Shavers-Hornaday et al. 1997). Waheed et al. (2015) grouped barriers into five categories and suggested ways to overcome some of them, including education, involving a culturally competent person, having appropriately translated materials that avoid stigmatizing language, and being sensitive to culture and norms. Attending to cultural norms and beliefs helps ensure that evidence-based interventions are acceptable to the women to whom they are offered.

Training Staff on the Intervention and Monitoring Fidelity

Training staff to fidelity is critical if the intervention is to approach the effectiveness shown in the clinical trial. We recommend using a "train-the-trainer" model in which one person from the institution is trained to fidelity and then trains his or her colleagues (Hoagwood et al. 2018). For the randomized trial, six interventionists were first-year students in a clinical psychology graduate program with no therapeutic experience and one was a licensed clinical social worker assigned to the NICU. These individuals were trained in an intensive 1-day session by the program developers. The purpose of each session, its goals, and the individual activities were discussed. The rationale behind the skills to be taught was also thoroughly discussed, as were strategies for building rapport and possible responses to any upsetting thoughts and feelings expressed by mothers. Sessions were discussed in groups of two, interventionists were grouped in pairs of two, and then the content of each session was role-played, with the intervention developers circulating to provide feedback and suggestions.

Following the intensive day of training, each of the interventionists was asked to complete and record the six-session intervention with two friends or family members. The audiotapes were reviewed for establishment of rapport, ease of interaction, offering of appropriate support, and the key elements to be addressed in each session. Following this, the interventionists were debriefed about their experience, had each recording reviewed with them, and had any questions answered. We had, a priori, set a threshold for fidelity at 0.85, and all interventionists achieved this level (Shaw et al. 2014a). Interventionists recorded all sessions with their first three study participants, and these sessions were reviewed by the program developers. After reviewing all the sessions for each interventionist's first three participants, we randomly selected one in five of the next study participants assigned to each interventionist to review and rate for fidelity. Fidelity remained high throughout the study and, given that the fidelity checklists for each session are highly structured, interrater reliability of fidelity was also high (intraclass correlation coefficient range 0.78–0.80; $P<0.001$). Additionally, study staff met every other week to discuss implementation challenges, appropriate responses to upsetting maternal issues, and administrative matters (Shaw et al. 2013).

The challenges for staff training are considerable. First, a member of the staff who will serve as an interventionist must become proficient in the intervention. Studying the manual, practicing the intervention, and scoring each practice session are critical. To help establish program fidelity and integrity, Stanford University and LPCH will establish a training and support program under the auspices of Richard Shaw and Sarah Horwitz for NICUs interested in implementing our program. Second, staff who are willing to commit time to be trained and deliver the intervention need to be recruited and trained. Finally, a system for the ongoing monitoring of fidelity must be developed to ensure drift does not occur. Recording sessions, scoring them, and discussing the scores in supervisory sessions are critical if the intervention is to be effective.

Knowing the Intervention "Worked"

Although fidelity to an evidence-informed practice is critical to ensure effectiveness, knowing whether the intervention actually decreased mothers' symptoms is equally important. There are many reasons in addition to drift for why an intervention may not be effective when applied outside of an experimental setting. Although they are the gold standard for establishing efficacy and effectiveness (internal validity), randomized trials suffer from a lack of external validity. This essentially means that the results may not generalize to individuals who differ from the study population (Deaton and Cartwright 2018). A treatment tested in a randomized clinical trial may have an effect, but that effect applies to the study sample and may not apply to individuals who differ from those in the study population (Summers-Trio et al. 2019). Thus, the group of women to whom the intervention is being delivered differs in some significant way from the study population in which it was tested.

Additionally, in a randomized trial, the protocol is strictly adhered to, considerable effort is made to ensure that subjects are not lost to follow-up, and fidelity is rigorously monitored. In routine clinical practice, aggressive measures to prevent loss to follow-up are usually not possible given the demands of busy clinical settings. As a result, women may not receive all sessions of the intervention, thus diminishing its effects. Similarly, even with fidelity monitoring, the diverse needs of NICU mothers may make portions of the intervention difficult or impossible to deliver. Therefore, when implementing this intervention, it would be prudent to readminister the screening instruments to the first group of women who complete the intervention. If decreases in symptoms occur, continuing to deliver the intervention makes good clinical sense. If symptoms do not decrease, we suggest that those responsible for delivering the intervention examine both whether the women with whom they are undertaking the intervention differ in significant ways from the women who participated in the clinical trial and whether their fidelity to the session content reached the level reported in the trial (Shaw et al. 2013, 2014b). If the clinical population of women differs in important ways from the study population, then the intervention may need to be modified to address issues of the clinical population that were not addressed in the intervention. If the fidelity is suboptimal, rigorous retraining is necessary.

Future Directions

Given the documented decrease in the effectiveness of evidence-based interventions when delivered outside a carefully controlled experimental trial, documenting symptom changes and maternal satisfaction with the intervention in multiple settings is important. For interventions to be truly effective, they must be usable in routine clinical settings. Therefore, changes in symptom data from NICUs not involved in the original effectiveness trial are the real test of whether clinical staff's time should be redirected to deliver this intervention. If effective, it can make mothers' lives better, improve their ability to interact with their infants so the infants maximize their potential, and may prevent some of the unnecessary use of expensive health care (Horwitz et al. 2015; Shaw et al. 2013).

In addition to documenting whether this intervention is effective in usual-care settings, two augmentations to the original intervention could improve the lives of infants born prematurely. The original intervention showed no effect on mothers' perceptions of their child's vulnerability (Horwitz et al. 2015): both groups showed decreases. Although this decrease was greater in mothers who received the intervention, the difference between groups did not achieve statistical significance (Horwitz et al. 2015). Thinking through why this intervention was not effective in changing perceptions, we concluded that although it included educational material on infant vulnerability, the *perception* of the infant as vulnerable was not addressed in any of the cognitive restructuring activities. Thus, an intervention specifically addressing infant vulnerability had to be developed and tested, such as that described in Chapter 7.

A second important addition to the original intervention is sessions for fathers. Because of the rigor required of a randomized trial, our interest in testing the intervention with mothers regardless of their marital status, and the likely bias that could result from involving only some fathers, fathers were excluded from participating in the original intervention. In our early discussions with NICU staff, they accurately observed that fathers often had to return to work or care for other children and therefore spent less time than mothers in the NICU. Because of the time commitment of the intervention, we knew its format would not be appropriate for fathers, but we learned from comments made to the interventionists by both fathers and mothers that many fathers also experienced considerable anxiety, would welcome support, and would appreciate learning the restructuring techniques being taught to mothers. Therefore, an intervention for fathers has been developed and is being piloted. This intervention and a detailed discussion of issues facing fathers were presented in Chapter 3. Adding both these new services to the intervention developed for mothers of preterm infants will improve the functioning of these parents and their infants.

References

Aarons GA, Sommerfeld DH: Leadership, innovation climate, and attitudes toward evidence-based practice during a statewide implementation. J Am Acad Child Adolesc Psychiatry 51(4):423–431, 2012

Aarons GA, Hurlburt M, Horwitz SM: Advancing a conceptual model of evidence-based practice implementation in public service sectors. Adm Policy Ment Health 38(1):4–23, 2011a

Aarons GA, Sommerfeld DH, Willging CE: The soft underbelly of system change: the role of leadership and organizational climate in turnover during statewide behavioral health reform. Psychol Serv 8(4):269–281, 2011b

Aarons GA, Green AE, Trott E, et al: The roles of system and organizational leadership in system-wide evidence-based intervention sustainment: a mixed-method study. Adm Policy Ment Health 43(6):991–1008, 2016

American College of Nurse Midwives: Position Statement: Depression in Women. Silver Spring, MD, American College of Nurse Midwives, 2003

American College of Nurse Midwives: Position Statement: Depression in Women. Silver Spring, MD, American College of Nurse Midwives, 2013

American College of Obstetricians and Gynecologists: Committee opinion no. 453: screening for depression during and after pregnancy. Obstet Gynecol 115(2 Pt 1):394–395, 2010

American Psychiatric Association: Trauma- and stressor-related disorders, in Diagnostic and Statistical Manual of Mental Disorders, 5th Edition. Arlington, VA, American Psychiatric Association, 2013, pp 265–290

Aytekin A, Yilmaz F, Kuguoglu S: Burnout levels in neonatal intensive care nurses and its effects on their quality of life. Aust J Adv Nurs 31(2):39, 2013

Beck AT, Steer RA: Beck Anxiety Inventory Manual. San Antonio, TX, Psychological Corporation, 1993

Beck AT, Steer RA, Brown GK: Manual for the Beck Depression Inventory–II. San Antonio, TX, Psychological Corporation, 1996

Bride BE: Prevalence of secondary traumatic stress among social workers. Social Work 52(1):63–70, 2007

Brown G, Marshall M, Bower P, et al: Barriers to recruiting ethnic minorities to mental health research: a systematic review. Int J Methods Psychiatr Res 23(1):36–48, 2014

Cella D, Lai JS, Nowinski CJ, et al: Neuro-QOL: brief measures of health-related quality of life for clinical research in neurology. Neurology 78(23):1860–1867, 2012

Damschroder LJ, Aron DC, Keith RE, et al: Fostering implementation of health services research findings into practice: a consolidated framework for advancing implementation science. Implement Sci 4(1):50, 2009

Deaton A, Cartwright N: Understanding and misunderstanding randomized controlled trials. Soc Sci Med 210:2–21, 2018

Demier RL, Hynan MT, Harris HB, Manniello RL: Perinatal stressors as predictors of symptoms of posttraumatic stress in mothers of infants at high risk. J Perinatol 16(4):276–280, 1996

Dessy E: Effective communication in difficult situations: preventing stress and burnout in the NICU. Early Hum Dev 85(10):S39–S41, 2009

Earls MF, Yogman MW, Mattson G, et al: Incorporating recognition and management of perinatal depression into pediatric practice. Pediatrics 143(1):e20183260, 2019

Figley CR: Compassion fatigue: toward a new understanding of the costs of caring, in Secondary Traumatic Stress: Self-Care Issues for Clinicians, Researchers, and Educators. Edited by Stamm BH. Baltimore, MD, Sidran Press, 1995, pp 3–28

Garland AF, Brookman-Frazee L, Hurlburt MS, et al: Mental health care for children with disruptive behavior problems: a view inside therapists' offices. Psychiatr Serv 61(8):788–795, 2010

Greenhalgh T, Robert G, Macfarlane F, et al: Diffusion of innovations in service organizations: systematic review and recommendations. Milbank Q 82(4):581–629, 2004

Hoagwood K, Olin SS, Storfer-Isser A, et al: Evaluation of a train-the-trainers model for family peer advocates in children's mental health. J Child Fam Stud 27(4):1130–1136, 2018

Horwitz SM, Leibovitz A, Lilo E, et al: Does an intervention to reduce maternal anxiety, depression and trauma also improve mothers' perceptions of their preterm infants' vulnerability? Infant Ment Health J 36(1):42–52, 2015

Hynan MT, Mounts KO, Vanderbilt DL: Screening parents of high-risk infants for emotional distress: rationale and recommendations. J Perinatol 33(10):748, 2013

Institute of Medicine: Crossing the Quality Chasm: A New Health System for the 21st Century. Washington, DC, National Academies Press, 2001

Jenkins SR, Baird S: Secondary traumatic stress and vicarious trauma: a validational study. J Trauma Stress 15(5):423–432, 2002

Joinson C: Coping with compassion fatigue. Nursing 22:116–121, 1992

Kroenke K, Spitzer RL, Williams JB: The PHQ-9: Validity of a brief depression severity measure. J Gen Intern 16:606–613, 2001

LeCook B, Hou SS, Lee-Tauler SY, et al: A review of mental health and mental health care disparities research: 2011–2014. Med Care Res Rev 76(6):683–710, 2019

Lilo EA, Shaw RJ, Corcoran J, Storfer-Isser A: Does she think she's supported? Maternal perceptions of their experiences in the neonatal intensive care unit. Patient Exp J 3(1):15–24, 2016

Maslach C, Jackson SE, Leiter MP, et al: Maslach Burnout Inventory, Vol 21. Palo Alto, CA, Consulting Psychologists Press, 1986, pp 3463–3464

Meadors P, Lamson A, Swanson M, et al: Secondary traumatization in pediatric healthcare providers: compassion fatigue, burnout, and secondary traumatic stress. Omega (Westport) 60(2):103–128, 2010

Olin SS, Nadeem E, Gleacher A, et al: What predicts clinician dropout from state-sponsored managing and adapting practice training. Adm Policy Ment Health 43(6):945–956, 2016

Peebles-Kleiger MJ: Pediatric and neonatal intensive care hospitalization as traumatic stressor: implications for intervention. Bull Menninger Clin 64(2):257, 2000

Profit J, Sharek PJ, Amspoker AB, et al: Burnout in the NICU setting and its relation to safety culture. BMJ Qual Saf 23(10):806–813, 2014

Rogers EM: Diffusion of Innovations, 5th Edition. New York, Free Press, 2003

Shavers-Hornaday VL, Lynch CF, Burmeister LF, Torner JC: Why are African Americans under-represented in medical research studies? Impediments to participation. Ethn Health 2(1–2):31–45, 1997

Shaw RJ, St John N, Lilo E, et al: Prevention of traumatic stress in mothers with preterm infants: a randomized controlled trial. Pediatrics 132(4):e886–e894, 2013

Shaw RJ, Lilo EA, Storfer-Isser A, et al: Screening for symptoms of postpartum traumatic stress in a sample of mothers with preterm infants. Issues Ment Health Nurs 35(3):198–207, 2014a

Shaw RJ, St John N, Lilo E, et al: Prevention of traumatic stress in mothers of preterms: 6-month outcomes. Pediatrics 134(2):e481–e488, 2014b

Summers-Trio P, Hayes-Conroy A, Singer B, Horwitz RI: Biology, biography, and the translational gap. Sci Transl Med 11(479), 2019

Tawfik DS, Sexton JB, Kan P, et al: Burnout in the neonatal intensive care unit and its relation to healthcare-associated infections. J Perinatol 37(3):315, 2017

Van Mol MM, Kompanje EJ, Benoit DD, et al: The prevalence of compassion fatigue and burnout among healthcare professionals in intensive care units: a systematic review. PLoS One 10(8):e0136955, 2015

Wagner C: Moral distress as a contributor to nurse burnout. Am J Nurs 115(4):11, 2015

Waheed W, Hughes-Morley A, Woodham A, et al: Overcoming barriers to recruiting ethnic minorities to mental health research: a typology of recruitment strategies. BMC Psychiatry 15(1):101–112, 2015

Waller G, Turner H: Therapist drift redux: why well-meaning clinicians fail to deliver evidence-based therapy, and how to get back on track. Behav Res Ther 77:129–137, 2016

White D: The hidden costs of caring: what managers need to know. The Health Care Manager 25(4):341–347, 2006

Index

Page numbers printed in **boldface** type refer to tables or figures.